Cambridge Monographs on Cancer Research

Cyclopenta[a]phenanthrenes

Cambridge Monographs on Cancer Research

Scientific Editors
M. M. Coombs, Imperial Cancer Research Fund Laboratories, London
J. Ashby, Imperial Chemical Industries, Macclesfield, Cheshire

Executive Editor
H. Baxter, formerly at the Laboratory of the Government Chemist, London

Books in this Series
Martin R. Osborne and Neil T. Crosby *Benzopyrenes*

Cyclopenta[a]phenanthrenes

Polycyclic aromatic compounds structurally related to steroids

MAURICE M.COOMBS
TARLOCHAN S.BHATT
Imperial Cancer Research Fund, London

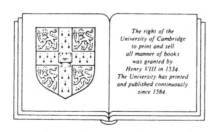

The right of the
University of Cambridge
to print and sell
all manner of books
was granted by
Henry VIII in 1534.
The University has printed
and published continuously
since 1584.

CAMBRIDGE UNIVERSITY PRESS
Cambridge
New York New Rochelle
Melbourne Sydney

CAMBRIDGE UNIVERSITY PRESS
Cambridge, New York, Melbourne, Madrid, Cape Town, Singapore, São Paulo, Delhi

Cambridge University Press
The Edinburgh Building, Cambridge CB2 8RU, UK

Published in the United States of America by Cambridge University Press, New York

www.cambridge.org
Information on this title: www.cambridge.org/9780521301237

First published 1987
This digitally printed version 2008

A catalogue record for this publication is available from the British Library

Library of Congress Cataloguing in Publication data

Coombs, Maurice M.
  Cyclopenta(a)phenanthrenes: polycyclic aromatic
  compounds structurally related to steroids.

  (Cambridge monographs on cancer research)
  Includes bibliographies and index.
  1. Cyclopentaphenanthrene – Derivatives.
  2. Carcinogens. I. Bhatt, Tarlochan S. II. Title.
  III. Series. [DNLM: 1. Carcinogens. 2. DNA –
  metabolism. 3. Gonanes. QU 85 C775c]
  RC268.7.C95C66 1987   616.99'4071   86–34339

ISBN 978-0-521-30123-7 hardback
ISBN 978-0-521-10192-9 paperback

This book is dedicated to the memory of our colleague and friend
Dr David Campbell Livingston, 1936–1983,
late of the Chemistry Laboratory, Imperial Cancer Research
Fund, London.

Contents

Abbreviations employed in this book

Journal titles

Acta Crystallogr.   Acta Crystallographica
Acta Unio Int. Cancrum   Acta Unio Internationalis contra Cancrum
Adv. Lipid Res.   Advances in Lipid Research
Am. J. Cancer   American Journal of Cancer
Am. J. Physiol.   American Journal of Physiology
An. Asoc. Quim, Argent.   Anales de la Associacion Quimica Argentina
Annalen   Justus Liebigs Annalen der Chemie
Arch. Biochem. Biophys.   Archives of Biochemistry and Biophysics
Arch. Geselwulstforsch.   Archiv für Geselwulstforschung
Aust. J. Chem.   Australian Journal of Chemistry
Ber.   Berichte der Deutschen Chemischen Gesellschaft
Biochem. J.   Biochemical Journal
Biochim. Biophys. Acta   Biochimica et Biophysica Acta
Biomed. Mass Spectrom.   Biomedical Mass Spectrometry
Br. J. Cancer   British Journal of Cancer
Br. Med. J.   British Medical Journal
Bull. Acad. Polon. Sci., Sér. Sci. Chim.   Bulletin de l'Academie Polonaise de
   Sciences, Série des Sciences Chimique
Cancer Biochem. Biophys.   Cancer Biochemistry and Biophysics
Cancer Lett.   Cancer Letters
Cancer Res.   Cancer Research
Can. J. Chem.   Canadian Journal of Chemistry
Chem. Abst.   Chemical Abstracts
Chem. Ber.   Chemische Berichte
Chem. Ind. (London)   Chemistry and Industry (London)
Chem. Geol.   Chemical Geology
Collect. Czech. Chem. Commun.   Collection of Czech Chemical
   Communications

C. R. Hebd. Séances Acad. Sci.   Comptes rendus Hebdomadaires des Séances de l'Academie des Sciences

C. R. Hebd. Séances Acad. Sci. Sér. C   Comptes rendus Hebdomadaires des Séances de l'Academie des Sciences, Séries C, Séries Chimiques

Dokl. Bolg. Acad. Nauk   Doklady Bolgarshoi Akademii Nauk

Edinburgh Med. J.   Edinburgh Medical Journal

FEBS Lett.   Federation of European Biochemical Societies Letters

Fed. Proc.   Federation of American Societies for Experimental Biology, Proceedings

Geochim. Cosmochim. Acta   Geochimica et Cosmochimica Acta

Helv. Chim. Acta   Helvetica Chimica Acta

Indian J. Phys.   Indian Journal of Physics

Int. Abst. Surg.   International Abstracts of Surgery

Int. J. Cancer   International Journal of Cancer

Izv. Akad. Nauk S.S.S.R. Otdel. Khim. Nauk   Izvestiya Akademii Nauk S.S.S.R. Otdelenii Khimicheskikh Nauk

J. Am. Chem. Soc.   Journal of the American Chemical Society

J. Am. Med. Assoc.   Journal of the American Medical Association

J. Biol. Chem.   Journal of Biological Chemistry

J. Chem. Phys.   Journal of Chemical Physics

J. Chem. Soc.   Journal of the Chemical Society

J. Chem. Soc., Chem. Commun.   Journal of the Chemical Society, Chemical Communications

J. Heterocyclic Chem.   Journal of Heterocyclic Chemistry

J. Indian Chem. Soc.   Journal of the Indian Chemical Society

J. Labelled Compd. Radiopharm.   Journal of Labelled Compounds and Radiopharmaceuticals

J. Org. Chem.   Journal of Organic Chemistry

J.N.C.I.   Journal of the National Cancer Institute

Mitt. Geb. Lebensmittelunter. Hyg.   Mitteilungen aus dem Gebeite der Lebensmitteluntersuchung und Hygiene

Mutation Res.   Mutation Research

Nucleic Acids Res.   Nucleic Acids Research

Proc. Am. Pet. Inst.   Proceedings, American Petroleum Institute

Proc. Nat. Acad. Sci. U.S.A.   Proceedings of the National Academy of Sciences of the United States of America

Proc. R. Soc. (London), A   Proceedings of the Royal Society of London, Series A

Prog. Exp. Tumor Res.   Progress in Experimental Tumor Research

Science   Science (Washington, D.C.)

Tetrahedron Lett.   Tetrahedron Letters

Trans. Faraday Soc.   Transactions of the Faraday Society

Yale J. Biol. Med.   Yale Journal of Biology & Medicine

Z. Ernaehungswiss.   Zeitschrift für Ernaehungswissenschaft

Z. *Krebsforsch.*   Zeitschrift für Krebsforschung
Z. *Kristallogr.*   Zeitschrift für Kristallographie
Z. *Naturforsch.*   Zeitschrift für Naturforschung
Z. *Physiol. Chem.*   Zeitschrift für Physiologische Chemie
Zh. *Obshch. Khim.*   Zhurnal Obshchei Khimii

Some other common abbreviations

Å   Ångstrom unit (10^{-10} metre)
bp   boiling point
Ci   Curie (3.7×10^{10} nuclear transformations/second)
Et   ethyl (C_2H_5)
h   hour
hplc   high-pressure liquid chromatography
Hz   Hertz (frequency unit, $1\,cm^{-1} \cong 3 \times 10^{10}\,Hz$)
J   coupling constant (in Hz)
L   litre
Me   methyl
min   minute
mL   millilitre ($10^{-3}\,L$)
mp   melting point
m/z   ratio of mass to charge
n   normal
NADPH   nicotinamide-adenine dinucleotide phosphate, reduced
n_D refractive index (at sodium D-line)
nm   nanometre (10^{-9} metre)
nmr   nuclear magnetic resonance
ppm   parts per million
s   second, singlet
S.D.   standard deviation
sec.   secondary
tert. tertiary
tlc   thin-layer chromatography
Tris   tris(hydroxymethyl)aminomethane hydrochloride (buffer)
α_D optical rotation (at sodium D-line)
δ chemical shift (in ppm from tetramethylsilane)
λ_{max} ultraviolet maxima (in nanometres)
ν_{max} infrared maxima (in microns, μm)
μL   microlitre ($10^{-6}\,L$)
μm   micron (micrometre, 10^{-6} metre)

Acknowledgements

There has been an interest in cyclopenta[a]phenanthrenes in the laboratories of the Imperial Cancer Research Fund in London for 20 years, beginning with G. F. Marrian's suggestion of a possible metabolic route leading to the complete aromatization of steroids. We wish to acknowledge the continued generous financial support afforded by this organization throughout this period.

We are also indebted to all those listed below whom we have been fortunate to have as collaborators on this project, and who have contributed so many ideas and years of hard work.

Imperial Cancer Research Fund
Peter Abbott
Jeffrey Allen
Francis Crawley
Frances Crew
Charles Croft
Cynthia Dixon
Stanley Fisher
Sheila Furn
John Gilbert
Stephen Hadfield
Maureen Hall
Andrea Harper
S. Bala Jaitly
Joseph Jiricny
Michael Jones
Anna-Maija Kissonerghis
Campbell Livingston
Andrew McEwen
Odarty Ribeiro
James Richards

Veronica Siddle
Clive Smith
Murugesu Thanikasalam
David Thomas
Colin Vose
Jill Welsh
Stretton Young

Northern Polytechnic, London
Alexandra Clayton
Kim Hendrick
Mary McPartlin
Jill Trotter

Fox Chase Center, Philadelphia
Jenny Glusker
Setsuo Kashino
Richard Peck
David Zacharias

Wistar Institute, Philadelphia
Leila Diamond
John DiGiovanni
Francis Kruszewski

University College, Swansea
Dianne Kelly
James Parry
J. L. Wiebers

University of Surrey
John Elvidge
John Jones
Jeremy Russell
Alan Wiseman

King's College, London
Alex Drake

University of Uppsala, Sweden
Kirsten Lindahl-Kiessling
Inga Karlberg

We are also greatly indebted to Audrey Becket who typed the manuscript of this book and helped us in many ways with its preparation.

Authors' preface

Extensive world-wide studies in cancer epidemiology throughout most of this century have led to a generally accepted view that as much as 80–90% of all human cancer has its origins in environmental factors in our diet and lifestyle. Although in most cases several factors are likely to combine to produce a particular disease, the real significance of the above conclusion is its corrollary, that identification and elimination of these environmental factors should reduce the incidence of the disease. During this time period the incidence of most forms of cancer has remained essentially constant with one notable exception, lung cancer. Mortality from this disease has risen inexorably to its present epidemic proportions during the last seventy years and now accounts for the death of some 26 000 men and 15 000 women each year in England and Wales alone. There is now no doubt that this is a direct result of cigarette smoking, and it is reliably predicted that abandonment of the habit would reduce this death rate ten-fold. The causes of other major forms of cancer, such as breast cancer in women and colon cancer in both sexes, have proved to be much more elusive. Their origins are probably complex and they are more difficult to study because there are no natural 'controls' as there are with lung cancer, where direct comparisons may be made between smokers and non-smokers. All possibilities for their causation are now under active consideration, and among them the influence of endogenous carcinogens generated by aberrant metabolism within the host is unknown, but cannot be discounted. It is now established that carcinogens of varied types are elaborated by both plants and microorganisms, and there seems to be no *a priori* reason why animals should not be similarly afflicted. Since most cancers are primarily diseases of old age it would seem unlikely that there would be strong evolutionary pressure against this happening. The idea that carcinogens, arising from steroids by incorrect metabolism, might be important in the induction of human cancer was a view commonly held in the past, but which has been neglected in recent times.

Over fifty years ago, at the very outset of research into chemical carcinogenesis, the potent polycyclic aromatic hydrocarbon carcinogen 3-methylcholanthrene was prepared by simple chemical transformations from a bile acid derivative. The correct structures for the bile acids and sterols were themselves established at about the same time, and the synthesis of this carcinogen took on an exaggerated importance in the minds of scientists. The enduring idea that methylcholanthrene formed by incorrect bile acid or sterol metabolism in the body might prove to be a cause of human cancer led to numerous attempts to identify this carcinogen in tumours and other tissues, but without success. The reason for this failure now seems obvious because experience has shown that cyclization of the sterol side chain does not occur to provide a fifth fused ring. Instead this side-chain tends to be lost with migration of the angular methyl groups, leading to compounds of the simpler four-ring cyclopenta[a]phenanthrene series. These compounds thus possess the same basic carbon ring system as the steroids, but lack the angular methyl groups which characterize the latter. They are therefore capable of complete dehydrogenation to fully aromatic phenanthrene derivatives, and compounds of this type do in fact occur widely in petroleum and in oil-bearing shales as well as in river and lake sediments; they are also found in cooking oils that have been overheated. Advances in our understanding of oestrogen biosynthesis and metabolism have moreover suggested a plausible route by which cyclopenta[a]phenanthrenes might be formed in the body, but so far no attempts have been made to test this possibility. The need for further investigations in this area using modern techniques is now apparent, because numerous cyclopenta[a]phenanthrenes have since been synthesized and some have been shown to be strong carcinogens; similar in potency to the classical polycyclic hydrocarbon carcinogen benzo[a]pyrene.

This book is concerned with the occurrence, chemical synthesis, physical and chemical properties, and biological attributes of cyclopenta[a]phenanthrenes. These are discussed in detail, as is their history which is intimately connected with the establishment of the correct structure of steroids. Interesting structure /carcinogenicity relationships, similar to those found among related polycyclic aromatic systems such as the chrysenes and benzo[a]anthracenes, are examined in relation to the metabolism of these compounds and the interactions of their metabolites with biological macromolecules. The book also lists physical data for nearly 350 cyclopenta[a]phenanthrene derivatives and contains exhaustive references to the original literature. It is hoped that it will provide a useful point of departure for those concerned with the possibility of the involvement of cyclopenta[a]phenanthrenes in the aetiology of human disease.

M.M.C.
T.S.B.

1

Introduction

Six possible isomers can be formed by fusion of a cyclopentane ring with the angular tricyclic aromatic hydrocarbon phenanthrene, as shown in Fig. 1. Of these the [a] isomer occupies a special position because it possesses the same carbon ring system as members of the large and important group of natural products, the steroids. Indeed, cyclopenta[a]phenanthrenes became of importance during the elucidation of the structures of these natural products over 50 years ago. At about the same time it first became evident that carcinogenic properties were associated

Fig. 1

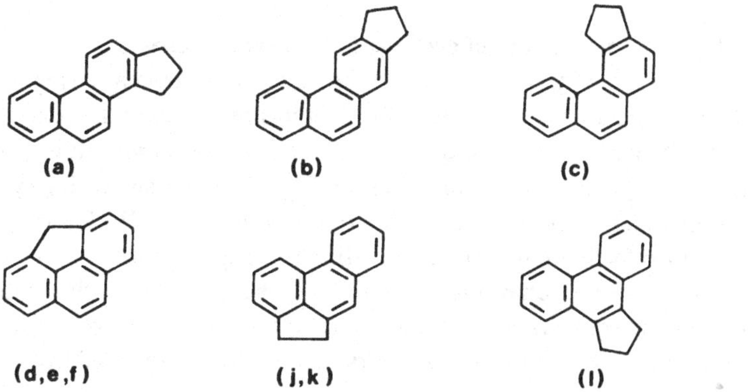

Phenanthrene

(a)

(b)

(c)

(d,e,f)

(j,k)

(l)

with many polycyclic aromatic hydrocarbons which result from incomplete combustion of most carbonaceous materials, and that the great majority of these could also be considered as derived from phenanthrene. The coincidence in time between the fruition of these two quite independent lines of research led many to feel that there might be a connection between them, and for a time there was considerable interest in the possible relationship between these two classes of compounds. Although most of the carcinogenic polycyclic aromatic hydrocarbons discovered at that time contained four or more fused benzene rings, the simpler cyclopenta[a]phenanthrenes with the same carbon skeleton as the C_{18} and C_{19} steroids (with the exception of the angular methyl groups in these steroids) were also examined, and these studies have continued until the present day.

In writing this monograph the purpose is to review the subject fully including both the earlier work as well as the more recent developments. A careful search has been made in *Chemical Abstracts* back to 1907, but a problem has been encountered in that the term 'cyclopenta[a]phenanthrene' includes numerous partially hydrogenated derivatives which are better considered as steroids. In general we have neglected these if they include in their structure angular methyl groups, unless they have some direct relevance to the phenanthrene-derived compounds which are the main topic here. This work now spans more than half a century and in reviewing it almost inevitably some omissions will have occurred; the authors wish to apologize for these in advance. In the text individual compounds are assigned arabic numbers (**in heavy type**) sequentially so that they can be referred to without ambiguity, and the structures of most are shown in the figures. The latter and also the tables are numbered sequentially throughout the monograph, but literature references are collected at the end of each chapter in alphabetical and chronological order.

1.1   Nomenclature of cyclopenta[a]phenanthrenes

In common with many other polycyclic aromatic ring systems, the nomenclature of cyclopenta[a]phenanthrenes has undergone changes since the early work, and this will lead to confusion unless it is dealt with here. Originally compound (1) in Fig. 2 was named 1,2-cyclopentenophenanthrene and was numbered as shown **1(A)**. With the advent of the more facile method of designating the edge of each ring by a letter, as shown for phenanthrene in Fig. 1, the prefix denoting the fused five-membered ring becomes cyclopenta[a]; however, cyclopenta[a]phenanthrene itself now refers to the fully unsaturated hydrocarbon

of which (2) is the 17*H*-isomer. 15*H*-cyclopenta[a]phenanthrene is therefore compound (3), and the compound (1) containing only one double
bond in the five-membered ring is correctly named 16,17-dihydro-15*H*-
cyclopenta[a]phenanthrene. In the older literature these two unsaturated
hydrocarbons, (2) and (3), were named $\Delta^{1'(2')}$ and $\Delta^{2'(3')}$-1,2-cyclopent-
dienophenanthrene, respectively. When the position of the 'extra'
hydrogen atom (on the carbon not doubly bonded) is fixed by a substituent, for example by the ketone oxygen atom in the ketone (4), its
position need not be designated; e.g., the correct name for this ketone is
15,16-dihydrocyclopenta[a]phenanthren-17-one or 15,16-dihydro-17-
oxocyclopenta[a]phenanthrene. Numbering of the ring system follows
the steroid convention as indicated on formula 1(B) in Fig. 2. The term
cyclopenta[a]phenanthrene is therefore properly reserved for the fully
unsaturated compounds containing a double bond in the five-membered
ring. However, in this monograph it will be also used more loosely as a
general term for compounds such as (1)-(4) of both types, except of
course, in formal chemical names.

1.2 Cyclopenta[a]phenanthrenes, steroids, and carcinogenic polycyclic hydrocarbons

Sterols isolated from plant and animal tissues and the bile acids
from animal bile had been studied for over a century when in 1928
Windaus and Wieland received the Nobel Prize for their outstanding
work on these natural products. Extensive degradative experiments
utilizing the classical methods of organic chemistry, purification by

Fig. 2

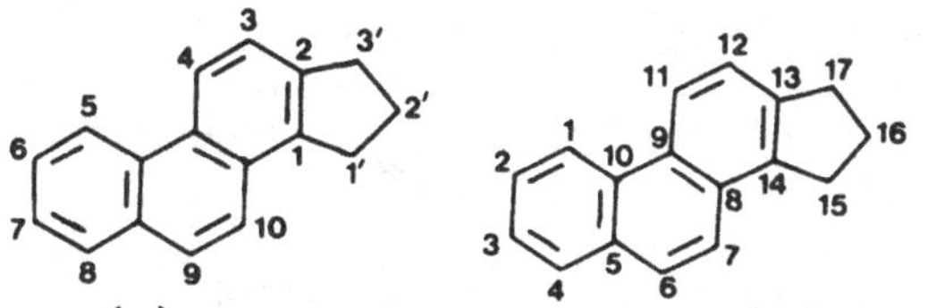

(A) 1 (B)

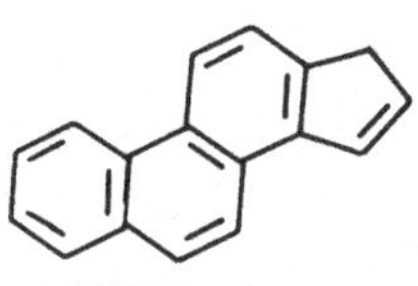

17*H*
2

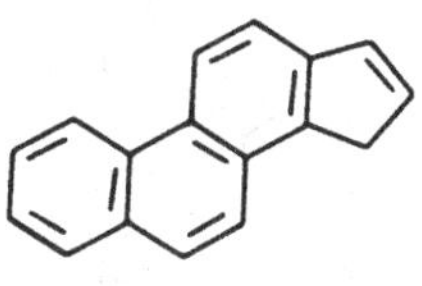

15*H*
3

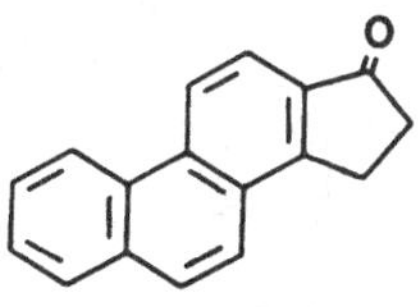

-17-one or 17-oxo-
4

crystallization to a constant melting point or constant optical rotation and identification by elemental analysis, were unassisted by the chromatographic and spectroscopic techniques so widely used today. By 1928 these experiments had culminated in the structures shown in Fig. 3 for the bile acid deoxycholic acid and the typical sterol cholesterol. However, in 1932 these formulae were criticized on what at that time were quite esoteric grounds. In an X-ray crystallographic investigation of the vitamin D precursor ergosterol Bernal (1932b) determined its molecular dimensions to be $7.2 \times 5 \times 17$–20 Å, and pointed out that these figures did not fit well with those ($8.5 \times 7 \times 18$ Å) calculated for this sterol from the Wieland–Windaus structure. This supported a previous observation based on the results of experiments with surface films of sterols by Adam and Rosenheim (1929). Several years previously Diels *et al.* (1927) had obtained chrysene (**5**) and two other unidentified hydrocarbons by dehydrogenation of sterols by prolonged heating at 360°C with selenium, but it was at that time generally considered that these drastic conditions might well lead to deep-seated rearrangements within the molecule, so that the products would be of little use as indicators of structure. Discarding this view, Rosenheim and King (1932) proposed the novel structure (**6a**) for deoxycholic acid based on perhydrochrysene, and Bernal (1932a) calculated that an analogous structure for ergosterol would have the dimensions ($7.5 \times 4.5 \times 20$ Å), in good agreement with those found. Within a few months chemical considerations led to the revised structure (**6b**) for deoxycholic acid based on perhydrocyclopenta[a]phenanthrene; this formula has stood the test of time and is accepted

Fig. 3

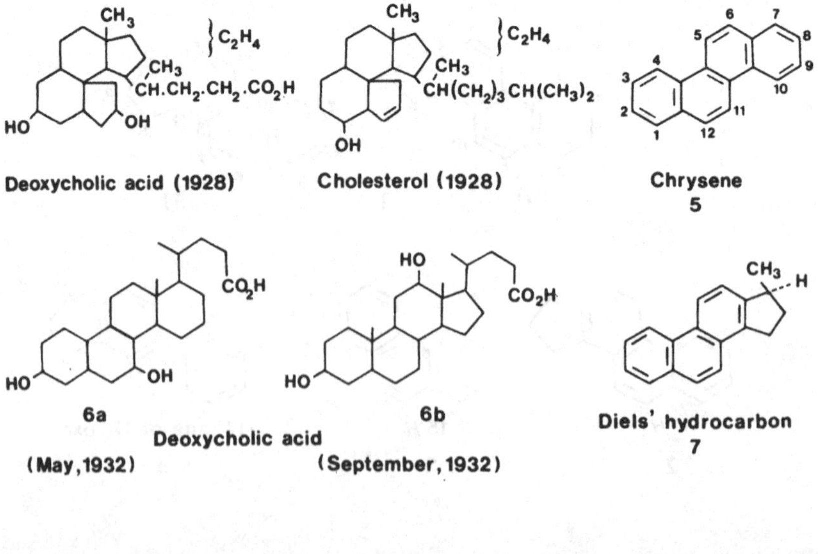

Deoxycholic acid (1928)   Cholesterol (1928)   Chrysene
5

6a   6b   Diels' hydrocarbon
7

Deoxycholic acid

(May, 1932)   (September, 1932)

today. In order to confirm this new structure for the bile acids and sterols the other hydrocarbons obtained by Diels, particularly the one melting at 124–125°C, were reinvestigated. This hydrocarbon, which has since become known as Diels' hydrocarbon, was originally obtained, together with chrysene and another hydrocarbon $C_{25}H_{24}$, by selenium dehydrogenation of cholesterol and cholesteryl chloride; it was also isolated from the products of similar dehydrogenation of ergosterol and cholic acid. The following year Rosenheim and King (1933) proposed that Diels' hydrocarbon was 16,17-dihydro-17-methyl-15H-cyclopenta[a]phenanthrene (7) on the basis of its ultraviolet spectrum, another use of a novel technique in those early days. The problem was taken up by several groups and all three (15-, 16-, and 17-methyl) hydrocarbons as well as the parent hydrocarbon 16,17-dihydro-15H-cyclopenta[a]phenanthrene (1) were synthesized. It was not, however, until 1935 that Diels' hydrocarbon was finally and unambiguously assigned structure (7) by careful comparison with the synthetic specimen (Hillemann, 1935), thus finally confirming the steroid ring structure previously arrived at on quite different grounds.

At the same time momentous discoveries were being made in the field of carcinogenesis. Over 100 years ago occupational skin cancer was reported among oil and tar workers both in Germany (von Volkmann, 1875) and in Scotland (Bell, 1876). Attempts to induce skin tumours in animals by topical application of these materials failed at first, but success was finally achieved by two Japanese workers, Yamagiwa and Ichikawa (1915). They succeeded where others had failed by persisting in their treatment, thus simulating human exposure; they found that tumours could be induced on the ears of rabbits by repeated, frequent applications of coal tar over a protracted period. It was then discovered that the dorsal skin of mice offered a more convenient test system, and using this technique a systematic search for the active carcinogenic agent in coal tar was initiated under the direction of Sir Ernest Kennaway at the Royal Cancer Hospital, London (for a short history of this work see Kennaway, 1955). It was soon established that carcinogenic tars resulted from the pyrolysis of many carbon-containing materials as widely different as cholesterol, yeast, human hair and tissue, and even acetylene. It was also noted (Hieger, 1930) that all tars contained characteristic lines in their fluorescence spectra similar to those displayed by the polycyclic aromatic hydrocarbon benz[a]anthracene (Fig. 4), which is itself essentially non-carcinogenic. These lines, however, were of shorter wavelength in benz[a]anthracene, suggesting that the carcinogenic compound giving the characteristic lines was of similar type, but of higher molecular weight. The homologue dibenz[a,h]anthracene first prepared by Clar (1929) now holds the distinction of being the first pure chemical compound to be shown to be carcinogenic, as demonstrated by Kennaway and Heiger (1930). The Royal Cancer Hospital group then undertook the fractionation of two tons of gas-works pitch and, using the fluorescence spectrum as a guide, eventually (Cook *et al.*, 1933) obtained seven grams of yellow crystals consisting mainly of benzo[a]pyrene. This polycyclic aromatic hydrocarbon was found to be a potent carcinogen in the mouse skin-painting test, more active than dibenz[a,h]anthracene and having a fluorescence spectrum closely similar to that previously observed to be associated with carcinogenicity in the crude tars. Later work established that most polycyclic aromatic carcinogens were derived from the angular system of phenanthrene, whereas its linear isomer anthracene did not generally give rise to biologically active derivatives.

In the same year another carcinogenic polycyclic aromatic hydrocarbon was isolated, not from tar but from the products of pyrolysis of a steroid. During the elucidation of the structure of the cholic acids, the degradation product 12-ketocholanic acid (**8**) was found to undergo cyclization and decarboxylation at 330°C to yield dehydronorcholine (**9**). Dehydrogenation of this hydrocarbon with selenium led to loss of the two angular methyl groups and aromatization of the four six-membered rings to give 3-methylcholanthrene (Wieland and Dane, 1933) which was subsequently shown to be an even more potent carcinogen than benzo[a]pyrene (Cook and Hazelwood, 1933, 1934). This simple,

Fig. 4

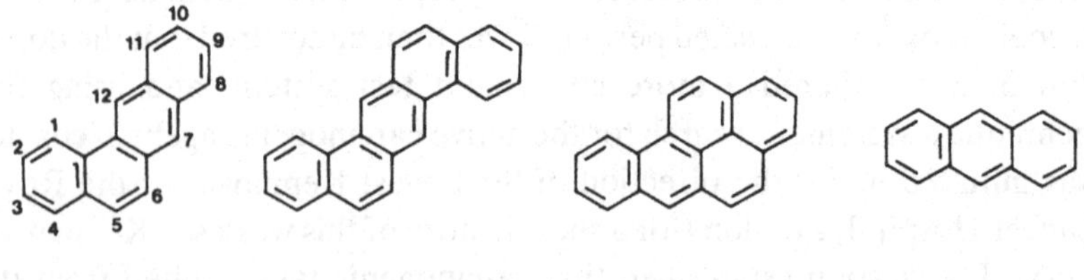

benz[a]
anthracene

dibenz [a,h]
anthracene

benzo [a]
pyrene

anthracene

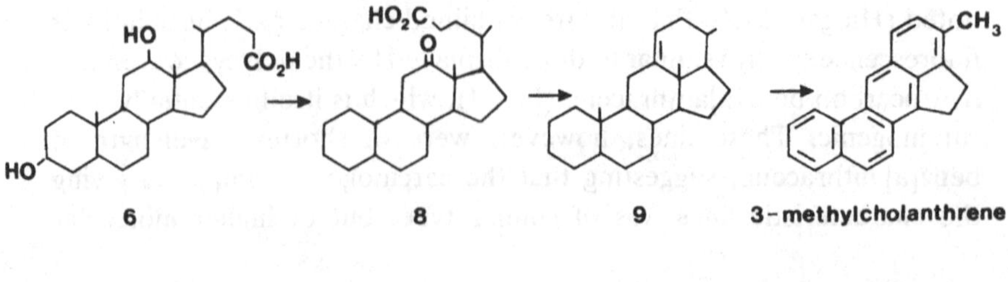

6

8

9

3-methylcholanthrene

straightforward four-step transformation of a natural steroid into a potent carcinogen was important on several grounds. Firstly, selenium dehydrogenation was accompanied by the loss of the angular methyl groups, but the ring system remained intact. Thus it became more probable that the cyclopenta[a]phenanthrene skeleton of Diels' hydrocarbon correctly represented the steroid ring system. Secondly, the position of the carbon side chain was established at C-17 in cholic acids and thus through chemical correlations in all the sterols, as well as in other physiologically important steroids such as the progestogens and corticoids to be discovered later. Finally, this remarkable preparation of a carcinogen from a natural steroid for a time led to the feeling that an important and exciting breakthrough in our understanding of the origin of human cancer was at hand. For example, Fieser (1936) in his book *Chemistry of Natural Products Related to Phenanthrene* wrote,

> 'While proof is entirely lacking, it appears possible that many forms of cancer may originate in the metabolic production of methylcholanthrene or related substances from the bile acids, or perhaps from the sterols or sex hormones, of the body'.

Fifty years later we have to say that this possibility has not been realized, although it has not been disproved. There have been a number of new twists to the story among which the cyclopenta[a]phenanthrenes find an important place. The chemistry and biological attributes of these compounds have been studied extensively partly because of their close relationship with the steroids, but also because of the attraction of this possibility of the endogenous formation of carcinogens from normal steroid hormones.

Early work on the synthesis of cyclopenta[a]phenanthrenes was largely aimed at proving, through the provision of pure synthetic specimens of known structure, the nature of the steroid dehydrogenation products. It was soon established that Diels' hydrocarbon, its 15- and 16-methyl isomers, and the parent hydrocarbon (1) (Fig. 2) were not carcinogenic (Hartnell, 1951). Interest then centred on the possibility of the formation of cholanthrenes from steroids under conditions approximating to physiological (Inhoffen, 1953). The discovery of the C_{18} and C_{19} steroid hormones lacking a side chain at C-17, required to provide the extra carbon atoms for construction of the fifth ring, seemed to rule these out as precursors, although Fieser (1941) suggested that 17-ketones might condense with biological ketoacids to provide the necessary atoms. Parallel with this, work on the synthesis and testing of numerous polycyclic aromatic hydrocarbons went on apace, and it rapidly became clear that nearly all these were based upon a phenanthrene ring system. Moreover, methyl substituents often had a dramatic effect in increasing the activity of weakly carcinogenic hydrocarbons. Thus the feeble carcinogenicity of chrysene (Fig. 3) is considerably enhanced by methyl substitution at C-5, whereas substitution at other ring positions has little effect (Dunlap and Warren, 1943). In the benz[a]anthracene (Fig. 4) series the hydrocarbon itself is essentially inactive, whilst carcinogenic activity of the monomethylbenz[a]anthracenes decreases in the order 7-Me > 12-Me > 9-Me (Cook and Kennaway, 1938); 7,12-dimethylbenz[a]anthracene (DMBA) is one of the most potent carcinogens known (Bachmann *et al.*, 1938). It therefore became of importance to study the eight possible derivatives of 16,17-dihydro-15*H*-cyclopenta[a]phenanthrene (1) bearing methyl groups on the aromatic rings. Butenandt (1942) began by synthesizing the 6-methyl derivative from the androgen dehydroandrosterone (3-hydroxyandrost-5-en-17-one); during the following decade he and his group obtained the rest of the isomers by total synthesis and tested them for carcinogenicity in the mouse skin-painting test (Butenandt and Dannenberg, 1953). All were inactive with the exception of the 7- and 11-methyl hydrocarbons which were extremely weak carcinogens, thus strengthening the opinion held at that time that four aromatic rings were essential for high potency. In later work Dannenberg showed that introduction of a double bond into the five-membered D-ring also led to weak activity in the absence of methyl substitution. He found (Dannenberg, 1970) that dehydrogenation of sterols with high-potential quinones led to compounds of this class.

1.3   Oestrogens and cyclopenta[a]phenanthrenes

Continuing this short account of those exciting and eventful early years we turn to the female sex hormones, the oestrogens. A convenient and reliable assay for oestrogenic activity was devised by Allen and Doisy (1923) based on the ability of the test compound to induce oestrus in castrated female mice, as indicated by characteristic morphological changes in the cells lining the vagina. Using this test it was discovered that human pregnancy urine was a good source of oestrogenic activity, and six years later two groups led by Doisy (1929) in America and Butenandt (1929) in Germany isolated the main oestrogenic hormone, oestrone (Fig. 5). This hormone differs from most other steroids in possessing a phenolic A-ring and in lacking the angular methyl group at C-10. Soon afterwards a second, less active oestrogen, oestriol, was obtained from the same source by Marrian (1930) in England, while in France, Girard *et al.* (1932) using the water-solubilizing ketone reagent (trimethylaminoacetohydrazine hydrochloride) which now bears his name fractionated over 50 000 L of pregnant mares' urine to isolate the naphtholic oestrogen equilenin.

During work aimed at establishing the structure of oestrone, the methyl ether of this hormone was submitted to Wolff–Kishner reduction to yield the 17-deoxy derivative (**10**) (Fig. 5) which on selenium dehydrogenation yielded 16,17-dihydro-3-methoxy-15*H*-cyclopenta[a]phenanthrene (**11**) identical with a synthetic specimen (Cook and Girard, 1934). Again selenium dehydrogenation led to elimination of the angular methyl group, but retention of the ring system. On the other hand, when oestrone methyl ether was treated with the methyl Grignard reagent and the resulting tertiary alcohol (**12**) was dehydrogenated the product was the 17,17-dimethyl derivative (**14**), not as expected the 17-monomethyl compound (**17**) or either of its 15- and 16-methyl isomers, all of which were synthesized for comparison (Cohen *et al.*, 1935). Thus migration of the angular methyl group occurs during dehydrogenation and dehydration of this carbinol (**12**). The reason for this would appear to be the

Fig. 5

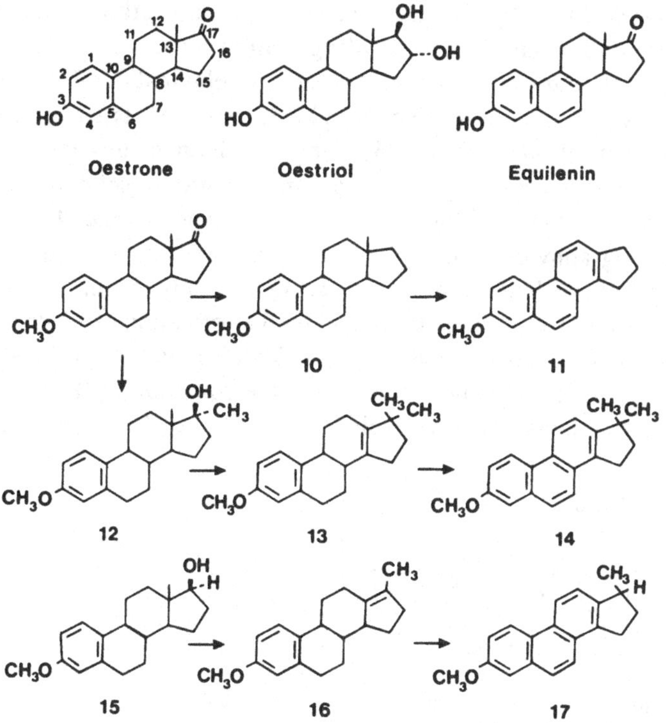

Oestrone   Oestriol   Equilenin

10   11

12   13   14

15   16   17

presence of the hydroxyl group vicinal to the quaternary carbon at C-13, because migration also occurs when oestradiol methyl ether (**15**) is similarly dehydrogenated to yield 16,17-dihydro-3-methoxy-17-methyl-15*H*-cyclopenta[a]phenanthrene (**17**). Migration also occurs when these alcohols are dehydrated under less drastic conditions to give the 17,17-dimethyl- and 17-methyl-18-nor-steroids (**13**) and (**16**), respectively. The structure of equilenin was also confirmed by selenium dehydrogenation of the tertiary alcohol derived from the methyl ether (analogous to **12**) to furnish 15,16-dihydro-17,17-dimethyl-3-methoxycyclopenta[a]phenanthrene (**14**).

In the body oestrogens are biosynthesized from male sex hormones, the androgens. This was conclusively proved when it was shown that ^{14}C-labelled testosterone was converted into [^{14}C]oestradiol (Heard *et al.*, 1955; Baggett *et al.*, 1955). Aromatization of the A-ring in the androgen androst-4-ene-3,17-dione (**18**) (Fig. 6) requires the loss of the C-19 methyl group together with two of the hydrogen atoms at C-1 and C-2. Meyer (1955*a*) isolated the 19-hydroxy derivative (**19**) as a metabolite of this androgen, and showed that on incubation with enzyme preparations from the adrenal gland, the ovary, and the placenta it gave rise to oestrogens more readily than the original hormone (Meyer, 1955*b*). It is now established that further oxidation at this carbon gives the 19-aldehyde (**20**) from which one hydrogen atom at C-2 is lost by enolization and the other at C-1 by concerted oxidative elimination of the aldehyde group as formic acid to give the phenol oestrone as shown in Fig. 6 (Stevenson *et al.*, 1985). Working on human urinary oestrogen metabolites at Edinburgh, Marrian and his group isolated a new and unusual oestrone metabolite from pregnancy urine by partition chromatography on Celite. This compound was characterized (Loke *et al.*, 1959) as 18-hydroxyoestrone (**21**) by its ready loss of formaldehyde when treated with dilute alkali, and by the formation of 18-noroestrone characterized as its methyl ether (**22**) identical with a synthetic sample (Loke *et al.*, 1958) (Fig. 7). At that time compound (**21**) was unique, being the first instance of a steroid hydroxylated at C-18. Later, of course,

Fig. 6

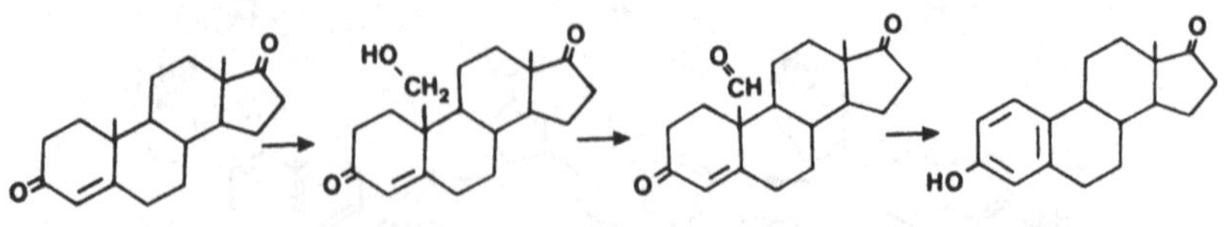

18   19   20

it was found that similar 18-hydroxylation occurs during the biosynthesis of the adrenocortical hormone aldosterone when the substrate is probably corticosterone (Eisenstein, 1967). Thus 18-hydroxylation is established as a normal adrenal function, at least for C_{21} steroids. After his move to London at about this time to take up the position of Director of Research at the Imperial Cancer Research Fund, Marrian pointed out to one of the present authors (M.C.) that should elimination of the 18-methyl group from oestrone occur *in vivo*, there would arise the possibility of complete aromatization of the steroid to 15,16-dihydro-3-hydroxycyclopenta[a]phenanthren-17-one (23). An oestrogen, equilenin, was already known with both A- and B-rings aromatic, but aromatization of ring-C in this compound is normally blocked by the angular 18-methyl group. Furthermore, 3-deoxyequilenin (25) had been isolated from mares' pregnancy urine by two groups (Marker and Rohrmann, 1939; Prelog and Fuhrer, 1945) under conditions which apparently precluded its formation as an artefact. The structure of this compound was later confirmed by its synthesis from equilenin (Bachmann and Dreiding, 1950); they submitted the steroid to the Bücherer reaction to obtain its 3-amino analogue, the diazonium salt of which was reduced with hypophosphorous acid to give the 3-deoxy compound with properties identical with those of 3-deoxyequilenin isolated from natural sources. The biosynthesis of this compound is unknown, but if it is formed like normal 3-oxygenated steroids via lanosterol, presumably elimination of this oxygen must occur before the final aromatization step takes place. In yeast squalene cyclization first gives enzyme-bound lanosta-8,24-diene which is subsequently 3-hydroxylated (Barton and Moss, 1966). If the enzyme-bound, fully cyclized hydrocarbon became free before the final step it could conceivably give rise to 3-deoxy steroids. It is interesting that

Fig. 7

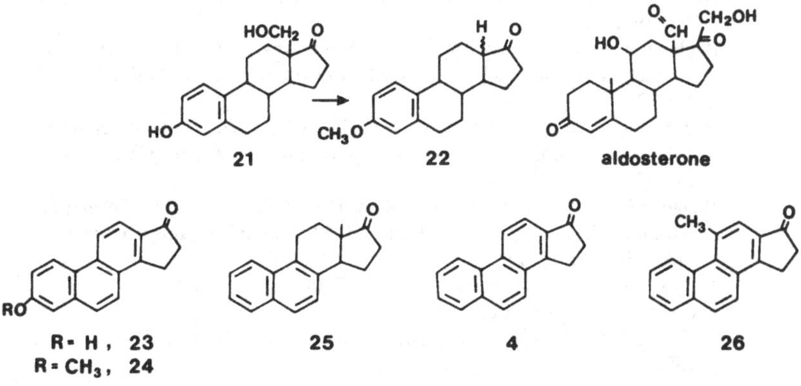

equilenin itself is apparently not derived from oestrone by further biological dehydrogenation (Gallagher *et al.*, 1958). Non-oxidative cyclization of squalene to several triterpenes which lack oxygen at C-3 is well known, but has been little investigated (Manitto, 1981). Elimination of the 18-methyl group and C-ring aromatization in the 3-deoxy compound (25) would furnish the parent ketone 15,16-dihydrocyclopenta[a]phenanthren-17-one (4).

It was therefore decided to synthesize both these cyclopenta[a]phenanthren-17-ones (4) and (23) in order to examine them for both oestrogenic and carcinogenic activity. In addition, preparation of the series of 17-ketones corresponding to Butenandt's isomeric methyl hydrocarbons was also undertaken. When it was discovered that the 11-methyl-17-ketone (26) (15,16-dihydro-11-methylcyclopenta[a]phenanthren-17-one) was a strong carcinogen (Coombs and Croft, 1966), much more potent than the corresponding hydrocarbon tested by Butenandt, interest in cyclopenta[a]phenanthrenes was renewed; work in this area has continued until the present day, and numerous related 17-oxocyclopenta[a]phenanthrenes have been synthesized and tested for mutagenic and carcinogenic activity. Recent work has been aimed at understanding the observed structure/activity relationships in terms of the metabolism of these compounds and their ability to modify biological macromolecules. In quite another sphere a number of cyclopenta[a]phenanthrene derivatives have very recently been shown to occur naturally in petroleum and other mineral oils, as well as in river and lake sediments, thus again giving rise to renewed interest in this series of compounds.

1.4   References

Adam, N. K. & Rosenheim, O. (1929). The structure of surface films. Part XIII. Sterols and their derivatives. *Proc. R. Soc. (London)*, **A126**, 25–34.

Allen, E. & Doisy, E. A. (1923). An ovarian hormone. *J. Am. Med. Assoc.*, **81**, 819–21.

Bachmann, W. E., Kennaway, E. L. & Kennaway, N. M. (1938). The rapid production of tumours by two new hydrocarbons. *Yale J. Biol. Med.*, **11**, 97–102.

Bachmann, W. E. & Dreiding, A. S. (1950). Conversion of d-equilenin into its 3-amino analog. Synthesis of d-desoxyequilenin. *J. Am. Chem. Soc.*, **72**, 1329–31.

Baggett, B., Engel, L. L., Savard, K. & Dorfman, R. I. (1955). Formation of estradiol-17β-C^{14} from testosterone-3-C^{14} by surviving human ovarian slices. *Fed. Proc.*, **14**, 175–6.

Barton, D. H. R. & Moss, G. P. (1966). Squalene cyclisation in yeast. *J. Chem. Soc., Chem. Commun.*, 261–2.

Bell, J. (1876). Paraffin epithelioma of the scrotum. *Edinburgh Med. J.*, **22**, 135–7.

Bernal, J. D. (1932a). Carbon skeleton of the sterols. *Chem. Ind. (London)*, **51**, 466.

Bernal, J. D. (1932b). Crystal structures of vitamin D and related compounds. *Nature (London)*, **129**, 277–8.

Butenandt, A. (1929). Uber 'Progynon' ein krystallisiertes weibliches Sexualhormon. *Naturwissenschaften*, **17**, 879.

Butenandt, A. & Suranyi, L. A. (1942). Uberfuhrung von Steroidhormonen in Methylhomologe des Cyclopentenophenanthren. *Ber.*, **75B**, 597–606.

Butenandt, A. & Dannenberg, H. (1953). Untersuchungen über die krebserzeugende Wirksamheit der Methylhomologen des 1,2-Cyclopentenophenanthrens. *Arch. Geschwulstforsch.*, **6**, 1–7.

Clar, E. (1929). Zur kennis merkerniger aromatischer Kohlenwasserstoffe und ihr Abkommlinge. 1 Mitt.: Dibenzanthracene und ihr Chinone, *Ber.*, **62**, 350–9.

Cohen, A., Cook, J. W. & Hewett, C. L. (1935). The synthesis of compounds related to the sterols, bile acids, and oestrus-producing hormones. Part VI. Experimental evidence of the complete structure of oestrin, equilin and equilenin. *J. Chem. Soc.*, 445–55.

Cook, J. W. & Girard, A. (1934). Dehydrogenation of oestrin. *Nature (London)*, **133**, 377–8.

Cook, J. W. & Hazelwood, G. A. D. (1933). The conversion of a bile acid into a hydrocarbon derived from 1:2-benzanthracene, *Chem. Ind. (London)*, **11**, 758–9.

Cook, J. W. & Hazelwood, G. A. D. (1934). The synthesis of 5:6-dimethyl-1:2-benzanthraquinone, a degradation product of deoxycholic acid. *J. Chem. Soc.*, 428–33.

Cook, J. W., Hewett, C. L. & Hieger, I. (1933). The isolation of a cancer-producing hydrocarbon from coal tar. Parts I and II. *J. Chem. Soc.*, 395–8.

Cook, J. W. & Kennaway, E. L. (1938). Chemical compounds as carcinogenic agents. *Am. J. Cancer*, **33**, 50–97.

Coombs, M. M. & Croft, C. J. (1966). Carcinogenic derivatives of cyclopenta[a]phenanthrene. *Nature (London)*, **210**, 1281–2.

Dannenberg, H. (1970). Vollstandige Dehydrierung von Sterinen und Steroiden mit Chinonen. *Synthesis*, **2**, 74–81.

Diels, O., Gadke, W. & Kording, P. (1927). Uber die Dehydrierung des Cholesterins. *Annalen*, **459**, 1–26.

Doisy, E. A., Veler, C. D. & Thayer, S. (1929). Folliculin from urine of pregnant women. *Am. J. Physiol.*, **90**, 329–30.

Dunlap, C. E. & Warren, S. (1943). The carcinogenic activity of some new derivatives of aromatic hydrocarbons. I. Compounds related to chrysene. *Cancer Res.*, **3**, 606–7.

Eisenstein, A. B. (1967). *The Adrenal Cortex*, p. 72. Churchill: London.

Fieser, L. F. (1936). Cancer producing hydrocarbons. In *Chemistry of Natural Products Related to Phenanthrene*, Chap. 3. Reinhold: New York.

Fieser, L. F. (1941). Univ. of Pennsylvania, Bicent. Conf., Philadelphia.

Gallagher, T. F., Kraychy, S., Fishman, J., Brown, J. B. & Marrian, G. F. (1958). A comparison of methods for the analysis of estrone, estradiol, and esteriol in extract of human urine. *J. Biol. Chem.*, **233**, 1093–6.

Girard, A., Sandulesco, G., Fridenson, A. & Rutgers, J. J. (1932). Sur une nouvelle hormone sexuelle cristallisé. *C. R. Hebd. Séances Acad. Sci.*, **195**, 981.

Hartnell, J. L. (1951). *Survey of compounds which have been tested for carcinogenic activity.* US Public Health Service Publ. No. 149, p. 184.

Heard, R. D. H., Jellinck, P. H. & O'Donnell, V. J. (1955). Biogenesis of the estrogens: the conversion of testosterone-4-C^{14} to estrone in the pregnant mare. *Endocrinology*, **57**, 200–4.

Hieger, I. (1930). The spectra of cancer-producing tars and oils and of related substances. *Biochem. J.*, **24**, 505–11.

Hillemann, H. (1935). Uber die identitat von γ-methyl-1,2-cyclopentenophenanthren mit dem dielsschen Kohlenwasserstoff $C_{18}H_{16}$. *Ber.*, **68**, 102–5.

Inhoffen, H. H. (1953). The relationship of natural steroids to carcinogenic aromatic compounds. In *Progress in Organic Chemistry*, vol. 2, p. 131. New York.

Kennaway, E. L. (1955). The identification of carcinogenic compounds in coal tar. *Br. Med. J.*, **ii**, 744–52.

Kennaway, E. L. & Heiger, I. (1930). Carcinogenic substances and their fluorescence spectra. *Br. Med. J.*, **i**, 1044.

Loke, K. H., Marrian, G. F., Johnson, W. S., Meyer, W. L. & Cameron, D. D. (1958). Isolation and identification of 18-hydroxyoesterone from the urine of pregnant women. *Biochim. Biophys. Acta*, **28**, 214.

Loke, K. H., Marrian, G. F. & Watson, E. J. D. (1959). The isolation of a sixth Kober chromogen from the urine of pregnant women and its identification as 18-hydroxyoestrone. *Biochem. J.*, **71**, 43–8.

Manitto, P. (translated by Sammes, P. G.) (1981). *Biosynthesis of Natural Products*, pp. 285–6. Chichester: Ellis Horwood Ltd.

Marker, R. E. & Rohrmann, E. (1939). The steroid content of mare's pregnancy urine. *J. Am. Chem. Soc.*, **61**, 2537–46.

Marrian, G. F. (1930). The chemistry of oestrin. III An improved method of preparation and the isolation of active crystalline material. *Biochem. J.*, **24**, 435–45.

Meyer, A. S. (1955*a*). 19-Hydroxylation of 4-androstene-3,17-dione and dehydroepionaloesterone by bovine adrenals. *Experientia*, **11**, 99–102.

Meyer, A. S. (1955*b*). Conversion of 19-hydroxy-Δ^4-androstene-3,17-dione to estrone by endocrine tissue. *Biochim. Biophys. Acta*, **17**, 441–2.

Prelog, von V. & Fuhrer, J. (1945). Uber die Isolierung von 3-Deoxy-equilenin aus dem Harn trachtiger Stuten. *Helv. Chim. Acta*, **28**, 583–90.

Rosenheim, O. & King, H. (1932). The ring-system of sterols and bile acids. *Chem. Ind. (London)*, **51**, 464–6.

Rosenheim, O. & King, H. (1933). Ring-system of sterols and bile acids. V. Constitution of ergosterol and its irradiation product. *Chem. Ind. (London)*, **52**, 299–300.

Stevenson, D. E., Wright, J. N. & Akhtar, M. (1985). Synthesis of 19-functionalised derivatives of 16α-hydroxytestosterone: mechanistic studies on oestriol biosynthesis. *J. Chem. Soc., Chem. Commun.*, 1078–80.

von Volkmann, R. (1875). *Beitrage zur Chiragie*. Leipzig.

Wieland, H. & Dane, E. (1933). Untersuchungen über die Konstitution der Gallensausen. *Z. physiol. Chem.*, **219**, 240.

Yamagiwa, K. & Ichikawa, K. (1915). Experimentelle Studie über die Pathogenese der Epithelialgeschwulst. *Mitt. med. Fak.*, Tokio, **15**, 295.

2

Chemical synthesis of cyclopenta[a]phenanthrenes: hydrocarbons

2.1   Early synthesis of hydrocarbons in connection with steroids

As has already been outlined, syntheses of cyclopenta[a]phenan-
threnes lacking oxygen substitution in ring-D were originally undertaken
50 years ago to provide rigid structural proof for steroid dehydrogenation
products. These syntheses were greatly assisted by previous investigations on the preparation of phenanthrene derivatives by Haworth and his
school in connection with elucidation of the structures of the resin acids
(Fieser, 1936). The parent hydrocarbon 16,17-dihydro-15H-cyclopen-
ta[a]phenanthrene (1) was obtained by both Kon (1933) and by Ruzicka
et al. (1933) by essentially the same route, outlined in Fig. 8. Condensation of 2-(1-naphthyl)ethyl bromide with ethyl cyclopentanone-2-carbox-
ylate gave the β-keto-ester (40) which was decarboxylated, and the

Fig. 8

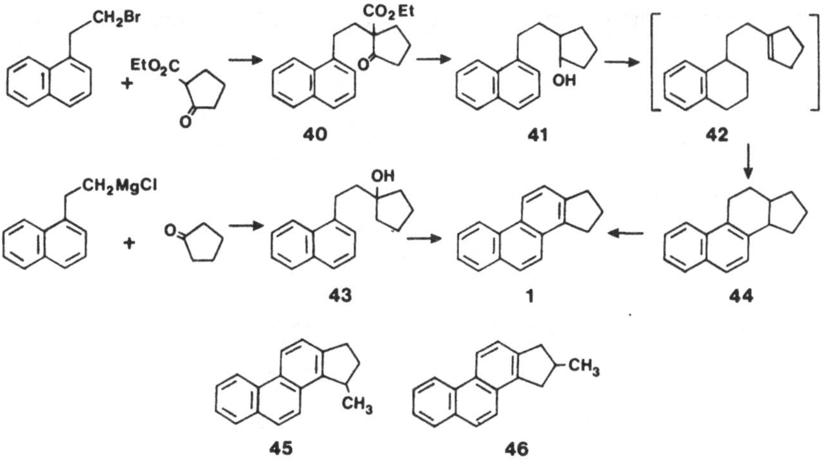

resulting ketone was reduced to the secondary alcohol (41). This was cyclized to the tetracyclic compound (44), without isolation of the intermediate cyclopentene (42), by heating it with phosphorus pentoxide, and the synthesis was completed by dehydrogenation with selenium. Ruzicka discovered that the final hydrocarbon (1) could be obtained directly by heating the keto-ester (40) with sulphuric acid. A somewhat different route was followed by Cook and Hewett (1933) who were interested in this compound in connection with their work on polycyclic aromatic hydrocarbon carcinogens. These workers first obtained the tertiary alcohol (43) by treating cyclopentanone with the Grignard reagent from 2-(1-naphthyl)-ethyl chloride, and this was cyclized directly to the final cyclopenta[a]phenanthrene with hot sulphuric and acetic acids. In both cases the unsaturated hydrocarbon (42) was probably an intermediate in these cyclizations because it could be formed from either of the alcohols (41) or (43) by dehydration under mild conditions. Presumably the sulphuric acid acts as an oxidizing agent in these reactions to remove the extra hydrogen atoms after dehydrating the alcohol and forming the carbonium ion. By employing the two isomeric 4-methyl and 5-methyl homologues of ethyl cyclopentanone-2-carboxylate Ruzicka also synthesized the 15- and 16-methyl derivatives (45 and 46, respectively) of the parent hydrocarbon; both proved to be distinctly different from Diels' hydrocarbon (7) obtained from sterol dehydrogenations. In later work Cook and Hewett (1934) investigated the cyclization of the naphthylethylcyclopentene (42) with aluminium chloride and stannic chloride, isolating two spirans in addition to the expected product. The spiran rings in these two hydrocarbons were unstable to the high-temperature conditions during selenium dehydrogenation which aromatized them to chrysofluorene and 2-methylpyrene as shown in Fig. 9. Spiran formation was suppressed by placing a methyl group at the other

Fig. 9

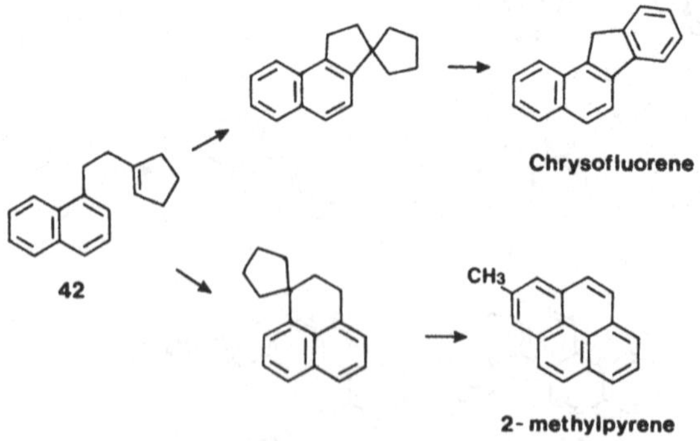

Chrysofluorene

42

CH₃

2- methylpyrene

end of the double bond in (**42**). Thus in a synthesis of Diels' hydrocarbon (**7**) (Harper *et al.*, 1934) shown in Fig. 10, 2,5-dimethylcyclopentanone was treated with the Grignard reagent from 2-(1-naphthyl)ethyl bromide to give the tertiary carbinol (**47**), which on being heated with phosphorus pentoxide led to a good yield of the cyclized product (**48**). The angular methyl group was eliminated, but the 17-methyl group was retained on selenium dehydrogenation to yield Diels' hydrocarbon (**7**). A year earlier Bergmann and Hillemann (1933) had obtained the same compound for the first time, from 2-acetylnaphthalene by way of a Reformatsky reaction with methyl bromoacetate, followed by reduction of the double bond, hydrolysis, ring closure, and Clemmensen reduction of the 15-ketone (**49**) (Fig. 10). Both samples melted at 125°C, like Diels' hydro-carbon itself, but for a time there was some confusion between this compound and the parent hydrocarbon (**1**), although the latter melted some 10 degrees higher. The two compounds cannot be distinguished readily from their elementary compositions:

Calculated for $C_{18}H_{16}$: C, 93.1; H, 6.9%
Calculated for $C_{17}H_{14}$: C, 93.5; H, 6.5%

owing to the limits of accuracy of combustion analysis (Ruzicka and Thomann, 1933); also mixed melting points failed to be helpful in this instance. In order to resolve this question, Hillemann (1935) prepared another sample of the hydrocarbon, this time by the method of Harper, and carefully compared the purified material with Diels' hydrocarbon with which it proved to be identical. In particular the synthetic sample gave a characteristic nitroso compound, mp 238–239°C, identical with that given by Diels' hydrocarbon, whereas the hydrocarbon (**1**) did not, as had been noted by Diels previously (Diels and Clar, 1934). Thus the structure of Diels' hydrocarbon was settled at last.

Another synthesis of Diels' hydrocarbon, together with its 17-ethyl and 17-isopropyl derivatives, was described by Riegel *et al.* (1943) (Fig. 11).

Fig. 10

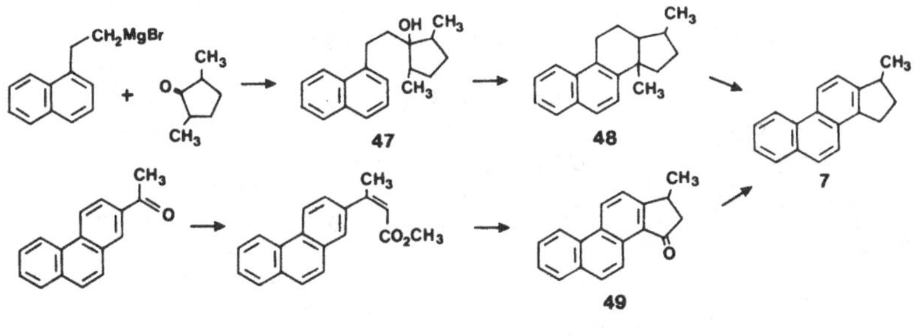

The 3-acylphenanthrenes were converted in three steps into the propionic acids which were cyclized to yield the 15-ketones (**49** and **50**). The 17-alkyl-16,17-dihydro-15*H*-cyclopenta[a]phenanthrenes (**7**, **52**, and **53**) were then obtained by reduction. The 17-ethyl hydrocarbon (**52**) was also isolated in 40% yield from selenium dehydrogenation of pregnanediol at 300–350°C (Schöntube and Janak, 1968). A similar synthesis of Diels' hydrocarbon via its 15-ketone was reported by Tatta and Bardhan (1968). Condensation of diethyl 2-(1-naphthyl)-ethylmalonate with ethyl crotonate in the presence of base, followed by hydrolysis and decarboxylation gave the di-acid (**54**). Ring closure was effected with 85% sulphuric acid, and the resulting ketone was reduced and aromatized by being heated with sulphur; the overall yield was over 70%. Cyclization of the acid chloride to give the 17-methyl-15-ketone (**49**) was accomplished with aluminium chloride in nitrobenzene; reduction of this ketone gave Diels' hydrocarbon (**7**). The authors pointed out three advantages of this synthetic route: (i) the easy availability of starting materials; (ii) good yields throughout; and (iii) the avoidance of dehydrogenation in the final stage of the synthesis.

This first phase of cyclopenta[a]phenanthrene synthesis concluded with the synthesis of several methoxycyclopenta[a]phenanthrenes in connection with structural studies on the oestrogens, as discussed in Chapter 1. For the synthesis of 16,17-dihydro-3-methoxy-15*H*-cyclopenta[a]phenanthrene (**11**) (Fig. 12) the Grignard reagent, prepared from the chloride (**55**), itself secured in six steps from 2-naphthylamine, was added to 2-methylcyclopentanone; dehydration of the resulting alcohol gave the cyclopentene which was cyclized with aluminium chloride to the angular methyl compound (**56**). The angular methyl group was elimin-

Fig. 11

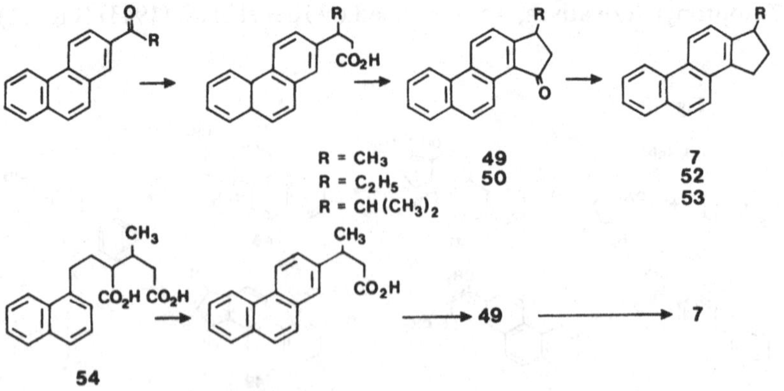

R = CH₃   **49**   **7**
R = C₂H₅   **50**   **52**
R = CH(CH₃)₂   **53**

54

ated as usual on selenium dehydrogenation to furnish the desired 3-methoxy hydrocarbon (**11**) (Cohen *et al.*, 1935). The overall yield from 2-aminonaphthalene was only 0.02%, but the pure sample was identical with the sample prepared by selenium dehydrogenation of 17-deoxy-oestrone methyl ether. The 17,17-dimethyl derivative (**14**) was obtained in an analogous manner from 2,5,5-trimethylcyclopentanone, as was the 17-methyl compound (**17**) from 2,5-dimethylpentanone. For the preparation of the 16- and 15- isomers (**57** and **58**) the bromide corresponding to (**55**) was condensed with ethyl 4-methyl- and 5-methylcyclopentanone-2-carboxylate, respectively, following the original synthesis shown in Fig. 10. The 4- and 6-methoxy isomers (**59**), (**61**), and (**62**) were prepared by Kon and Ruzicka (1935) in an analogous manner from the corresponding methoxy-1-naphthylethyl bromides. The 3-methoxy hydrocarbon (**11**) was obtained in better yield by a different route (Chuang *et al.*, 1939). Condensation of the acid chloride of the methoxynaphthylbutyric acid with the sodium salt of 2-acetyl-diethyl-succinate gave the diketo–diester (**64**) which on ring closure with sodium ethoxide and decarboxylation

Fig. 12

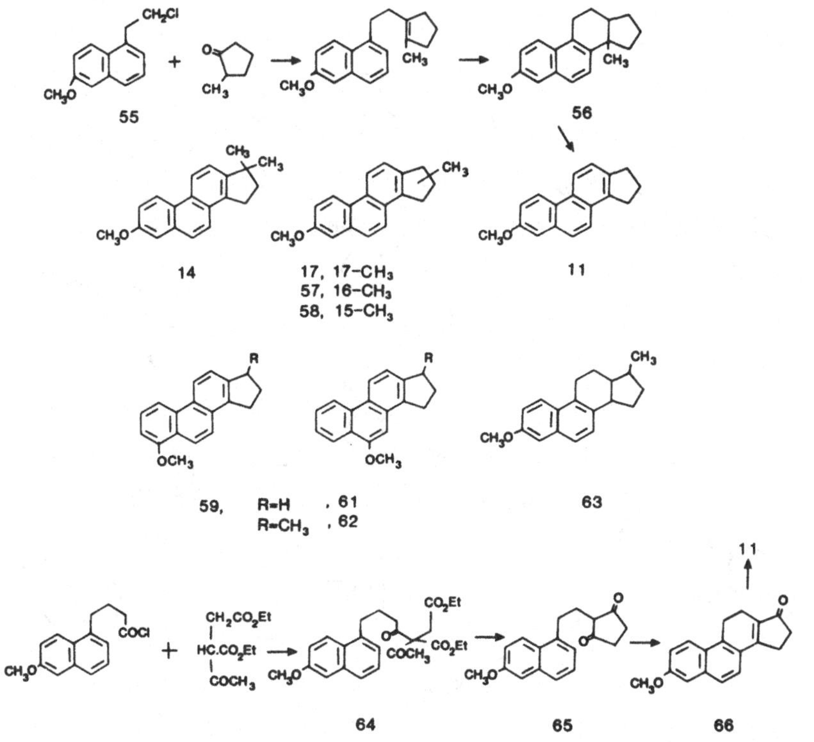

yielded the 1,3-cyclopentanedione (**65**). Cyclization of the latter with phosphorus pentoxide then gave 3-methoxy-11,12,15,16-tetrahydro-cyclopenta[a]phenanthren-17-one (**66**), converted by Clemmensen reduction and selenium dehydrogenation to the desired 3-methoxy hydrocarbon (**11**). The 3-methoxy-17-methyl compound (**17**) was later obtained from the corresponding 17-ketone via a Grignard reaction (Coombs, 1966), and by dehydrogenation of a byproduct (**63**) isolated from the demethylation of oestrone methyl ether by fusion with pyridinium hydrochloride at 200°C (Hoffsommer *et al.*, 1966). The way in which these methoxycyclopenta[a]phenanthrenes were used to establish the structures of oestrone and equilenin have been discussed in Chapter 1 (see Fig. 5).

2.2   Syntheses of the isomeric aryl methyl hydrocarbons

The next synthetic phase, in which all the possible monomethyl and several dimethyl derivatives of 16,17-dihydro-15*H*-cyclopenta[a]phenanthrene were prepared, led to the first detection of carcinogenicity among compounds of this class. However, the first step in this direction was taken in connection with the structure of the cardiac

Fig. 13

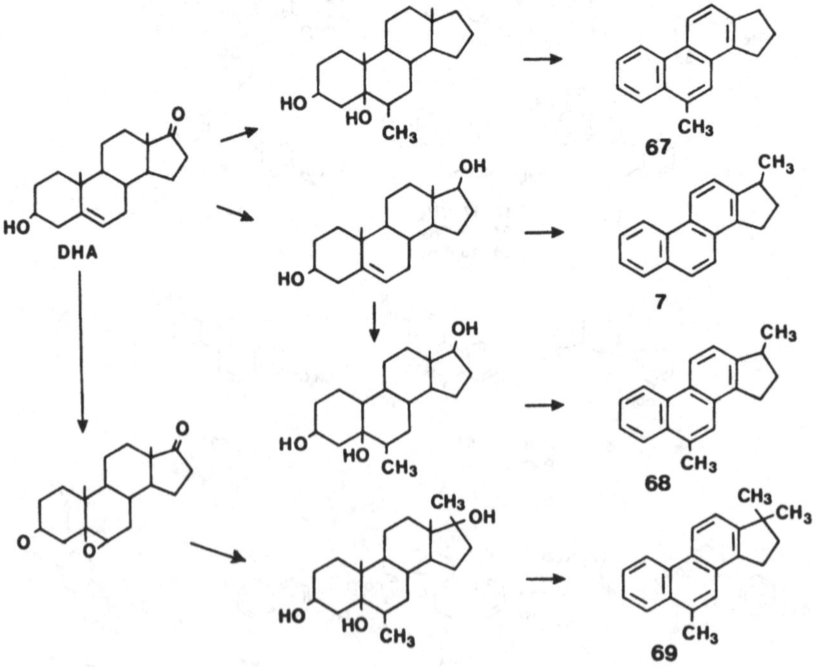

aglycone strophanthidin. Like the sterols, this gave Diels' hydrocarbon on selenium dehydrogenation, although a suggested formula for the aglycone should have led to its 6-methyl homologue (**68**) (Fig. 13). Both this cyclopenta[a]phenanthrene and the 6-monomethyl derivative (**67**) were synthesized by Gamble and Kon (1935) from 1-(4-methyl-1-naph-thyl)-ethyl bromide and the requisite cyclopentanone following the general method of Harper (see Fig. 10). Neither compound was identical with Diels' hydrocarbon and the suggested formula for strophanthidin had to be abandoned. The same two compounds together with the 6,17,17-trimethyl analogue (**69**) were later obtained by Butenandt and Suranyi (1942) from the androgen dehydroepiandrosterone (DHA, 3-hydroxy-androst-5-en-17-one). The 6-methyl group was introduced into the steroid by opening the 5,6-epoxide, prepared by oxidizing the 5(6)-double bond with perbenzoic acid, by means of methyl magnesium iodide. Introduction of the 17-methyl group was achieved by using the known propensity of the steroid 18-methyl group vicinal to a hydroxyl group to migrate to C-17 during selenium dehydrogenation. Diels' hydrocarbon (**7**) was also synthesized by dehydrogenation of 3,17-dihydroxyandrost-5-ene, omitting the epoxidation step. Yet two more cyclopenta[a]phenanthrenes were synthesized while establishing the structure of the plant sapogenin, sarsasapogenin (Kon and Woolman, 1939) (Fig. 14). To locate the hydroxyl group in this molecule the alcohol was oxidized to the ketone and the position of the oxygen was marked by converting it to the tertiary carbinol, methylsarsasapogenin, by treatment

Fig. 14

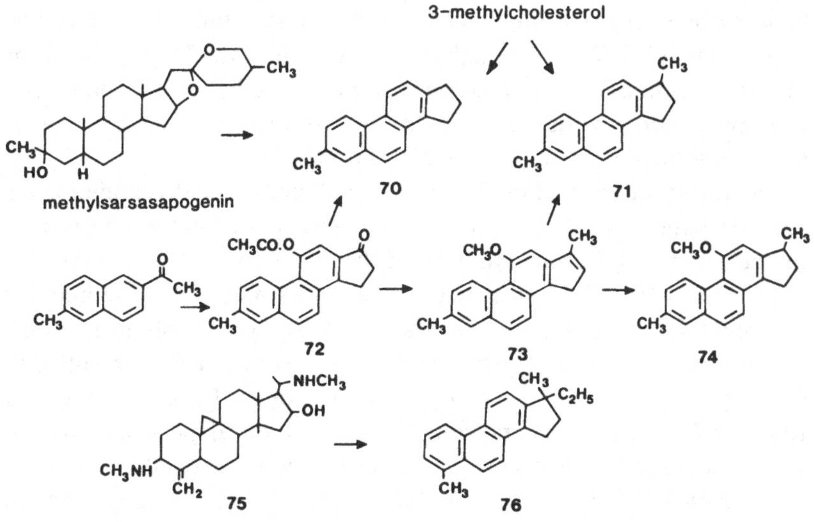

3-methylcholesterol

methylsarsasapogenin

70

71

72

73

74

75

76

with methyl magnesium iodide. Dehydrogenation gave a hydrocarbon thought to be 16,17-dihydro-3-methyl-15H-cyclopenta[a]phenanthrene (70), rather than the initially expected 3,17-dimethyl analogue (71). In order to confirm this, both these hydrocarbons were prepared as outlined in Fig. 14. 2-Acetyl-6-methylnaphthalene was transformed into 11-acetoxy-15,16-dihydro-3-methylcyclopenta[a]phenanthren-17-one (72) by Robinson's method (discussed later in this chapter), and the derived methyl ether was treated with the methyl Grignard reagent to give 3,17-dimethyl-11-methoxy-15H-cyclopenta[a]phenanthrene (73), dehydration of the intermediate tertiary carbinol having occurred readily during the reaction. Mild hydrogenation of this compound saturated the 16(17)-double bond yielding the dihydro derivative (74), while prolonged, vigorous catalytic reduction (Adams catalyst in acetic acid at 80–85°C for some days) of both the 11-acetoxy-17-ketone (72) and the 11-methoxy-16(17)-ene (73) removed the oxygen functions and partially reduced the aromatic rings. The crude reduction products were heated at 320°C with equal weights of 10% palladized charcoal, and the hydrocarbon fractions were isolated by percolation of petroleum extracts through columns of activated alumina. The 3-methyl hydrocarbon (70), which was obtained in about 20% yield, was found to be identical with the dehydrogenation product of methylsarsasapogenin, showing that migration of the 18-methyl group to C-17 does not always occur during dehydrogenation of steroids. The 3,17-dimethyl hydrocarbon (71) was obtained in a similar way from (73) by vigorous reduction followed by dehydrogenation, and was shown to be identical with a major product from dehydrogenation of 3-methylcholestanol; a minor product appeared to be the 3-methyl hydrocarbon (70). During elucidation of the structure of the alkaloid cyclobuxine $C_{25}H_{42}ON_2$, thought to possess the formula (75) shown in Fig. 14, selenium dehydrogenation yielded 15,16-dihydro-4,17-dimethyl-17-ethyl cyclopenta[a]phenanthrene (76) (Brown and Kupchan, 1962) thus confirming the nature of the carbon skeleton.

The rest of the methyl isomers and a number of dimethyl homologues were prepared by Butenandt and his co-workers by total synthesis over the next 10 years. For the synthesis of the 11-methyl and 11,12-dimethyl derivatives (83 and 87, respectively) use was made of a method for cyclopenta[a]phenanthrene synthesis elaborated by Robinson in his extensive work directed at the synthesis of steroids and which resulted in an early total synthesis of an equilenin stereoisomer. In number XXI of a remarkable series of papers from Oxford entitled 'Experiments on the synthesis of substances related to the sterols' published in the *Journal of the Chemical Society*, Robinson (1938) adapted a little-known reaction discovered by Kehrer and Igler (1899) to the naphthalene series (Fig. 15). The furfurylidene derivative of 1-acetyl-naphthalene (**77**), obtained in high yield by base-catalysed condensation of 1-acetyl-naphthalene with furfuraldehyde, on being boiled with ethanolic hydrochloric acid yielded the diketoheptanoic acid (**78**). The mechanism of this intriguing reaction, in which the furan ring is opened by the formal addition of two molecules of water, is obscure; however, the acid is obtained reproducibly in about 50% yield, the other product being a black insoluble tar. Intramolecular ring closure of the side chain brought about by hot 2% potassium hydroxide gave the naphthylcyclopentenone acetic acid (**79**) which was itself cyclized to yield 11-acetoxy-15,16-dihydrocyclopenta[a]phenanthren-17-one (**80**) by boiling it with acetic anhydride. Both these cyclizations occur essentially quantitatively and the whole sequence provides an elegant entry into the cyclopenta[a]phenanthrene series.

Butenandt *et al.* (1946*a*) modified this route by first converting the cyclopentenone (**79**) into the cyclopentane (**81**) by mild hydrogenation of the tetrasubstituted double bond (Koebner and Robinson, 1938), followed by heating the derived semicarbazone with sodium ethoxide at 180°C (Fig. 15). Cyclization in this acid is less facile because it is not favoured by the driving force provided by the creation of a new aromatic ring; it was achieved by treating the acid chloride of (**81**) with aluminium chloride to give the ketone (**82**) in about 50% yield. The 11-methyl group was introduced by a Grignard reaction with methyl magnesium iodide; dehydration and dehydrogenation with platinized charcoal at 300–310°C

Fig. 15

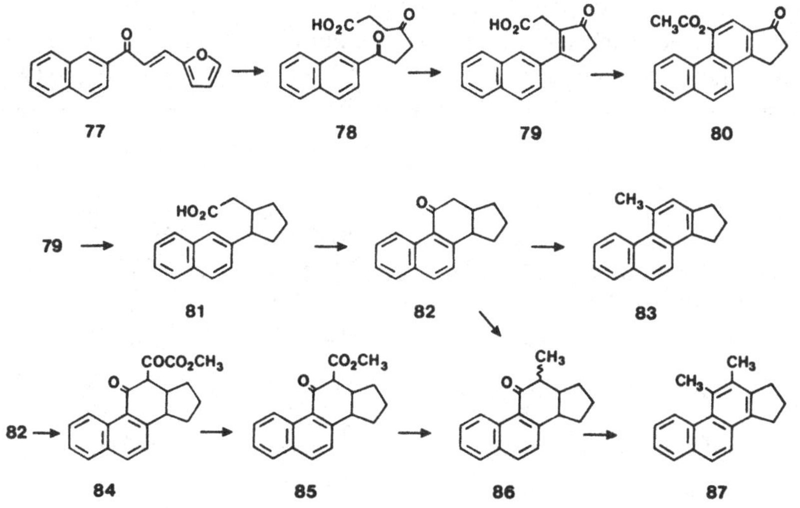

then led to 16,17-dihydro-11-methyl-15H-cyclopenta[a]phenanthrene
(**83**). Methylation at C-12 in the 11-ketone (**82**) was achieved in two ways;
direct methylation with methyl iodide and potassium *tert.*-butoxide
yielded a monomethyl derivative (**85**) of mp 85–86°C. Alternatively,
condensation of the ketone (**82**) with dimethyloxalate in the presence of
sodium methoxide, followed by pyrolysis of the glyoxalate (**84**) on glass
powder at 180°C gave the 12-carboxylic ester (**85**); base-catalysed
methylation of the latter with methyl iodide and decarboxylation of the
intermediate led to a stereo-isomeric 12-methyl-ketone, mp 117–118°C,
which could be converted into the lower-melting isomer with aqueous
methanolic potassium hydroxide. Treatment of (**86**) with methyl lithium
and dehydration–dehydrogenation of the intermediate tertiary carbinol
finally yielded 16,17-dihydro-11,12-dimethyl-15H-cyclopenta[a]phenan-
threne (**87**). The 12-methyl hydrocarbon was also prepared in low yield
from the 12-methyl-11-ketone (**86**) by way of Clemmensen reduction,
and proved to be identical with a specimen prepared by another route
(see below).

This general synthetic route to cyclopenta[a]phenanthrenes was also
employed for the synthesis of the 7-methyl isomer (Butenandt *et al.*,
1949*a*), starting from 2-acetyl-3-methyl-5,6,7,8-tetrahydronaphthalene
(**88**) (Fig. 16). This was converted into the furfurylidene derivative (**89**)
which underwent acid-catalysed furan ring opening to the heptanoic acid
(**90**). However, on ring closure with dilute potassium hydroxide
Butenandt reported that the cyclopentenone acetic acid (**91**) was
accompanied by the furan propionic acid (**95**) (although in the
experimental part of their paper, under the description of the acid (**90**)
they state, 'In manchen Ansatzen wurde ein Gemisch der Dioxoheptan-
saure und der nachstehend beschrieben Furan-propionsaure erhalten').
In connection with the synthesis of the 17-ketone corresponding to (**94**)
Coombs and Jaitly (1971) repeated the acid treatment of the fur-

Fig. 16

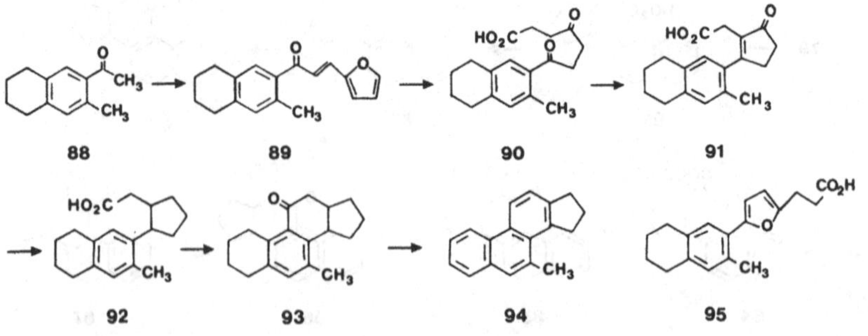

88   89   90   91

92   93   94   95

furylidene compound (89), obtaining similar amounts of the furan acid (95) and the required heptanoic acid (90); however, cyclization of the latter with dilute alkali led exclusively to (91). The reason for this apparent discrepancy is not known. The German preparation continued by vigorous catalytic reduction of (91), saturating the double bond and removing the ketone oxygen to yield the acid (92). Cyclization of the corresponding acid chloride with stannic chloride to the ketone (93) (70.5%), Clemmensen reduction of the latter, and dehydrogenation gave 16,17-dihydro-7-methyl-15*H*-cyclopenta[a]phenanthrene (94).

Another intermediate (96) discovered by Robinson during the early approaches to steroid synthesis was adopted by Butenandt for the preparation of several other cyclopenta[a]phenanthrenes (Fig. 17). This ketone was obtained by Hawthorne and Robinson (1936) by condensation of tetralone with acetylcyclopent-1-ene in the presence of sodium amide. Elimination of the ketone oxygen by heating the semicarbazone with sodium ethoxide and a trace of hydrazine hydrate, followed by dehydrogenation provided a new synthesis of 16,17-dihydro-15*H*-cyclopenta[a]phenanthrene (1) (Butenandt *et al.*, 1946c). Introduction of a methyl group at C-12 by treatment of the ketone (96) with methyl magnesium iodide, followed by dehydration and dehydrogenation gave the 12-methyl hydrocarbon (97). In a similar manner 7-methyltetralone

Fig. 17

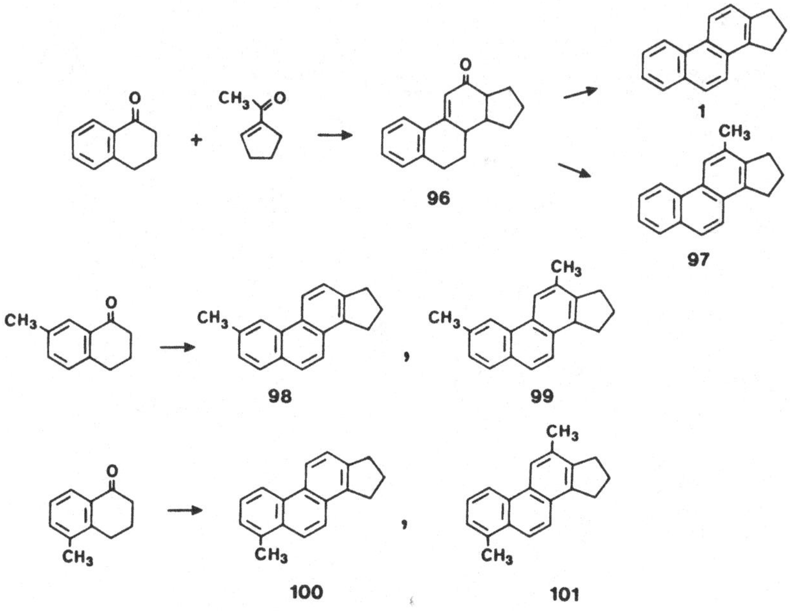

gave rise to the 2-methyl and 2,12-dimethyl compounds (**98** and **99**, respectively), while the 4-methyl (**100**) and 4,12-dimethyl (**101**) isomers were prepared from 5-methyltetralone (Butenandt *et al.*, 1949*b*).

Oxidation of the parent hydrocarbon (**1**) with chromic acid did not lead, as expected for a phenanthrene derivative, to the 6,7-quinone (Butenandt *et al.*, 1946*b*). Instead oxidation occurred at the five-membered ring to afford the 15-ketone (**102**) (Fig. 18) previously synthesized by Bachmann (1935). On the other hand, osmium tetroxide added across the 6,7-double bond in the hydrocarbon (**1**) to yield the 6,7-*cis*-dihydrodiol (**103**), mild oxidation of which with chromic acid in acetic acid solution gave the desired quinone (**104**). Reaction of this quinone with an excess of methyl magnesium iodide followed by heating the product with a mixture of zinc chloride and zinc dust then furnished 16,17-dihydro-6,7-dimethyl-15*H*-cyclopenta[a]phenanthrene (**105**) in 12.5% yield based on the quinone.

For the synthesis of the 1-methyl hydrocarbon (**107**) (Butenandt *et al.*, 1950) 1-bromo-8-methylnaphthalene, obtained in several steps from 1,8-diaminonaphthalene (Fieser and Seligman, 1939), was treated with

Fig. 18

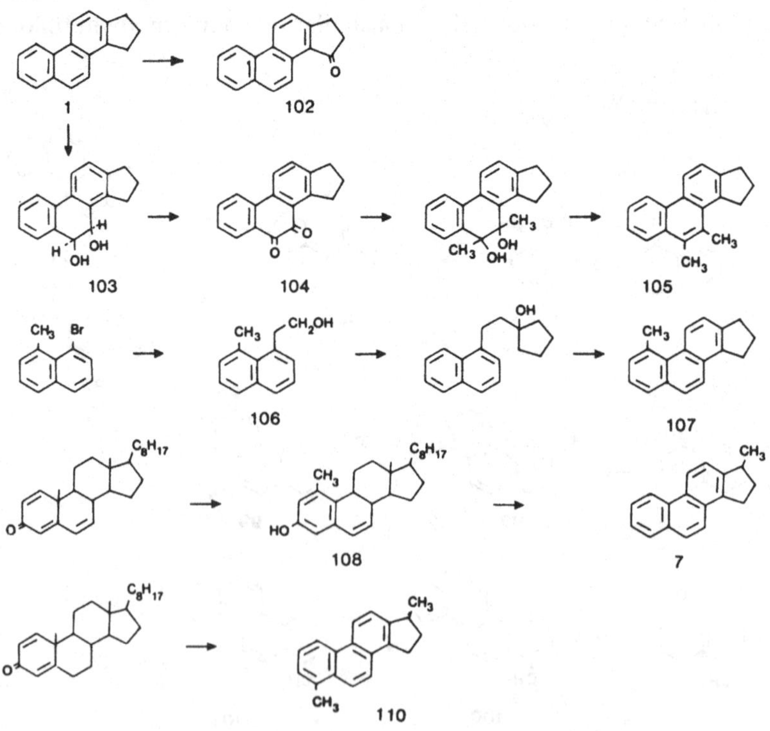

phenyl lithium at −10°C and ethylene oxide was added to yield the naphthylethyl alcohol (106). The scheme then followed the original method of Cook and Hewett (1933) shown in Fig. 8. In the final cyclization, addition of some acetic anhydride together with acetic and sulphuric acids was found markedly to improve the yield of 16,17-dihydro-1-methyl-15H-cyclopenta[a]phenanthrene (107). In its absence a second hydrocarbon, $C_{18}H_{20}$ having a naphthalene chromophore, was also isolated. 1-Methyl compounds are also obtainable from steroids by migration of the 19-methyl group to C-1 by the dienonephenol rearrangement (Kirk and Hartshorn, 1969). Thus 1-methyl-19-norcholesta-1,3,5(10),6-tetraen-3-ol (108) is readily available from cholesta-1,4,6-trien-3-one by treatment with hot acid. Dehydrogenation of this compound with selenium was accompanied, however, by loss of the 1-methyl group with formation of Diels' hydrocarbon (7) (Butenandt *et al.*, 1954). A dimethyl hydrocarbon thought to be 16,17-dihydro-1,17-dimethyl-15H-cyclopenta[a]phenanthrene was obtained earlier (Inhoffen *et al.*, 1949) by similar dehydrogenation of cholesta-1,4-dien-3-one or its rearrangement product, but was later shown to be the 4,17-isomer (110). Butenandt's synthesis of the 1-methyl hydrocarbon concluded the acquisition of the 11 possible monomethyl hydrocarbons derived from 16,17-dihydro-15H-cyclopenta[a]phenanthrene. A number of 17-methyl hydrocarbons carrying in addition aryl methyl groups were later obtained from 17-ketones via the Grignard reaction; these are discussed in the next section.

Three syntheses of 16,17-dihydro-15H-cyclopenta[a]phenanthrenes have been described employing the Diels–Alder reaction to construct this ring system (Fig. 19). Sen Gupta and Bhattacharyya (1954) condensed 1-vinylnaphthalene with cyclopentane-1,2-dicarboxylic acid anhydride in boiling xylene to obtain a crystalline adduct thought to be (111). Treatment with alkali or acid converted it to the naphthyl isomer (112) which resisted dehydrogenation with selenium. Conversion of this to its calcium salt followed by heating the latter with lime caused decarboxylation, and the crude product could then be dehydrogenated to the parent hydrocarbon (1). In the second approach Tamayo and Martin (1952) formed ring-B by condensation of 4-vinylindan (113) with *p*-benzoquinone. The starting material was obtained from 4-chloroindan *via* the lithium derivative which reacted with ethylene oxide to yield 4-(2-hydroxyethyl)indan, readily dehydrated to (113). Condensation of this with *p*-benzoquinone at 100°C for 20 h gave the adduct (114) which was converted into the dihydroxy-tetrahydro compound (115) and thence into 16,17-dihydro-1,4-dihydroxy-15H-cyclopenta[a]phenanthrene (116). In the third method (Butz *et al.*, 1940) the acetylene (**117**) was heated together with maleic anhydride at 130°C to yield the crystalline adduct (**118**), mp 249–251°C, which could be converted into the parent hydrocarbon (**1**) in low yield by dehydrogenation over palladium on charcoal at an elevated temperature.

Yet another way of constructing the cyclopenta[a]phenanthrene system by finally closing ring-C was devised by Birch and Robinson (1944) (Fig. 20). Condensation of the 1-acetyl-3,4-dihydronaphthalenes (**119** and **120**) with lithium 2-isopropylcyclopentenone gave the diketones (**121** and **122**) which could be cyclized by sodium ethoxide to the 11-keto-12(13)-enes (**123** and **124**). Attempted methylation of (**123**) at the angular position (C-13) by addition of methyl magnesium iodide in the presence

Fig. 19

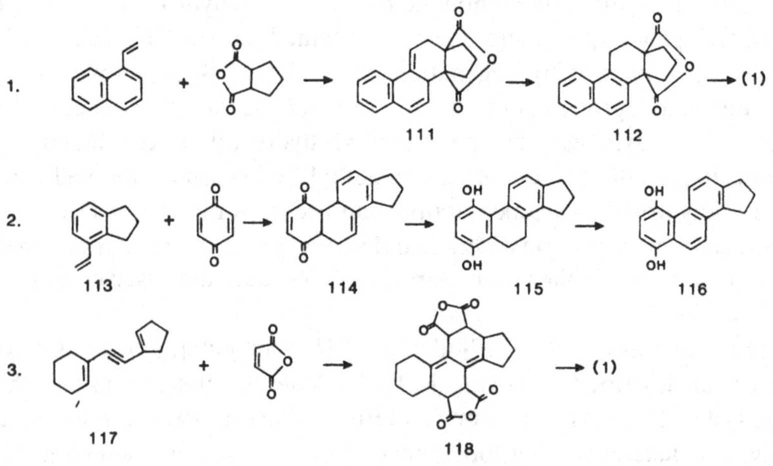

Fig. 20

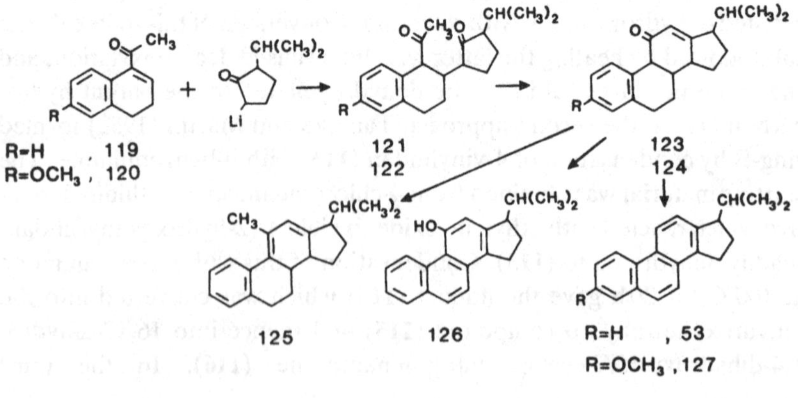

of cuprous bromide failed, giving instead the product of addition to the carbonyl group and dehydration (6,7,8,14,16,17-hexahydro-17-isopropyl-11-methyl-15*H*-cyclopenta[a]phenanthrene, **125**). Direct dehydrogenation of (**123**) with palladium on charcoal gave the 11-phenol (**126**) whilst reduction of both (**123**) and (**124**) with sodium and ethanol followed by selenium dehydrogenation led to 16,17-dihydro-17-isopropyl-15*H*-cyclopenta[a]phenanthrene (**53**) and its 3-methoxy derivative (**127**).

2.3 Hydrocarbons containing an extra double bond in ring-D (15*H*-and 17*H*-cyclopenta[a]phenanthrenes)

Although heating with either selenium or noble metal catalysts causes efficient dehydrogenation of the six-membered rings, a double bond is not introduced into the five-membered ring of the steroid or dihydrocyclopenta[a]phenanthrene systems by these reagents. This can, however, be readily accomplished starting from the ring-D ketones, the syntheses of which are described in Chapter 3. Thus treatment of 15,16-dihydrocyclopenta[a]phenanthren-15-one (**102**) and -17-one (**4**) with methyl magnesium iodide in boiling benzene, followed by chromatography of the products on active alumina yielded 15-methyl-17*H*-cyclopenta[a]phenanthrene (**128**) and its 17-methyl-15*H* isomer (**133**), respectively (Dannenberg *et al.*, 1960) (Fig. 21). These compounds were found to be carcinogenic in the mouse skin-painting test, rather more active than the very weakly carcinogenic 7- and 11-methyl-16,17-dihydro-15*H*-derivatives previously tested, and the question arose as to whether carcinogenicity would be higher in molecules containing both these structural features (Dannenberg, 1960). This was later found to be the case by Coombs and Croft (1969) who investigated the series of six 17-methyl-16(17)-enes (**133–138**) prepared from the corresponding 17-ketones by the same method (Coombs, 1966). Dannenberg noted that the formation of (**133**) was accompanied by the appearance of a dimer $C_{36}H_{28}$, and suggested the structure (**129**) for this substance. This was confirmed by Coombs by a nuclear magnetic resonance study; he also reported that the yield of the monomer varied appreciably with the structure of the ketone used as substrate, as shown in Table 1. Dimerization apparently occurred during chromatography although neutral alumina was employed, for the yield of the 11-methoxy-17-methyl-16(17)-ene (**138**) was only 18% when it was obtained in this way, whereas it was 85% when it was isolated directly by crystallization before chromatography. The yield was also low for the 12-methyl (**136**) and 11,12-dimethyl (**137**) compounds prepared by the general procedure.

Hydrogenation of the D-ring double bond occurred readily to give the corresponding dihydro derivatives (**7, 17, 139–142**), but the corresponding double bond in the dimer (**129**) was inert, as anticipated from its sterically hindered nature. Dannenberg also obtained the 17-methyl-16(17)-ene (**133**) when 15,16-dihydrocyclopenta[a]phenanthren-17-one

Fig. 21

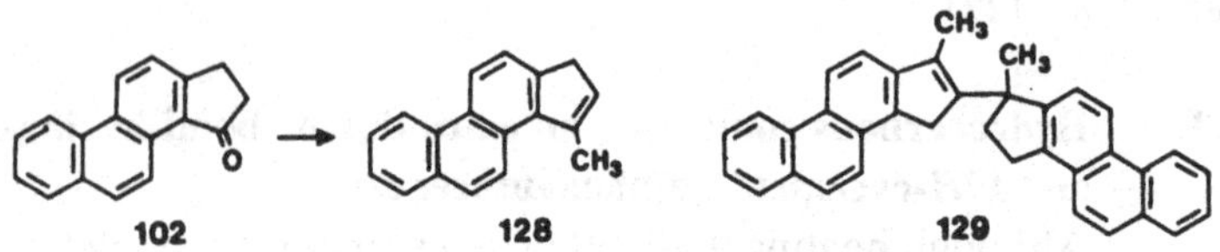

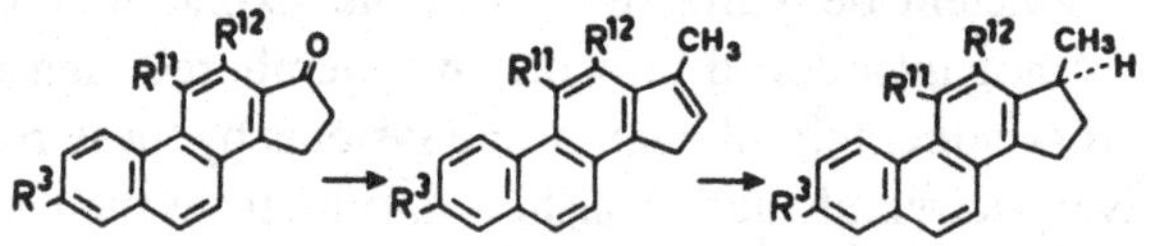

R^3	R^{11}	R^{12}			
H	H	H	4	133	7
OCH₃	H	H	24	134	17
H	CH₃	H	26	135	139
H	H	CH₃	130	136	140
H	CH₃	CH₃	131	137	141
H	OCH₃	H	132	138	142

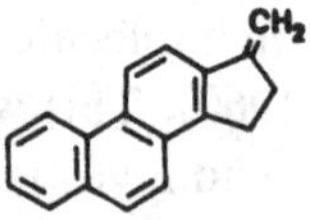

143

Table 1. *Yields of 17-methyl-15H-cyclopenta[a]phenanthrenes isolated after chromatography on alumina*

Compound	Yield (%)
unsubstituted (**133**)	60
3-methoxy (**134**)	55
12-methyl (**136**)	28
11-methyl (**135**)	74
11,12-dimethyl (**137**)	32
11-methoxy (**138**)	18

(4) was treated with the methyl Wittig reagent. Coombs, however, isolated the expected 17-methylene derivative (143) without difficulty, but showed that it isomerized very readily to (133) in the presence of traces of acid.

Two isomers of the parent hydrocarbon cyclopenta[a]phenanthrene can exist (Fig. 22), depending upon whether the ring-D double bond is at 16,17- (i.e., 15H) (3) or at 15,16- (i.e., 17H) (2). The theoretically possible third 16H-isomer (144) is unknown, although intermediates with this quinoid bond structure seem to be involved in certain reactions at ring-D (Chapter 3). The 17H-isomer, mp 164–165°C, was prepared by Badger *et al.* (1952) by elimination from the 15-benzoate (146) in boiling dimethylaniline and by Süss (1953) by decarboxylation of 17H-cyclopenta[a]phenanthrene-17-carboxylic acid (148). In an attempt to prepare the then-unknown 15H-isomer (3) Coombs (1966) reduced the 17-ketone (4) with sodium borohydride and converted the 17-alcohol into its *p*-toluene sulphonate (145). However, base-catalysed elimination from this ester in boiling collidine gave the 17H-isomer (2) of mp 164–165°C; the structure of this compound was confirmed by preparing it in the same manner from the 15-tosylate (147). Since the 16(17)-ene (3) had presumably been formed initially from the 17-tosylate (145) and had subsequently undergone isomerization at 170°C in the reaction mixture, use was made of dimethylsulphoxide as solvent for this elimination (Nace, 1959). After 30 min at 100°C in this solvent the hydrocarbon isolated in low yield by rapid chromatography on silica gel was different from (2); it was charac-

Fig. 22

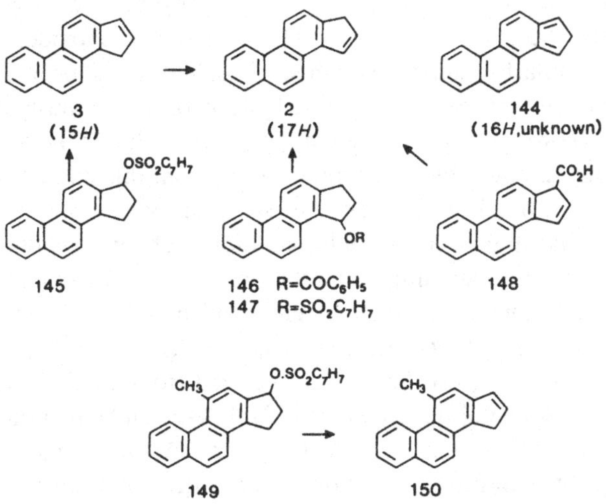

3
(15H)

2
(17H)

144
(16H,unknown)

145

146 R=COC₆H₅
147 R=SO₂C₇H₇

148

149

150

terized as the 16(17)-ene (**3**) by the similarity of its ultraviolet spectrum with that of 17-methyl-15*H*-cyclopenta[a]phenanthrene (**133**). In particular it lacked the small maximum at 239 nm characteristic of the 15(16)-ene chromophore. It was rapidly isomerized at 180°C, and even at 100°C when the elimination in dimethyl sulphoxide was prolonged; it melted at the same temperature as its 17*H*-isomer, no doubt due to the fact that it isomerized during heating up to 165°C. Kon (1933) had obtained an isomeric hydrocarbon, mp 182–183°C, by selenium dehydrogenation of the phosphoric acid cyclization product of the hydrocarbon (**42**) (Fig. 9) and thought it to be either 15*H*- or 17*H*-cyclopenta[a]phenanthrene, but this hydrocarbon was shown later to be chrysofluorene (Cook and Hewett, 1934). More recently Kotlyarevskii and Zanina (1961) isolated a compound of the same melting point and empirical formula from the products of pyrolysis of 1-(1,2,3,4-tetrahydro-1-hydroxy-1-naphthyl)-2(1-hydroxycyclopentyl)-acetylene over a magnesia–chromia–alumina catalyst at 400–500°C. They claimed it to be a 1,2-cyclopentadienophenanthrene by reference to Kon's paper, and by the fact that it consumed two atoms of hydrogen to yield 16,17-dihydro-15*H*-cyclopenta[a]phenanthrene. The structure of this compound is obscure, but it does not appear to be either 15*H*- or 17*H*-cyclopenta[a]phenanthrene. In a later study, Coombs and Hall (1973) treated 15*H*-cyclopenta[a]phenanthrene (**3**) with osmium tetroxide to obtain the *cis*-16,17-diol. Similar treatment of the 17*H*-isomer (**2**), prepared by elimination from the 17-tosylate by boiling with collidine as described above, unexpectedly gave two diols, the anticipated *cis*-15,16-diol and in addition the *cis*-16,17-diol identical with that obtained from the *15H*-hydrocarbon. When 17*H*-cyclopenta[a]phenanthrene, prepared from the 15-tosylate by elimination by the more gentle method (in dimethyl sulphoxide at 100°C for 1 h), was similarly oxidized only the *cis*-15,16-diol was formed. It was therefore evident that the sample of the hydrocarbon previously thought to be the 17*H*-isomer was in fact a mixture of the 15*H*- and 17*H*-hydrocarbons; the pure hydrocarbon differed from this mixture only in that the 239-nm band in its ultraviolet spectrum was somewhat more intense, and that it gave rise to only one diol. Dehydrogenation of 16, 17-dihydro-15*H*-cyclopenta[a]phenanthrene with 2,3-dichloro-5,6-dicyanobenzoquinone in boiling benzene furnished a good yield of the mixture of 15*H*- and 17*H*-hydrocarbons, as disclosed by the osmium tetroxide test. By contrast the tosylate derived from 16,17-dihydro-11-methyl-15*H*-cyclopenta[a]phenanthren-17-ol (**149**) on being boiled with collidine, gave only the 15*H*-hydrocarbon (**150**), 11-methyl-15*H*-cyclopenta[a]phenanthrene; it showed no ultraviolet absorption at

239 nm and gave only one diol with osmium tetroxide. It therefore seems that an 11-methyl group stabilizes the 16(17)-double bond in the five-membered ring in this compound.

Introduction of a double bond into the five-membered D-ring of 15,16-dihydrocyclopenta[a]phenanthrenes cannot be accomplished directly by dehydrogenation by selenium or noble metal catalysts, but dehydrogenation with high-potential quinones is successful in this respect. Dannenberg *et al.* (1956) found that the ultraviolet spectra of a mixture of cyclopenta[a]phenanthrenes isolated from the products of dehydrogenation of cholesterol with chloranil (tetrachloro-*p*-benzoquinone) in boiling xylene indicated the presence of compounds having an extra double bond in ring-D (Fig. 23). Under these conditions three new cyclopenta[a]phenanthrenes (**151**)–(**153**) were isolated in 32% yield. In all these the cholesterol side chain was retained, but the 18-methyl group had migrated to C-17 giving optically active products. In addition the 19-methyl group had been eliminated in the case of (**151**), but had migrated

Fig. 23

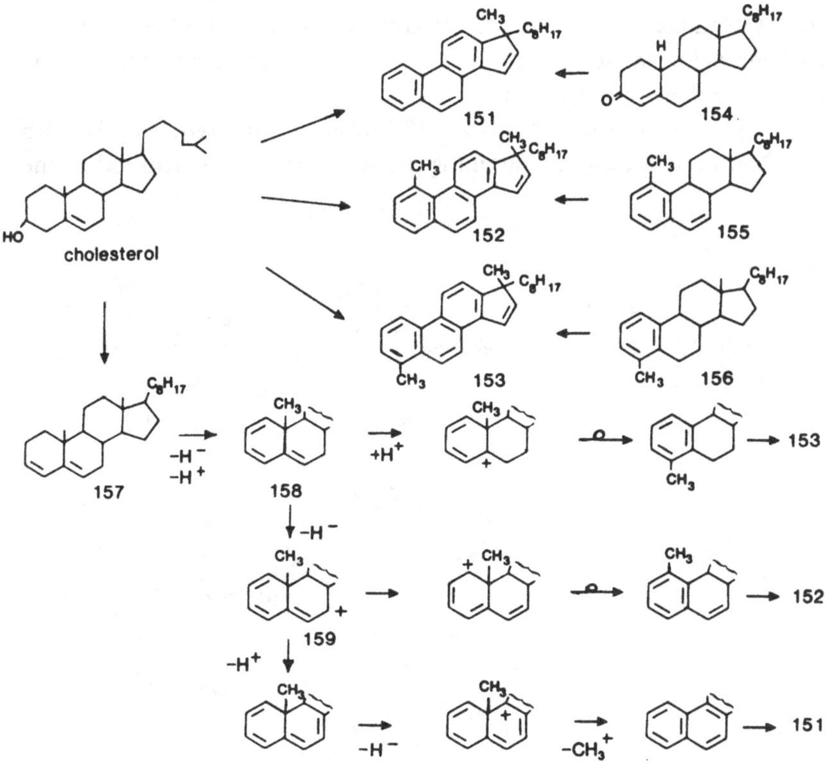

to C-1 in (152) and C-4 in (153). The structures of these hydrocarbons were confirmed by their preparation by similar dehydrogenation of 19-norcholesterol (154), 1-methyl-19-norcholesta-1,3,5(10),6-tetraene (155) (Dannenberg *et al.*, 1964), and 4-methyl-19-norcholesta-1,3,5-triene (156) (Dannenberg and Neumann, 1961) in yields ranging between 30 and 45%. The best yields and shortest reaction times were obtained with DDQ (2,3-dichloro-5,6-dicyanobenzoquinone) in boiling anisole. Quinone dehydrogenation reactions are known to involve a two-step ionic mechanism (Jackman, 1960). Abstraction of a hydride ion (H⁻) from cholesta-3,5-diene (157) by the quinone is followed by loss of a proton (H⁺) or carbonium ion (CH$_3^+$) with the formation of the hydroquinone and a double bond in the substrate (Fig. 23). Dannenberg (1970) proposed that this diene is first dehydrogenated to the 1,3,5-triene (158); addition of a proton then induces a diene–phenol type of rearrangement (symbolized by ⟶) leading eventually to the 4-methylcyclopenta[a]phenanthrene (153). Hydride abstraction from C-7 in this triene gives the carbonium ion (159) which undergoes another diene–phenol rearrangement to yield finally the 1-methyl hydrocarbon (152). Loss of a proton from (159) followed by hydride ion abstraction from C-9 in the 1,3,5,7-tetra-ene results in loss of the methyl group as a carbonium ion and formation of a naphthalene, finally converted to (151) by further dehydrogenations.

Dehydrogenation of 17β-methyl-$\Delta^{9(11)}$-testosterone (160) (Fig. 24) with DDQ in boiling dioxan containing *p*-toluene sulphonic acid led to the

Fig. 24

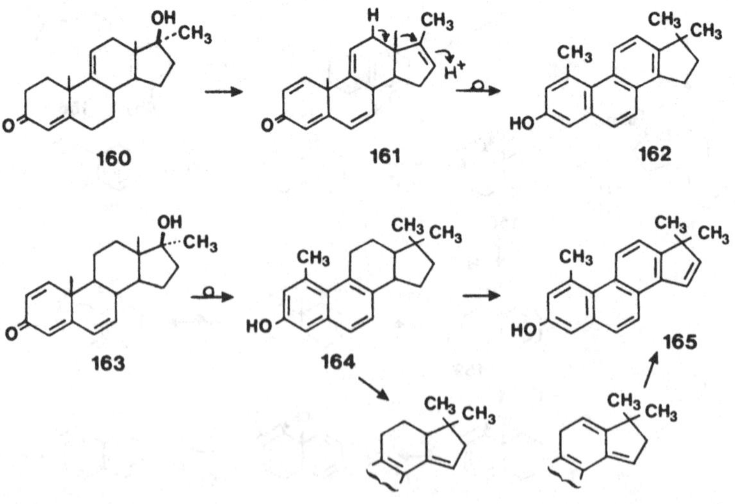

1,17,17-trimethyl-3-phenol (**162**) by way of the 1,4,6,9(11),16(17)-penta-
ene (**161**) (Brown and Turner, 1971). Isolation of a 16(17)-ene from a 17-
methyl-17-ol is unusual because dehydration is normally accompanied by
Wagner–Meewein rearrangement of the 18-methyl group to C-17. In this
case it was considered that relief of the usual 11β-H, 18-methyl diaxial
interaction of about 0.8 kcal/mol by the presence of the 9,11-double bond
accounts for this. The final step, involving a diene–phenol rearrangement
of the C-19 methyl group to C-1 as well as rearrangement of the C-18
methyl group to C-17, occurred simply by boiling the penta-ene (**161**)
with acetic anhydride and *p*-toluene sulphonic acid, possibly by the
mechanism shown, the last double bond being provided by aerial oxidation. By contrast the 1,4,6-trien-3-one (**163**) lacking the 9(11)-double
bond underwent the usual diene–phenol rearrangement to give the
naphthol (**164**), dehydrogenation of which with DDQ yielded a mixture
of (**162**) and the 15(16)-ene, 3-hydroxy-1,17,17-trimethylcyclopen-
ta[a]phenanthrene (**165**), probably via the sequence shown. This compound was not obtained from its 15,16-dihydro derivative (**162**) by
treatment with DDQ.

    Ring-D cleavage accompanied dehydrogenation of oestrone with
chloranil in a mixture of boiling dioxan and *tert.*-butanol (Cross *et al.*,
1963) (Fig. 25). Dehydrogenation proceeded *via* the 9(11)ene (**166**) to
yield the dihydrophenanthrene acid ester (**167**); this was not formed in
the absence of *tert.*-butanol. The 17,17-dicycloethylene ketal of oestrone

Fig. 25

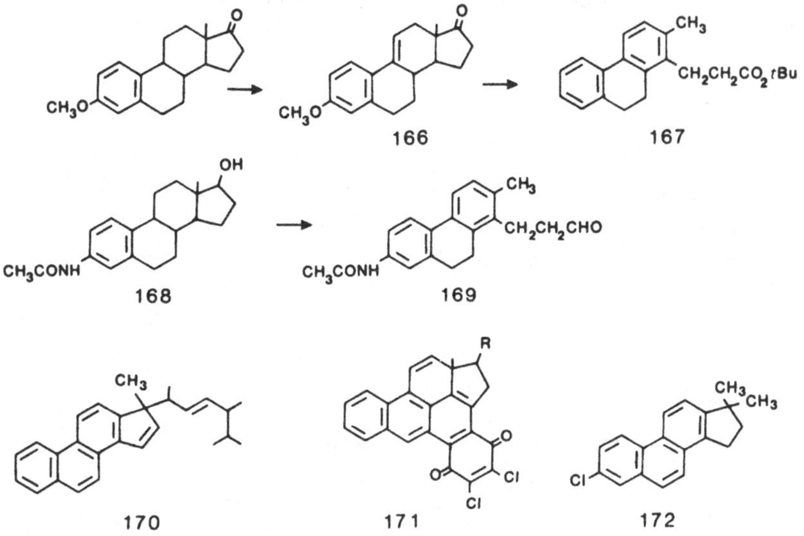

methyl ether gave a similar product in 77% yield under very mild
conditions with an excess of DDQ in benzene at room temperature for
5 min (Boots and Johnson, 1966). In the case of the 17β-ol (168) cleavage
occurred with the formation of the corresponding aldehyde (169) (Dannenberg, 1970). Quinone dehydrogenation is often accompanied by
Diels–Alder addition to yield quinones, and sometimes by chlorination.
Thus chloranil dehydrogenation of ergosterol gave, besides the expected
product 17-methyl-17-(1,4,5-trimethyl-2-hexenyl)-cyclopenta[a]phenan-
threne (170), also the product (171) of 7,15- addition of the quinone.
Similar dehydrogenation of 3β,17β-dihydroxy-17α-methylandrost-5-ene
gave 3-chloro-15,16-dihydro-17,17-dimethylcyclopenta[a]phenanthrene
(172) (Dannenberg and Hebenbrock, 1966).

A novel route to cyclopenta[a]phenanthrenes has recently been described by Lee-Ruff and co-workers based on the ready acid-catalysed ring
cleavage of cyclobutanones and cyclobutanols. Thus condensation of
cyclopentadiene with 1-naphthyl ketene, prepared *in situ* from 1-naph-
thylacetyl chloride and triethylamine in boiling benzene, gave the
cyclobutanone (173) (Fig. 26). Treatment of the latter with trifluoroacetic acid then led to 11,12,13,14-tetrahydro-17H-cyclopenta[a]phenan-
thren-12-one (174) by way of the enol cation or cyclopropyl cation in
about 75% yield (Lee-Ruff *et al.*, 1981). Reduction of the cyclobutanone
to the cyclobutanol (175) and acid treatment gave phenyl-1-naphthyl-
methane (60%), 13,14-dihydro-17H-cyclopenta[a]phenanthrene (176)
(25%), and 17H-cyclopenta[a]phenanthrene (2) (5%) (Lee-Ruff *et al.*,
1982). Both the tetrahydroketone (174) and the dihydrohydrocarbon
(176) were converted into (2) by conventional means.

Fig. 26

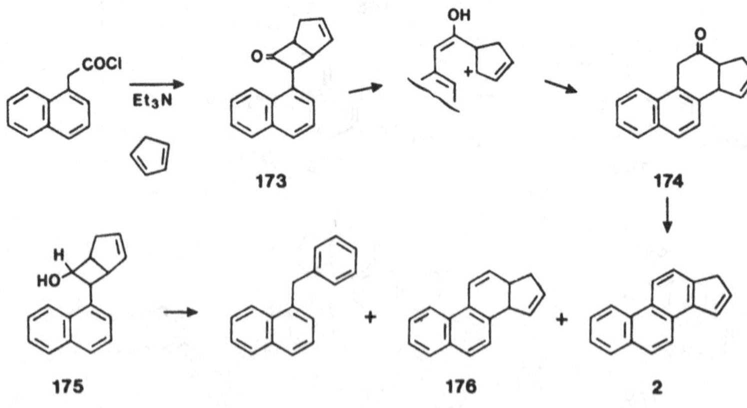

2.4 References

Bachmann, W. E. (1935). Synthesis of 1,2-cyclopentenophenanthrene and related compounds. *J. Am. Chem. Soc.*, **57**, 1381–2.

Badger, G. M., Carruthers, W. & Cook, J. W. (1952). New derivatives of 1:2-cyclopentenophenanthrene. *J. Chem. Soc.*, 4996–5000.

Bergmann, E. & Hillemann (1933). γ-methyl-1,2-cyclopentenophenanthrene. *Ber.*, **66**, 1302–6.

Birch, A. J. & Robinson, R. (1944). Experiments on the synthesis of substances related to steroids. Part XLIII. *J. Chem. Soc.*, 503–6.

Boots, S. G. & Johnson, W. S. (1966). Some observations on the steroid ring-D – fission C-aromatisation reaction. *J. Org. Chem.*, 31, 1285–7.

Brown, K. S. & Kupchan, S. M. (1962). The structure of cyclobuxine. *J. Am. Chem. Soc.*, **84**, 4590–1.

Brown, W. & Turner, A. B. (1971). Applications of high potential quinones. Part VII. The synthesis of steroidal phenanthrenes by double methyl migration. *J. Chem. Soc. (C)*, 2566–72.

Butenandt, A. & Suranyi, L. A. (1942). Uberfuhrung von Steroidhormonen in Methylhomologe des Cyclopentenophenanthrenes. *Ber.*, **75B**, 597–606.

Butenandt, A., Dannenberg, H. & von Dresler, D. (1946a). Methylhomologe des 1,2-cyclopentenophenanthrens, II. Mitteilung: Synthese des 3-methyl-, 4-methyl-, und 3,4-dimethyl-1,2-cyclopentenophenanthrens. *Z. Naturforsch.*, 1, 151–6.

Butenandt, A., Dannenberg, D. & von Dresler, D. (1946b). Methylhomologe des 1,2-cyclopentenophenanthrens, III. Mitteilung: Synthese des 9,10-dimethyl-1,2-cyclopentenophenanthrens. *Z. Naturforsch.*, 1, 222–6.

Butenandt, A., Dannenberg, H. & von Dresler, D. (1946c). Methylhomologe des 1,2-cyclopentenophenanthrens, IV. Mitteilung: Synthese des 6-methyl- und des 3,6-dimethyl-1,2-cyclopentenophenanthrens. *Z. Naturforsch.*, 1, 227–9.

Butenandt, A., Dannenberg, H. & von Dresler, D. (1949a). Methylhomologe des 1,2-cyclopentenophenanthrens, V. Mitteilung: Synthese des 10-methyl-1,2-cyclopentenophenanthrens. *Z. Naturforsch.*, **4b**, 69–76.

Butenandt, A., Dannenberg, H. & von Dresler, D. (1949b). Methylhomologe des 1,2-cyclopentenophenanthrens, VI. Mitteilung: Synthese des 8-methyl und 3,8-dimethyl-1,2-cyclopentenophenanthrens. *Z. Naturforsch.*, **4b**, 77–9.

Butenandt, A., Dannenberg, H. & Steidle, W. (1954). Methyl homologues of 1,2-cyclopentenophenanthrene. VIII. Experiments on the synthesis of 3′,5-dimethyl-1,2-cyclopentenophenanthrene. Selenium dehydrogenation of 1-methyl-19-norcholesta-1,3,5(10),6-tetraen-3-ol. *Z. Naturforsch.*, **9b**, 288–94.

Butenandt, A., Dannenberg, H., Bieneck, E. & Steidle, W. (1950). Methylhomologe des 1,2-cyclopentenophenanthren, VII. Mitteilung: Synthese des 5-methyl-1,2-cyclopentenophenanthrens. *Z. Naturforsch.*, **5b**, 405–9.

Butz, L. W., Gaddis, A. M., Butz, E. W. T. & Davis, R. E. (1940). The total synthesis of a non-benzenoid steroid. *J. Am. Chem. Soc.*, **62**, 995–6.

Chuang, C. K., Ma, C. M., Tien, Y. L. & Huang, Y. T. (1939). Synthetic studies in the sterol and sex hormone group. III. Synthesis of 7-hydroxy-3′-keto-3,4-dihydrocyclopenteno-1′,2′,1,2-phenanthrene. *Ber.*, **72**, 944–53.

Cohen, A., Cook, J. W. & Hewett, C. L. (1935). The synthesis of

compounds related to sterols, bile acids and oestrus-producing hormones.
Part VI. Experimental evidence of complete structure of oestrin, equilin,
and equilenin. *J. Chem. Soc.*, 445–55.

Cook, J. W. & Hewett, C. L. (1933). The synthesis of compounds related to
sterols, bile acids, and oestrus-producing hormones. Part 1. 1:2-
cyclopentenophenanthrene. *J. Chem. Soc.*, 1098–111.

Cook, J. W. & Hewett, C. L. (1934). The synthesis of compounds related to
the sterols, bile acids, and oestrus-producing hormones. Part II. The
formation of some tetracyclic hydroaromatic hydrocarbons. *J. Chem. Soc.*,
365–77.

Coombs, M. M. (1966). Potentially carcinogenic cyclopenta[a]phenanthrenes.
Part II. Derivatives containing further unsaturation in ring-D. *J. Chem.
Soc. (C)*, 965–8.

Coombs, M. M. & Croft, C. J. (1969). Carcinogenic
cyclopenta[a]phenanthrenes. *Prog. Exp. Tumor Res.*, **11**, 69–85.

Coombs, M. M. & Hall, M. (1973). Potentially carcinogenic
cyclopenta[a]phenanthrenes. Part VII. Ring-D diols and related
compounds. *J. Chem. Soc. Perkin Trans. I*, 1255–8.

Coombs, M. M. & Jaitly, S. B. (1971). Potentially carcinogenic
cyclopenta[a]phenanthrenes. Part V. Synthesis of 15,16-dihydro-7-
methylcyclopenta[a]phenanthren-1-one. *J. Chem. Soc. (C)*, 230–4.

Cross, A. D., Carpio, H. & Crabbe, P. (1963). Spectra and stereochemistry.
Part VI. A novel cleavage of ring D during dehydrogenation of oestrone
methyl ether. *J. Chem. Soc.*, 5539–42.

Dannenberg, H. & Neumann, H.-G. (1964). Dehydrogenation of steroids.
IX. Dependence of dehydrogenation with quinones on the quinone,
reaction medium, and steroid. *Annalen*, **675**, 109–25.

Dannenberg, H. (1960). Uber Beziehungen zwischen Steroiden und
krebserzungenden Kohlenwasserstoffe, II. Mitteilung. 1,2-
Cyclopentadieno-phenanthrene. *Z. Krebsforsch.*, **63**, 523–31.

Dannenberg, H. (1970). Vollstandige Dehydrierung von Sterinen und
Steroiden mit Chinonen. *Synthesis*, **2**, 74–81.

Dannenberg, H., Dannenberg-von Dresler, D. & Neumann, H.-G. (1960).
Dehydrierung von steroiden III. 1:2-Cyclopentadieno-phenanthrene.
Annalen, **636**, 74–87.

Dannenberg, H. & Hebenbrock, K. F. (1966). Dehydrierung von Steroiden.
XIII. Bildung dehydrierter Steroid-chloranil-Dienadditions-verbindungen.
Annalen, **700**, 106–9.

Dannenberg, H. & Neumann, H.-G. (1961). Dehydrierung von 4-methyl-
$\Delta^{1.3.5(10)}$-19-nor-cholestatrien mit chloranil. *Chem. Ber.*, **94**, 3085–94.

Dannenberg, H. & Steidle, W. (1954). Zur systematik der uv-absorption. II
Mitt. Die Methylhomologen des 1,2-cyclopentenophenanthrenes. *Z.
Naturforsch.*, **9b**, 294–7.

Dannenberg, H., Neumann, H.-G. & Dannenberg-von Dresler, D. (1964).
Dehydrogenation of steroids. VIII. Dehydrogenation of cholesterol with
chloranil. *Annalen*, **674**, 152–67.

Dannenberg, H., Scheurlen, H. & Dannenberg-von Dresler, D. (1956).
Notiz zur Dehydrierung von Cholesterin mit Chloranil. *Z. Physiol. Chem.*,
303, 282–5.

Diels, O. & Clar, E. (1934). Dehydrogenation of cholesterol and ergosterol
and the non-identity of the hydrocarbon $C_{18}H_{16}$ with 1,2-
cyclopentenophenanthrene. *Ber.*, **67B**, 113–22.

Fieser, L. F. (1936). *Chemistry of Natural Products Related to Phenanthrene*, chap. 2. Reinhold Publishing Corp.: New York.

Fieser, L. F. & Seligman, A. M. (1939). Synthetic routes to *meso* substituted 1,2-benzanthracene derivatives. *J. Am. Chem. Soc.*, **61**, 136–44.

Gamble, D. J. C. & Kon, G. A. R. (1935). Synthesis of polycyclic compounds related to sterols. Part III. 9-methyl- and 3′:9-dimethyl-cyclopentenophenanthrene. *J. Chem. Soc.*, 443–5.

Harper, S. H., Kon, G. A. R. & Ruzicka, F. C. J. (1934). Syntheses of polycyclic compounds related to the steroids. Part II. Diels' hydrocarbon $C_{18}H_{16}$. *J. Chem. Soc.*, 124–8.

Hawthorne, J. R. (1936). Experiments on the synthesis of substances related to sterols. Part XIII. Hydrocyclopentenophenanthrene derivatives. *J. Chem. Soc.*, 763–5.

Hillemann, H. (1935). Uber die Identitat von γ-methyl-1,2-cyclopentenophenanthren mit dem dielsschen Kohlenwasserstoff $C_{18}H_{16}$. *Ber.*, **68**, 102–5.

Hoffsommer, R. D., Taub, D. & Wendler, N. L. (1966). Rearrangement in the estrone series. *Chimia*, **20**, 251.

Inhoffen, H. H., Stoeck, G. & Kolling, G. (1949). The migration of the angular methyl group at carbon atom 10 in the steroids. Preparation of 1,17-dimethyl-15,16-dihydrocyclopenta[a]phenanthrene. *Chem. Ber.*, **82**, 263–6.

Jackman, L. M. (1960). Hydrogenation–dehydrogenation reactions. In *Advances in Organic Chemistry*, pp. 329–66. Interscience Pub.: New York.

Kehrer, E. A. & Igler, P. (1899). Ueber ein einfaches Verfahren zur Darstellung einbasischer 4.7-Diketosauren. *Ber.* **32**, 1176–80.

Kirk, D. N. & Hartshorn, M. P. (1969). *Steroid Reaction Mechanisms*, p. 277. Elsevier: Amsterdam.

Koebner, A. & Robinson, R. (1938). Experiments on the synthesis of substances related to sterols. Part XXII. Synthesis of x-norequilenin methyl ether. *J. Chem. Soc.*, 1994–7.

Kon, G. A. R. (1933). Synthesis of polycyclic compounds related to steroids. Part 1. *J. Chem. Soc.*, 1081–7.

Kon, G. A. R. & Ruzicka, F. C. J. (1935). Syntheses of polycyclic compounds related to the sterols. Part V. Methoxy and hydroxy derivatives of phenanthrene. *J. Chem. Soc.*, 187–92.

Kon, G. A. R. & Woolman, A. M. (1939). Sapogenins. Part III. The dehydrogenation products of methylsarsasapogenin and methylcholesterol. *J. Chem. Soc.*, 794–800.

Kotlyarevskii, L. & Zanina, A. S. (1961). Unsaturated hydrocarbons. XIV. Synthesis of polycyclic hydrocarbons by dehydroxylation of acetylene derivatives. *Zh. Obshch. Khim.*, **31**, 3206–14.

Lee-Ruff, E., Hopkinson, A. C. & Dao, Le H. (1981). Acid-catalysed rearrangements of cyclobutanones. VI. Synthesis of chrysenes and steroid-like substances. *Can. J. Chem.*, **59**, 1675–84.

Lee-Ruff, E., Hopkinson, A. C., Kazarians-Moghaddam, H., Gupta, B. & Katz, M. (1982). Acid catalysed rearrangement of cyclobutanols. Synthesis of chrysenes, cyclopenta[a]phenanthrenes, and diarylmethanes. *Can. J. Chem.*, **60**, 154–9.

Nace, H. R. (1959). The preparation of olefins from aryl sulfonate esters of alcohols. *J. Am. Chem. Soc.*, **81**, 5428–30.

Riegel, B., Gold, M. H. & Kubio, M. A. (1943). Synthesis of 3'-alkyl-1,2-cyclopentenophenanthrenes. *J. Am. Chem. Soc.*, **65**, 1772–6.

Robinson, R. (1938). Experiments on the synthesis of substances related to the sterols. Part XXI. A new synthesis of derivatives of keto*cyclo*pentenophenanthrene. *J. Chem. Soc.*, 1390–7.

Ruzicka, L. & Thomann, G. (1933). Polyterpene und polyterpenoide LXXIX. Zur konstitution des cholesterins und der gallensauren. *Helv. Chim. Acta*, **16**, 216–27.

Ruzicka, L., Ehmann, L., Goldberg, M. W. & Hosli, H. (1933). Synthesis of 1,2-cyclopentanophenanthrene, of its α- and β-methyl derivatives and of chrysene. *Helv. Chim. Acta*, **16**, 812–32.

Schöntube, E. & Janak, J. (1968). Analytical significance of dehydrogenation of steroids with selenium. Contribution to the problem of Diels' hydrocarbon content in products of steroid dehydrogenation. *Collect. Czech Chem. Comm.*, **33**, 193–209.

Sen Gupta, S. H. & Bhattacharyya, A. (1954). Synthesis of polynuclear hydrocarbons with fused cyclopentane ring. III. Application of the Diels–Alder reaction. *J. Indian Chem. Soc.*, **31**, 897–903.

Süss, O. (1953). Uber die Lichtreaktion der *o*-Chinondiazide; Photosynthese von Cyclopentadien-abkonimlingen. *Annalen*, **579**, 133–58.

Tamayo, M. L. & Martin, J. (1952). Derivatives of cyclopentenophenanthrene. I. The condensation of 1-vinyl hydrinene with *p*-benzoquinone. *Anales real Soc. espan. fis. y quim.*, **48b**, 693–8.

Tatta, K. R. & Bardhan, J. C. (1968). Synthesis of polycyclic compounds. Part VIII. Friedel–Crafts acylation with anhydrides of tricarboxylic acids. Synthesis of 16,17-dihydro-17-methyl-15*H*-cyclopenta[a]phenanthrene. *J. Chem. Soc. (C)*, 893–900.

Yamagiwa, K. & Ichikawa, K. (1915). Experimentelle Studie über Pathogenese der Epithelialgeschwulst. *Mitt. med. Fak., Tokio*, **15**, 295–344.

3

Chemical synthesis of cyclopenta[a]-
phenanthrenes: ring-D ketones

Early cyclopenta[a]phenanthrene syntheses were directed at the preparation of hydrocarbons and were not in the main readily adaptable to the synthesis of the corresponding ring-D ketones. However, parallel synthetic endeavour at that time was also aimed at the synthesis of 17-ketosteroids such as equilenin. Thus Bardhan (1936) condensed 2-(1-naphthyl)ethyl bromide with dimethyl 2-ketoadipate to give the product (177) which was cyclized with cold sulphuric acid to the dihydrophenanthrene (178) (Fig. 27). Formation of the five-membered ring by heating with acetic anhydride followed by decarboxylation at 210°C gave 11,12,15,16-tetrahydrocyclopenta[a]phenanthren-17-one (179). The last step of dehydrogenation to give the corresponding phenanthrene was not undertaken, but the structure of (179) was established by converting it by way of Clemmensen reduction and selenium dehydrogenation into the known hydrocarbon (1). A similar synthesis was reported by Bachmann et al. (1943); in this the final cyclization of the di-acid (178) was brought about under Dieckmann conditions with sodium methoxide in dry benzene. Bachmann and Kloetzel (1937) obtained the parent 17-ketone (4), 15,16-dihydro-cyclopenta[a]phenanthren-17-one by cyclization of the acid chloride of 3-(1-phenanthryl)propionic acid (180) with aluminium chloride in nitrobenzene at 0°C, several other cyclization methods having failed. This ketone, mp 195–196°C, was isolated in very low yield, the major product being its isomer (181) in which cyclization had occurred in the opposite direction. The isomeric 15-ketone (102) (15,16-dihydro-cyclopenta[a]phenenathren-15-one), mp 183–184°C, was the only product when the chloride of 3-(2-phenanthyl)propionic acid (182) was cyclized in nitrobenzene solution with stannic chloride at 80°C (Fig. 27). The structures of both these ketones were confirmed by reduction to the known hydrocarbon (1). Finally, the synthesis of the 15,17-diketone (185) was described by Fieser *et al.* (1936) who simply condensed dimethyl phenanthrene-1,2-dicarboxylate (183) with ethyl acetate in the presence of sodium, and hydrolysed and decarboxylated the product to give the pure diketone in 74% yield. 15,16-Dihydrocyclopenta[a]phenanthren-15,17-dione (185) melted at 240.5–241.5°C, and behaved as a typical diketone, dissolving in dilute alkali to give a red solution. It was recovered unchanged when the solution was immediately acidified, but on standing hydrolysis to a mixture of isomeric acetyl phenanthroic acids took place. 15,16-Dihydro-1,6-dimethoxy-cyclopenta[a]phenanthren-17-one (186) was also prepared in a similar manner (Fieser and Hershberg, 1936).

Two other syntheses of the 11,12-dihydro-17-ketone (179) have been described. Johnson and Petersen (1945) employed the Stöbbe reaction to

Fig. 27

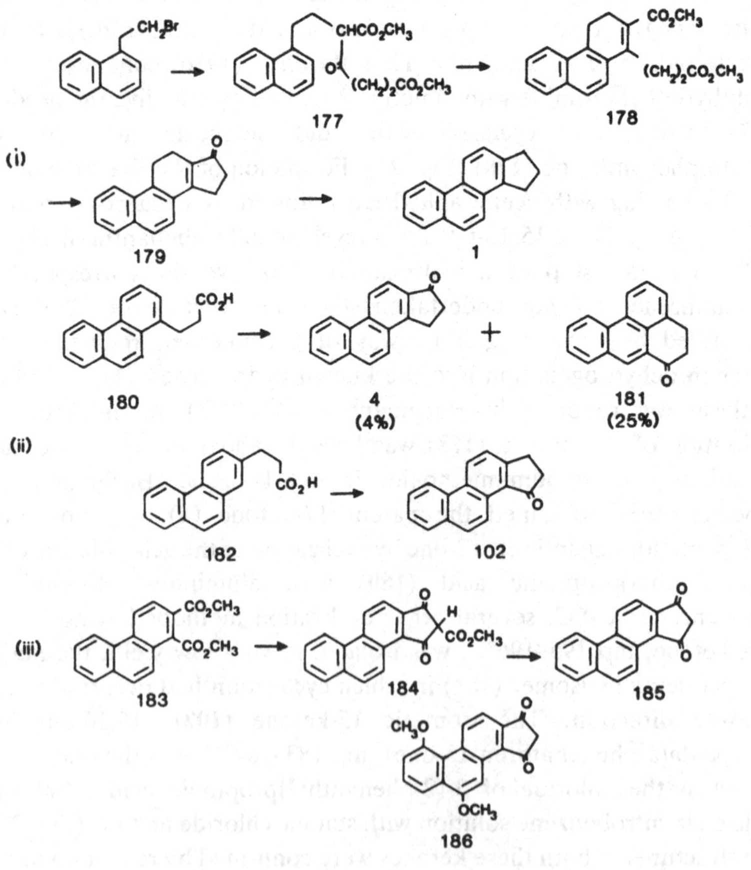

add ring-D to 1,2,3,4-tetrahydrophenanthren-1-one (187) as shown in Fig. 28; the final ring closure was effected with anhydrous zinc chloride in acetic acid. This method was later used extensively by Coombs and his co-workers for the preparation of methyl and other homologues. Bachmann and Holman (1951) used the same tetrahydrophenanthrene ketone (187) and its 3-methoxy derivative (188), but built up the three-carbon chain by a Reformatsky reaction with bromoacetic ester followed by Arndt–Eistert chain extension, and ring closure as before.

Robinson (1938) in searching for synthetic routes to 17-keto steroids devised the remarkable cyclopenta[a]phenanthrene synthesis already discussed in the previous chapter (see Fig. 29). In this reaction scheme closure of the six-membered ring-C in the precursors (79) and (189) (Robinson and Rydon, 1939) was brought about almost quantitatively by boiling them with acetic anhydride. The products (80) and (190),

Fig. 28

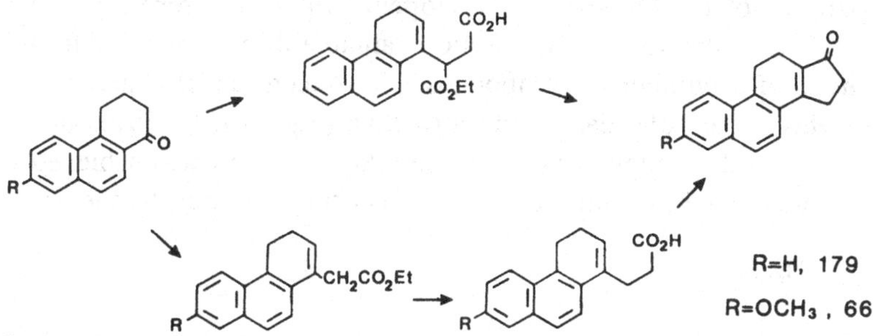

R=H, 187
R=OCH₃ ,188

R=H, 179
R=OCH₃ , 66

Fig. 29

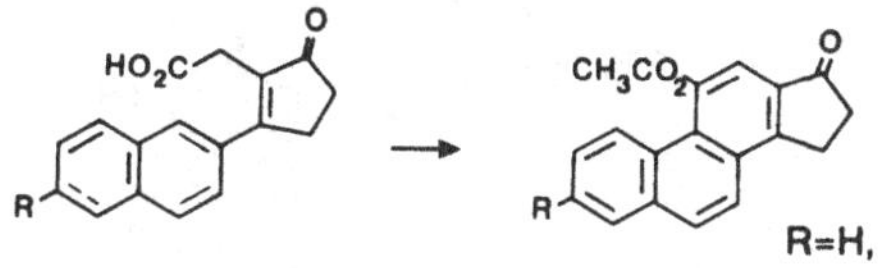

R=H, 79
R=OCH₃ ,189

R=H, 80
R=OCH₃ ,190

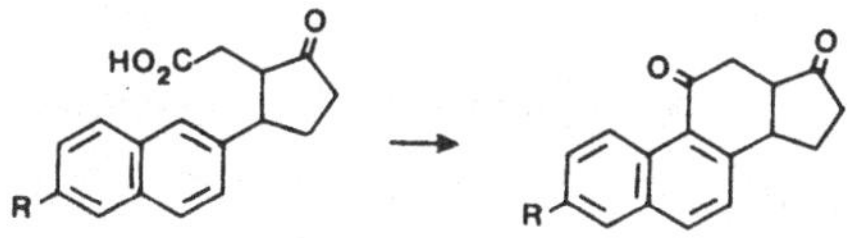

R=H, 191
R=OCH₃ ,192

R=H, 193
R=OCH₃ ,194

however, contained a phenolic acetate group at C-11, and methods for removing this without concomitant loss of the 17-oxygen function were unknown at that time. This problem was circumvented (Koebner and Robinson, 1938) by first reducing the 13(14)- double bond, then cyclizing the cyclopentanone acid (191) to give the 11,17-diketone (193). The two ketone groups in this compound differ markedly in reactivity, the 11-ketone being relatively inert owing to steric hindrance, and use was made of this property to eliminate the unwanted oxygen at C-11. Unfortunately, neither the reduction nor the cyclization proceed smoothly in this case; the catalytic reduction of the tetra-substituted double bond over palladium on charcoal is sluggish and over-reduction with loss of the 17-oxygen is difficult to minimize. Ring closure proceeds with difficulty; most conventional methods fail, but yields of about 40% can be obtained under strictly controlled conditions (exposure to polyphosphoric acid at 125°C for 3 min) (Birch *et al.*, 1945). The present authors experienced these difficulties when employing this route for the preparation of 17-ketones of the cyclopenta[a]phenanthrene series, but found that the diketone (193) was most valuable starting material for the synthesis of a number of compounds. Two recent developments have made this route potentially more attractive (Fig. 30). Cyclization of a closely related compound (195) to the diketone (196) was achieved in 65% yield (75% based on the recovered starting material) by the use of

Fig. 30

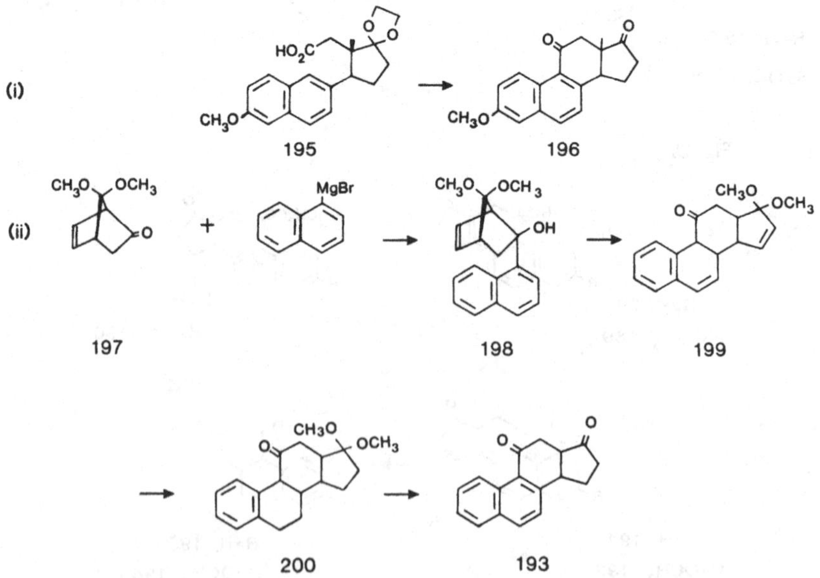

hydrogen fluoride in dry tetrahydrofuran (Posner *et al.*, 1979). Also the diketone (**193**) has been obtained (Jung and Hudspeth, 1978) by a new method. The bicyclic enone (**197**), readily obtainable in 67% yield in several steps from vinyl acetate and dimethoxytetrachlorocyclopentadiene, reacted with 1-naphthyl magnesium bromide to give a high yield of the exo-alcohol (**198**). Treatment of this in tetrahydrofuran with sodium amide caused a base-catalysed Cope rearrangement to the hexahydrocyclopenta[a]phenanthrene (**199**) in 75% yield. This compound was readily converted by partial hydrogenation, diketalization, and dehydrogenation into the diketone (**193**) *via* the decahydro compound (**200**). The C/D ring junction in this important diketone (**193**) is *trans* (Chinn *et al.*, 1962), and it has been resolved into its optically active (+) and (−) forms making use of stereospecific reduction with *Rhodotorula mucilaginosa* (Siewinski *et al.*, 1969). The diketone was first reduced to the diol with lithium aluminium hydride (Mejer and Kalinowska, 1969), then selectively oxidized back to the 17α- and 17β-hydroxy-11-ketones with chromium trioxide in pyridine. On fermentation of the 17α-hydroxy-ketone with this organism only half was reduced stereospecifically to the 17α, 11β-diol, which on re-oxidation yielded (+) (**193**); re-oxidation of the residual ketoalcohol led to (−) (**193**) of opposite and equal specific rotation. The melting point of both these optical isomers was 138°C, 20 degrees higher than that of the racemic diketone ordinarily encountered.

Following Marrian's suggestion regarding the possibility of aromatization of oestrone to its phenanthrene analogue already described in Chapter 1, a reappraisal of methods for the synthesis of 17-ketocyclopenta[a]phenanthrenes was undertaken. Robinson's 11,17-diketone (**193**) was initially taken as a point of departure (Fig. 31) (Coombs, 1965), and it was found that by heating it with 2-methyl-2-ethyl-1,3-dioxolan in the presence of a catalytic quantity of *p*-toluene sulphonic acid this diketone gave the oxo-ketal (**201**) in good yield. Prolonged heating led to the 11,17-diketal (**203**), but it was found that the benzylic ketal group in this compound was very sensitive to acid so that it could be readily converted back into the monoketal with a trace of hydrogen chloride in damp chloroform (Coombs, 1966). When this oxo-ketal (**201**) was reduced with sodium borohydride to the 11-ol and the latter was boiled with acetic acid containing hydrochloric acid in the presence of an excess of nitrobenzene 15,16-dihydrocyclopenta[a]phenanthren-17-one (**4**) was obtained directly in 86% yield melting at 197°C; after recrystallization it formed very pale yellow needles, melting at 203–204°C. In a similar way the 3-methoxy-oxo-ketal (**202**) furnished the methyl ether of the phenanthrene analogue of oestrone, 15,16-dihydro-3-methoxycyclopenta[a]phen-anthren-17-one (**24**), in the same yield. In the absence of nitrobenzene the yield of (**4**) was halved and the tetrahydro derivative (**205**) was also formed. A detailed examination of the reaction led to the conclusion that it proceeds via the enol by abstraction of hydrogen from C-14 as shown in Fig. 31. Nitrobenzene had been employed previously by Koebner and Robinson (1941) to induce aromatization of ring-C. Thus when the 11,17-diketone (**193**) was treated with sodium hydroxide in the presence of nitrobenzene the phenol 15,16-dihydro-11-hydroxycyclopenta[a] phenanthren-17-one (**206**) was formed directly, presumably via the enols by a similar mechanism. The tendency for dehydrogenation of ring-C to occur in suitable compounds was illustrated by these authors who found that the 16-benzylidene derivative of x-norequilenin methyl ether (**207**), dissolved in methanolic sodium hydroxide, on exposure to air for two days gave a bright yellow precipitate of 16-benzylidene-15,16-dihydro-3-methoxycyclopenta[a]phenanthren-17-one (**208**) by the formal loss of four hydrogen atoms from this ring.

In a similar manner (Fig. 32) treatment of the oxo-ketal (**201**) with methyl or ethyl magnesium iodide, or with *n*-butyl lithium (Coombs *et al.*, 1973), and submission of the products to acid in the presence of nitrobenzene led to good yields of the 11-methyl-, 11-ethyl-, and 11-*n*-butyl-derivatives (**26, 211**, and **212**). Methylation of the oxo-ketal (**201**)

Fig. 31

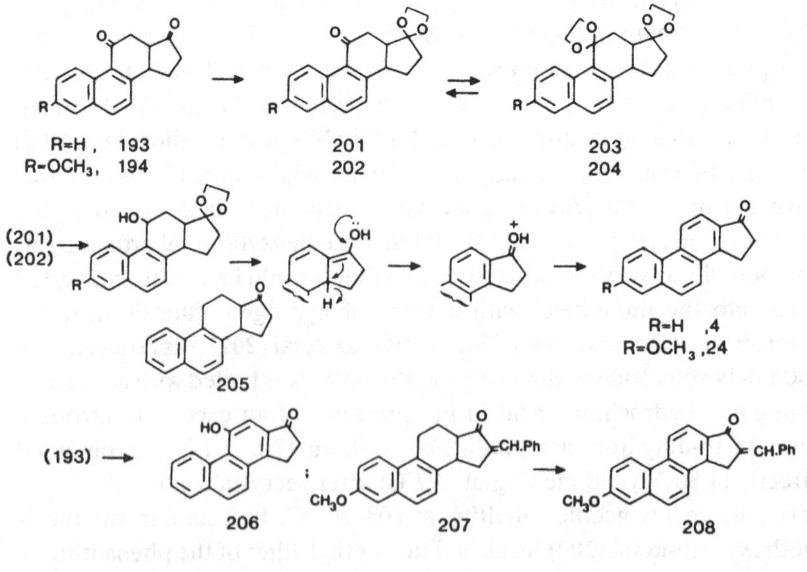

R=H , 193   201   203
R=OCH₃, 194   202   204

(201)
(202)

205

R=H ,4
R=OCH₃ ,24

(193) →

206   207   208

with methyl iodide in the presence of potassium *tert.*-butoxide gave a mixture of mono- and dimethyl derivatives (**209**) and (**210**), separated by column chromatography. Reduction of the 12-methyl-oxo-ketal (**209**) or treatment of it with methyl lithium followed by acid and nitrobenzene led to the 12-methyl- and 11,12-dimethyl-17-ketones (**130** and **131**), again in good yield. Treatment of the oxo-ketal (**201**) with the ylide from trimethylsulphonium iodide (Coombs *et al.*, 1975) and acidification of the intermediate epoxide to pH 3 afforded the diol (**213**) which was acetylated and dehydrated with phosphoryl chloride in pyridine. Quinone dehydrogenation of the product (**214**) and removal of the protecting groups finally yielded 15,16-dihydro-11-hydroxymethyl-cyclopenta[a]phenanthren-17-one (**215**). Condensation of the oxo-ketal (**201**) with ethyl formate in the presence of sodium ethoxide gave the bright yellow formyl-ketone (**216**) which was reduced to the diol with lithium aluminium hydride. When this diol was boiled with acetic acid containing hydrochloric acid and nitrobenzene, the 12-methyl-17-ketone (**130**) was formed together with the dimer (**217**).

Whilst this route was most successful for the preparations of 11- and 12-substituted-17-ketones, several difficulties beset its application to the

Fig. 32

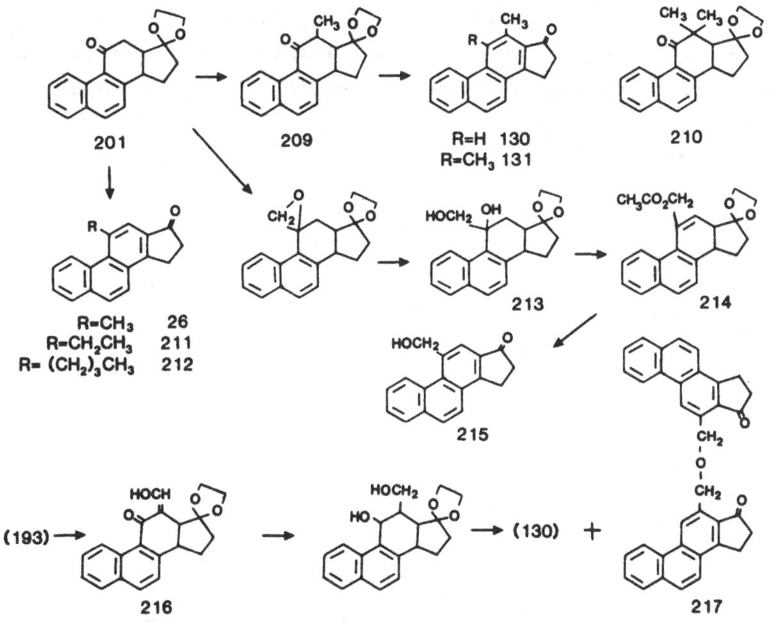

synthesis of 15,16-dihydro-7-methylcyclopenta[a]phenanthren-17-one (**230**) (Fig. 33). The furfurylidene derivative of 2-acetyl-3-methylnaphthalene (**218**) gave not only the expected dioxoheptanoic acid (**220**) on acid hydrolysis, but the naphthylfuran propionic acid (**223**) was also formed in similar yield (Coombs and Jaitly, 1971). The analogous methoxy compound (**219**) obtained from 2-acetyl-3-methoxynaphthalene gave mostly the furan acid (**224**) with only a small quantity of the dioxo acid (**221**), whereas the unsubstituted compound (**77**) gave the dioxo acid (**78**) almost exclusively (Coombs and Vose, 1975). An nmr study confirmed the previous suggestions (Butenandt *et al.*, 1949; Short and Rockwood, 1969) that a substitutent at C-3 in the naphthalene ring decreases conjugation between this ring system and the adjacent side chain by preventing co-planarity of these two systems. This in turn diminishes charge delocalization in the protonated intermediate (**225**) thereby promoting cyclization to the furan. The dioxo acid (**220**) underwent smooth ring-closure in dilute alkali to the cyclopentenone (**226**) in which again the methyl group prevents co-planarity of the naphthalene and cyclopentone rings. Hydrogenation of this compound gave a mixture of at least six products, and was not pursued further. Cyclization of (**226**) with boiling acetic anhydride occurred normally to give 11-acetoxy-15,16-dihydro-7-methylcyclopenta[a]phenanthren-17-one (**227**) in good yield. After several failures it was discovered that reduction of the corresponding diethylphosphate (**229**) with sodium in a mixture of tetrahydrofuran and liquid ammonia (Kenner and Williams, 1955) led to the desired 7-methyl-17-ketone (**230**), surprisingly in 47% yield. Presumably the

Fig. 33

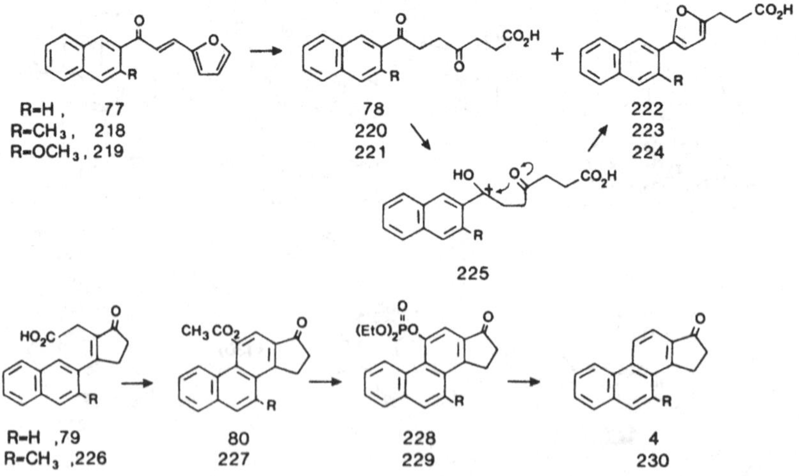

R=H ,   77
R=CH₃,   218
R=OCH₃, 219

78
220
221

222
223
224

225

R=H ,79
R=CH₃ ,226

80
227

228
229

4
230

ketone is protected as the enol during this reduction. When this scheme was applied to the synthesis of the unsubstituted ketone (**4**), the yield in the reduction of the phosphate (**228**) was 27%; overall the yield from the cyclopentenone acid (**79**) was 18%, similar to that obtained in the longer synthesis from this intermediate previously described (see Figs. 29 and 31). Desulphurization of the tosylate of 15,16-dihydro-11-hydroxy-cyclopenta[a]phenanthren-17-one with Raney nickel to the corresponding hydrocarbon was later reported (Kawarura *et al.*, 1974), but this procedure, of course, also removes the 17-carboxyl group.

Another kind of difficulty arose when syntheses of 1,2,3,4,15,16-hexhydrocyclopenta[a]phenanthren-17-one (**237**) and its 11-methyl homologue (**238**) were attempted using this general approach (Coombs and Bhatt, 1973) (Fig. 34). 6-Acetyl-1,2,3,4-tetrahydronaphthalene was converted into its furfurylidene derivative which with hot acid yielded the corresponding dioxoheptanoic acid without difficulty, and ring closure of this to give the cyclopentenone acid (**231**) occurred smoothly under alkaline conditions. Over-reduction was difficult to avoid during the hydrogenation of the double bond in this compound, and a better method of obtaining the desired cyclopentanone acid (**232**) was by reduction with lithium in liquid ammonia. The difficulty arose in the next cyclization step because, lacking the strong directing influence of a naphthalene ring system, ring closure occurred in both directions leading to the angular (**233**) and linear (**234**) diketones in the ratio 1:4. Cyclization of the cyclopentenone acid (**231**) with boiling acetic anhydride gave a similar mixture of angular (**235**) and linear (**236**) acetoxy ketones. The angular diketone (**233**) was converted into its 17-ketal which on being either reduced or treated with the methyl Grignard reagent, followed by

Fig. 34

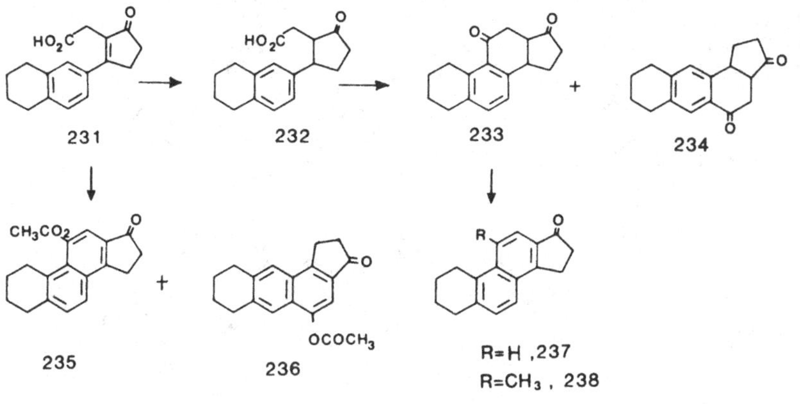

aromatization with nitrobenzene and acid, yielded the tetrahydro-17-ketones (237) and (238).

The above-described synthetic scheme is not convenient for the preparation of certain other ring-substituted 17-oxocyclopenta[a]phenanthrenes owing to the difficulty of obtaining suitably substituted 2-acetyl naphthalenes. Attention was therefore directed towards the method of Johnson and Petersen (1945) utilizing the Stöbbe reaction to build up the five-membered ring-D from suitable 1,2,3,4-tetrahydrophenanthren-1-ones. This method was also used by Riegel et al. (1948) for the synthesis of 12-substituted derivatives (Fig. 35). These authors condensed 1-naphthyl magnesium chloride with ethylidene, propylidene, and isobutylidene malonic diester and hydrolysed and decarboxylated the products to furnish the 3-alkyl-4-(1-naphthyl)butyric acids (239-241). Cyclization of the latter (phosphorus pentachloride and stannic chloride) gave the required three-ring ketones (242-245) which were converted into the half-esters (246-248) by means of the Stöbbe reaction with diethyl succinate in the presence of potassium *tert.*-butoxide. Closure of the five-membered ring (zinc chloride in acetic acid) followed by hydrolysis and decarboxylation gave the tetrahydro ketones (249-251), from which the 12-alkyl-15,16-dihydrocyclopenta[a]phenanthren-17-ones (130, 253, and 254) were obtained on dehydrogenation by heating with palladium on charcoal. Clemmensen reduction of these ketones gave the 12-alkyl hydrocarbons (97, 255, and 256) in which they were interested. This sequence was also employed by Woodward *et*

Fig. 35

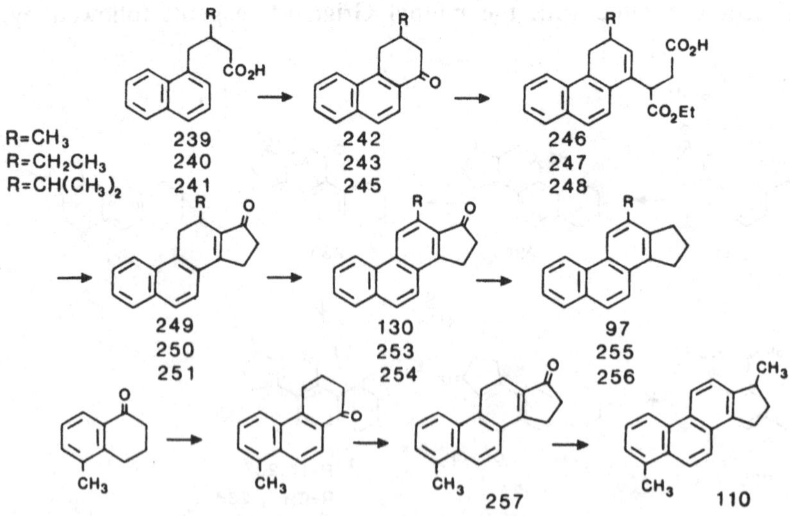

R=CH₃   239   242   246
R=CH₂CH₃ 240   243   247
R=CH(CH₃)₂ 241   245   248

249   130   97
250   253   255
251   254   256

257   110

al. (1953) to construct the 4,17-dimethyl hydrocarbon (**110**) from 5-methyl tetralone via 4-methyl-11,12,15,16-tetrahydro-cyclopenta[a]-phenanthren-17-one (**257**).

For the synthesis of the 2-, 3-, 4-, and 6-methyl- and 6-methoxy-17-ketones (Coombs *et al.*, 1970), the 2-methoxy-17-ketone (Coombs *et al.*, 1975), the 1-methyl, 7,11-dimethyl-, and 1,11-methano-17-ketones (Ribeiro *et al.*, 1983), and 1-methyl-4-hydroxy-17-ketone (Coombs *et al.*, 1985) the required 1,2,3,4-tetrahydrophenanthren-1-ones were prepared by several routes (Fig. 36). Thus reaction of Grignard reagents prepared

Fig. 36

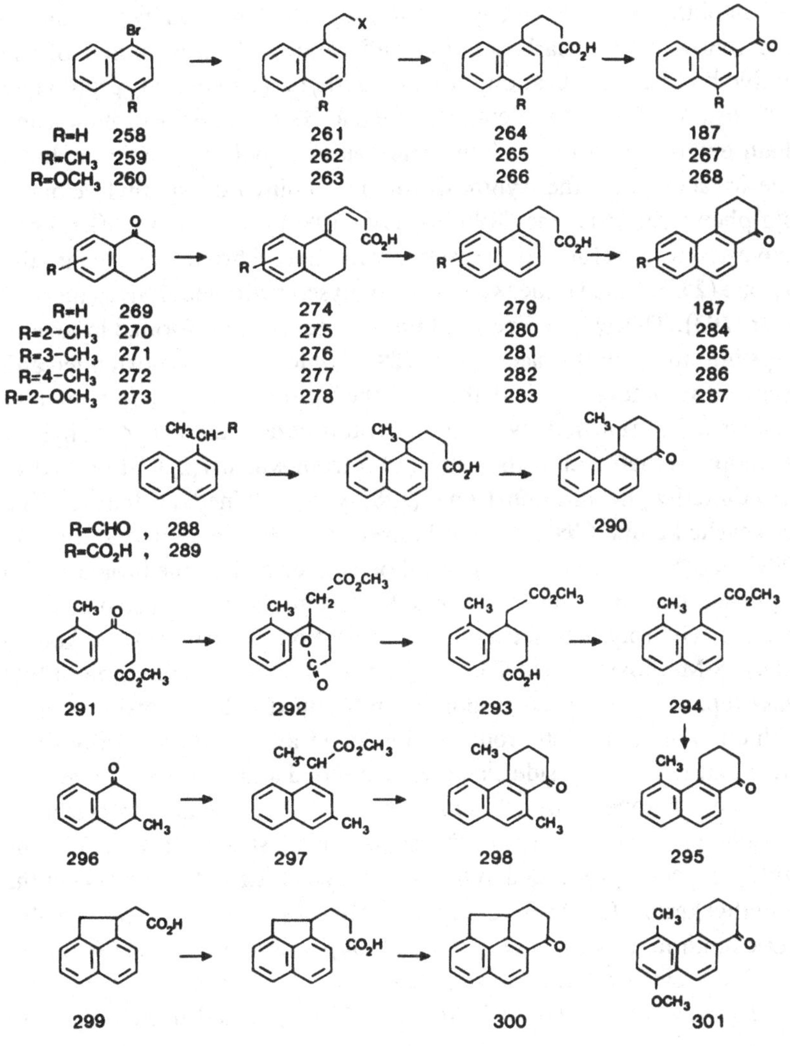

R=H	258
R=CH₃	259
R=OCH₃	260

261
262
263

264
265
266

187
267
268

R=H	269
R=2-CH₃	270
R=3-CH₃	271
R=4-CH₃	272
R=2-OCH₃	273

274
275
276
277
278

279
280
281
282
283

187
284
285
286
287

R=CHO , 288
R=CO₂H , 289

290

291   292   293   294

296   297   298   295

299   300   301

from the 1-bromonaphthalenes (258-260) with ethylene oxide gave the alcohols (261-263, X = OH), converted to the bromides (261-263, X = Br) with phosphorus tribromide and thence to the naphthyl butyric acids (264-266) by means of the malonic acid synthesis. Ring closure then gave the required tricyclic ketones (187, 267, and 268). In a second method the readily available 1-tetralones (269-273) reacted with methyl 3-bromo-crotonate under Reformatsky conditions to form the 2,4-dienoic acids (274-278); isomerization to the naphthyl acids (279-283) was achieved with palladium black at 280–300°C, followed by saponification. Cyclization as before gave the ketones (187 and 284-287). 1,2,3,4-Tetrahydro-4-methylphenanthren-1-one (290) was obtained either from 2-(1-naphthyl)-propionaldehyde (288) by condensation with malonic acid followed by decarboxylation and catalytic hydrogenation of the double bond and cyclization, or from methyl 2-(1-naphthyl)-propionate (289) by reduction to the alcohol, conversion of this into the bromide, and chain extension by the malonic acid route to yield the same naphthyl valeric acid. For the synthesis of 15,16-dihydro-1-methylcyclopenta[a]phenanthren-17-one (Ribeiro *et al.*, 1983) the keto-ester (291) was converted by a Reformatsky reaction with methyl bromoacetate into the lactone (292), which underwent acid-catalysed hydrogenolysis to the acid ester (293). This was cyclized and the ketone was transformed in several steps into the naphthyl acetic ester (294), which was chain-extended and cyclized as before to yield the tricyclic ketone. In a similar manner Reformatsky reaction with 3-methyltetralone (296) and ethyl 2-bromopropionate led to the ester (297) from which 1,2,3,4-tetrahydro-4,10-dimethylphenanthren-1-one (298) was obtained as before. The tetracyclic ketone (300) was synthesized from 3-acenaphthyl acetic acid (299) which was reduced to the alcohol, converted into the bromide with triphenylphosphine dibromide, and thence into the nitrile with potassium cyanide. Hydrolysis to the acid and cyclization gave the desired ketone (300). 8-Methoxy-5-methyl-1,2,3,4-tetrahydrophenanthren-1-one (301) was prepared from the corresponding tetralone by Reformatsky reaction with ethyl bromoacetate, followed by dehydration and aromatization to the naphthalene. The side chain was extended and cyclized as before.

These ketones were converted into 15,16-dihydrocyclopenta[a]phenanthren-17-ones by the sequence illustrated in Fig. 35. The Stöbbe reaction proceeded in fair to good yield, except in the case of the dimethyl ketone (298) where the yield of half-ester was poor; presumably steric hindrance by the *peri*-7-methyl group accounts for this. Closure of the five-membered ring was satisfactory provided strictly anhydrous conditions were maintained by the use of freshly fused zinc chloride in a mixture of acetic acid and acetic anhydride. Dehydrogenation, the final step in this synthesis, was best achieved with DDQ in boiling benzene or (probably better) by palladium in boiling *p*-cymene. The former method fails with the 11-methyl compounds, probably because the 11-methyl group is axial in the 11,12-dihydro- derivative and therefore does not possess a pair of *trans*-diaxial protons required for quinone dehydrogenation. Fifteen 17-ketones prepared in this way from 1,2,3,4-tetrahydrophenanthren-1-ones are summarized in Table 2.

The 1-methyl-17-ketone (**302**) was also obtained in very low yield from testosterone as shown in Fig. 37. Initially A-ring aromatization of a suitable steroid via the dienone–phenol rearrangement appeared to

Table 2. *15,16-Dihydrocyclopenta[a]phenanthren-17-ones prepared by the Stöbbe reaction*

	1,2,3,4-tetrahydro-phenanthrene	15,16-dihydrocyclopenta[a]-phenanthren-17-one
unsubstituted	(**187**)	(**4**)
1-CH$_3$	(**295**)	(**302**)
2-CH$_3$	(**284**)	(**303**)
3-CH$_3$	(**285**)	(**304**)
4-CH$_3$	(**286**)	(**305**)
6-CH$_3$	(**267**)	(**306**)
11-CH$_3$	(**290**)	(**26**)
2-OCH$_3$	(**287**)	(**307**)
6-OCH$_3$	(**268**)	(**308**)
7,11-(CH$_3$)$_2$	(**298**)	(**309**)
1,11-methano	(**300**)	(**310**)
1-CH$_3$-4-OCH$_3$	(**301**)	(**311**)
12-CH$_3$	(**242**)	(**130**)
12-CH$_2$CH$_3$	(**243**)	(**253**)
12-CH(CH$_3$)$_2$	(**245**)	(**254**)

Fig. 37

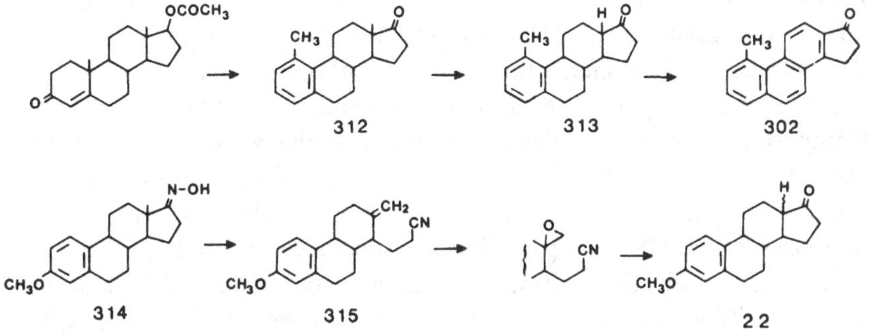

promise a convenient way of placing a methyl group at C-1 in a cyclopenta[a]phenanthrene. Testosterone acetate was transformed in four steps by known methods (Burgess *et al.*, 1962) into 1-methyloestra-1,3,5(10)-trien-17-one (**312**). After having rejected several possible methods for the elimination of the 18-methyl group, the method devised by Cohen *et al.* (1971) for the removal of a 4-methyl group from a tetracyclic triterpene was selected, and investigated first with the readily available oestrone methyl ether. Abnormal Beckmann rearrangement of the oxime (**314**) in dimethylsulphoxide with dicyclohexylcarbodimide and trifluoroacetic acid gave the cyano-ene (**315**) which was epoxidized with *m*-chloroperbenzoic acid. Cyclization of the epoxide with boron trifluoride in boiling toluene then afforded 18-noroestrone methyl ether (**22**) in 12.5% yield, from which both 13α and 13β epimers were isolated in the pure state (Coombs and Vose, 1974). When this reaction sequence was applied to the oxime of the steroid (**312**) its 18-nor derivative (**313**) was isolated in 14% yield, apparently as the single 13β epimer. Unfortunately, complete dehydrogenation of this compound with DDQ in boiling dioxan proceeded with difficulty, but a small amount of 15,16-dihydro-1-methylcyclopenta[a]phenanthren-17-one (**302**) identical with that prepared by total synthesis was isolated (Ribeiro *et al.*, 1983). Of no use practically, this transformation again stresses the close relationship between steroids and cyclopenta[a]phenanthrenes.

Isotopically labelled 15,16-dihydrocyclopenta[a]phenanthren-17-ones required for biochemical and biological studies were prepared (Fig. 38) by adapting the various methods already described. A methyl group labelled with either carbon-14 or tritium was readily introduced at C-11 by means of a Grignard reaction between the oxo-ketal (**201**) and the appropriately labelled methyl magnesium iodide followed by the usual aromatization procedure. The five-membered ring was also labelled at C-15 and C-16 with carbon-14 by the use of diethyl [2,3-^{14}C]succinate in the Stöbbe reaction (Coombs *et al.*, 1970). Reduction of the oxo-ketal (**201**) with tritiated sodium borohydride and removal of the easily exchangeable tritium gave the [11-^{3}H]alcohol (**317**) which yielded [11-^{3}H]-15,16-dihydrocyclopenta[a]phenanthren-17-one without further loss of label, showing that as expected the 11-hydroxyl group is axial in this alcohol. Comparatively low to moderate specific activities were obtainable by these methods. For higher specific activities (in excess of 1 Curie per millimole) catalytic debromination of readily available 15-bromo-17-ketones such as (**318**) over palladium on calcium carbonate in tritium gas readily gave 15-[^{3}H]-17-ketones at this activity. Even higher specific activities (5–30 Ci/mmol) were obtained by generally labelling with tritium by acid-catalysed exchange with [³H]acetic acid at 160°C over Adam's catalyst (Coombs, 1979). All positions were similarly labelled by this method with the exception of the sterically hindered bay region (C-1 and C-11), as disclosed by tritium nuclear magnetic spectroscopy (see Table 3). Tritium is readily lost from C-16 in these compounds by acid-catalysed exchange via the enol, but is stable at other positions under normal conditions (Russell *et al.*, 1985).

Badger *et al.* (1952) proposed an interesting route to 17-ketocyclopenta[a]phenanthrenes via ring-enlargement of the fluorenone (319) shown in Fig. 39. Treatment of this ketone with diazomethane in ether at room temperature, followed by addition of methanol and a trace of sodium carbonate gave the methoxyphenanthryl propionic ester in about 35% yield. Cyclization of the corresponding acid (320) with anhydrous hydrogen fluoride occurred, however, in the wrong direction to give the methoxy-ketone (321). In order to block this cyclization, the methoxyphenanthrene (320) was chlorinated with phosphorus pentachloride to the *o*-chloro-methoxy acid which on ring closure with phosphorus pentachloride and stannic chloride yielded 7-chloro-15,16-dihydro-6-methoxycyclopenta[a]phenanthren-17-one (322).

Fig. 38

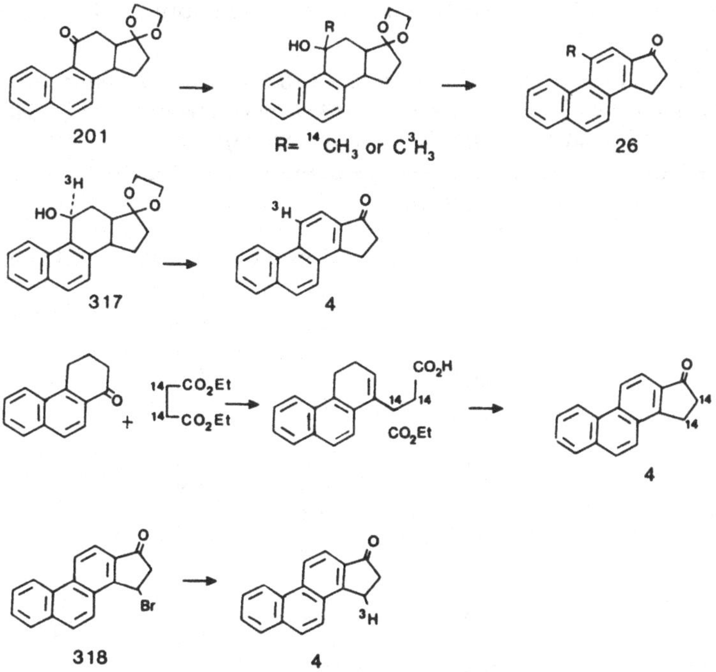

Another general method for the synthesis of cyclopenta[a]-phenanthrenes based on double acylation of naphthalenes has been described by Rahman and co-workers in several publications (Rahman and Perl, 1968; Rahman and Rodriguez, 1969, 1971; Rahman and Vuano, 1971). For example, ethyl 3-(2-naphthyl)propionate was acylated with succinic anhydride and aluminium chloride at C-6 to give the ketodiester (323) and was converted into the cyclopenta[a]-phenanthrenes (324), (325), (326), and (1) by standard methods. An attractive feature of this route is the good yield at each step, as shown in Fig. 39; many adaptations of this method can be visualized. A straight-forward preparation of 15,16-dihydro-15-phenyl-cyclopenta[a]phenan-thren-17-one (328) from 2-acetyl-naphthalene has also been reported (Shotter *et al.*, 1973). Conversion of the latter into the styryl ketone (327) in 91% yield was followed by cyclization with polyphosphoric acid at 130°C (47% yield). Treatment of the phenanthylhydroxypropionic acid (329) with 97% sulphuric acid gave 17-methyl-16-phenylcyclopen-ta[a]phenanthren-15-one (330) (Mladenova-Orlinova *et al.*, 1970).

A recent cyclopenta[a]phenanthren-17-one synthesis employs the Diels–Alder reaction to construct the C-ring (Corey and Estreicher, 1981). Reaction of 3-nitro-2-cyclopentenone with the dimethoxy-diene (331) in boiling toluene gave the adduct which, without isolation, was treated with 1,5-diazabicyclo-[4.3.0]non-5-ene forming 3,11-dimethoxy-

Table 3. *Distribution of tritium in 15,16-dihydrocyclopenta[a]-phenanthren-17-ones generally labelled by catalytic exchange with [³H]acetic acid as disclosed by tritium nmr spectroscopy*

Relative [³H] incorporation at:	Compound			
	unsubstituted	11-methyl	12-methyl	11,12-dimethyl
C-15	14.2	15.3	8.4	15.1
C-16	12.3	16.6	47.0	17.9
C-2	} 26.9	7.3	7.8	7.2
C-3		7.3	7.9	7.1
C-4	9.7	5.7	8.4	8.0
C-6	13.1	8.3	7.4	7.7
C-7	10.4	6.4	1.9	4.0
C-12	4.1	4.5	—	—
C-1	4.1	1.2	1.9	1.1
C-11	5.2	—	0	—
11-CH₃	—	27.4	—	} 31.9
12-CH₃	—	—	9.3	

6,7,15,16-tetrahydrocyclopenta[a]phenanthren-17-one (**332**) in 51%
yield. This approach clearly merits further attention.

Fig. 39

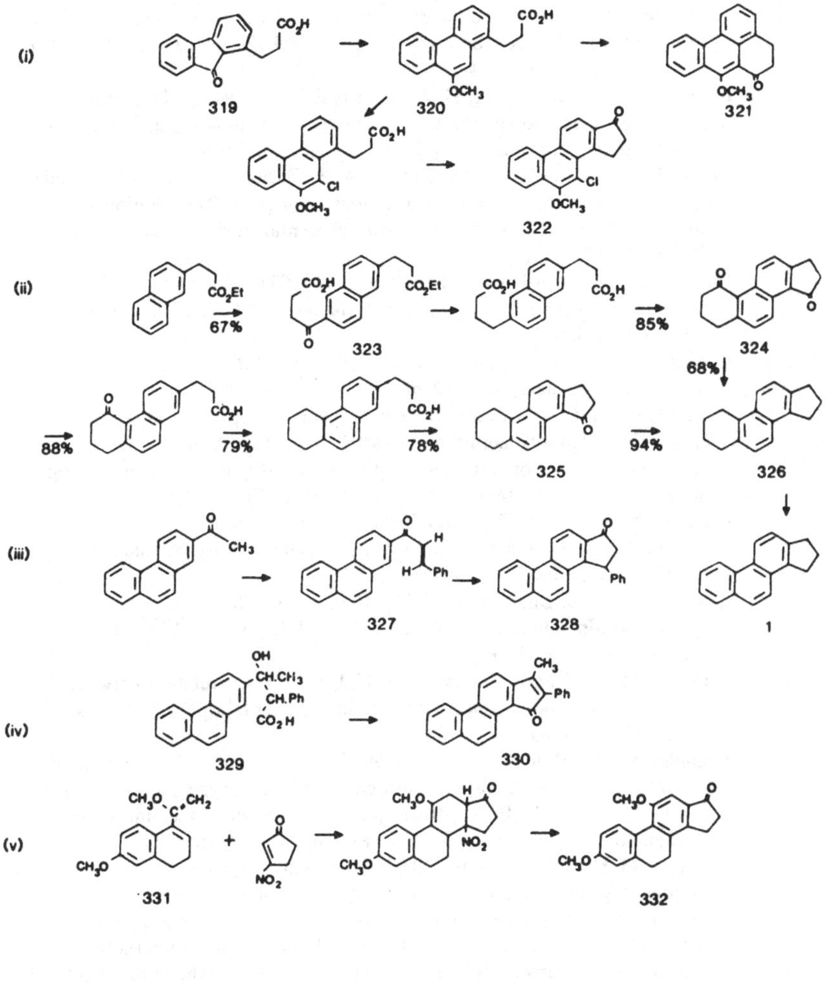

3.1   References

Bachmann, W. E., Gregg, R. A. & Pratt, E. F. (1943). Synthesis of
    compounds related to the sex hormones. *J. Am. Chem. Soc.*, **65**, 2314–18.

Bachmann, W. E. & Holman, R. E. (1951). Synthesis of compounds related
    to equilenin. *J. Am. Chem. Soc.*, **73**, 3660–5.

Bachmann, W. E. & Kloetzel, M. C. (1937). Phenanthrene derivatives. VII.
    The cyclization of β-phenanthrylpropionic acids. *J. Am. Chem. Soc.*, **59**,
    2207–13.

Badger, G. M., Carruthers, W. & Cook, J. W. (1952). New derivatives of
    1,2-cyclopentenophenanthrene. *J. Chem. Soc.*, 4996–5000.

Bardhan, J. C. (1936). Studies in the sterol–oestrone group. Part I. A synthesis of 3'-keto-3:4-dihydro-1:2-cyclopentenophenanthrene. *J. Chem. Soc.*, 1848–51.

Birch, A. J., Jaeger, R. & Robinson, R. (1945). The synthesis of substances related to the sterols. Part XLIV. dl-*cis* Equilenin. *J. Chem. Soc.*, 582–6.

Burgess, C., Burn, D., Ducker, J. W., Ellis, B., Feather, B., Hiscock, A. K., Leftwick, A. P., Mills, J. S. & Petrow, V. (1962). Modified steroid hormones. Part XXIX. Some 17α-chloroethynyl-17β-hydroxy-derivatives. *J. Chem. Soc. (C)*, 4995–5004.

Butenandt, A., Dannenberg, H. & von Dresler, D. (1949). Methylhomologe des 1,2-cyclopentenophenthrene. V. Mitteilung: Synthese des 10-methyl-1,2-cyclopentenophenanthrens. *Z. Naturforsch.*, **4b**, 69–76.

Chinn, L. J., Brown, E. A., Mikulec, R. A. & Garland, R. B. (1962). Studies in the total synthesis of steroids and their analogues. III. Additional products of *trans*-2-(alkoxyaryl)-5-oxocyclopentaneacetic acids. *J. Org. Chem.*, **47**, 1733–41.

Cohen, K. F., Kazlauskas, R. & Pinhey, J. T. (1971). A new method for removal of a 4-methyl group from triterpenes. *J. Chem. Soc., Chem. Commun.*, 1419–20.

Coombs, M. M. (1965). A new synthesis of 3'-oxo-1,2-cyclopentenophenanthrene. *Chem. Ind. (London)*, 270–1.

Coombs, M. M. (1966). Potentially carcinogenic cyclopenta[a]phenanthrenes (1,2-cyclopentenophenanthrenes). Part I. A new synthesis of 15,16-dihydro-17-oxo-cyclopenta[a]phenanthrene and the phenanthrene analogue of 18-noroestrone methyl ether. *J. Chem. Soc. (C)*, 955–62.

Coombs, M. M. (1979). Tritium labelling of carcinogenic cyclopenta[a]phenanthrenes at very high specific activity. *J. Labelled Comp. Radiopharm.*, **17**, 147–52.

Coombs, M. M. & Bhatt, T. S. (1973). Potentially carcinogenic cyclopenta[a]phenanthrenes. Part VI. 1,2,3,4-Tetrahydro-17-ketones. *J. Chem. Soc. Perkin Trans. I*, 1251–4.

Coombs, M. M., Bhatt, T. S. & Croft, C. J. (1973). Correlation between carcinogenicity and chemical structure in cyclopenta[a]phenanthrenes. *Cancer Res.*, **33**, 832–7.

Coombs, M. M., Hall, M., Siddle, V. A. & Vose, C. W. (1975). Potentially carcinogenic cyclopenta[a]phenanthrenes. Part X. Oxygenated derivatives of the carcinogen 15,16-dihydro-11-methylcyclopenta[a]phenanthren-17-one of metabolic interest. *J. Chem. Soc. Perkin Trans. I*, 265–70.

Coombs, M. M. & Jaitly, S. B. (1971). Potentially carcinogenic cyclopenta[a]phenanthrenes. Part V. Synthesis of 15,16-dihydro-7-methylcyclopenta[a]phenanthren-17-one. *J. Chem. Soc. (C)*, 230–4.

Coombs, M. M., Jaitly, S. B. & Crawley, F. E. H. (1970). Potentially carcinogenic cyclopenta[a]phenanthrenes. Part IV. Synthesis of 17-ketones by the Stöbbe condensation. *J. Chem. Soc. (C)*, 1266–71.

Coombs, M. M., Russell, J. C., Jones, J. R. & Ribeiro, O. (1985). A comparative examination of the *in vitro* metabolism of five cyclopenta[a]phenanthrenes of varying carcinogenic potential. *Carcinogenesis*, **6**, 1217–22.

Coombs, M. M. & Vose, C. W. (1974). A novel and convenient conversion of 17-ketosteroids into their 18-nor derivatives. *J. Chem. Soc., Chem. Commun.*, 602–3.

Coombs, M. M. & Vose, C. W. (1975). An n.m.r. spectral study of the acid hydrolysis of furfurylidene-2-acetylnaphthalenes using the shift reagent Eu(DPM)₃. *Chem. Ind. (London)*, 836–7.

Corey, E. J. & Estreicher, H. (1981). 3-Nitroalkenones, synthesis and use as reverse affinity cycloalkynone equivalents. *Tetrahedron Lett.*, **22**, 603–6.

Fieser, L. F., Fieser, M. & Hershberg, E. B. (1936). The synthesis of phenanthrene and hydrophenanthrene derivatives. VI. 1′,3′-Diketocyclopentenophenanthrenes. *J. Am. Chem. Soc.*, **58**, 2322–5.

Fieser, L. F. & Hershberg, E. B. (1936). The synthesis of phenanthrene and hydrophenanthrene derivatives. VII. 5,9-dimethoxy-1′,3′-diketo-1,2-cyclopentenophenanthrene. *J. Am. Chem. Soc.*, **58**, 2382–5.

Johnson, W. S. & Petersen, J. W. (1945). The Stöbbe condensation with 1-keto-1,2,3,4-tetrahydrophenanthrene. A synthesis of 3′-keto-3,4-dihydro-1,2-cyclopentenophenanthrene. *J. Am. Chem. Soc.*, **67**, 1366–8.

Jung, M. E. & Hudspeth, J. P. (1978). Anionic oxy-cope rearrangements with aromatic substrates in bicycle[2.2.1]heptene systems. Facile synthesis of *cis*-hydrindone derivatives, including steroid analogues. *J. Am. Chem. Soc.*, **100**, 4309–11.

Kawarura, M., Abe, K. & Hirami, Y. (1974). Synthesis of hydrocarbons by desulphurisation of 4-hydroxy-3′-keto-1,2-cyclopentenophenanthrene tosylate. *Kochi Joshi Daigaku Kujo, Shizen Kagaku Ben*, **22**, 19–23 (*Chem. Abst.*, **81**, 120303v).

Kenner, G. W. & Williams, N. R. (1955). A method of reducing phenols to aromatic hydrocarbons. *J. Chem. Soc.*, 522–5.

Koebner, A. & Robinson, R. (1938). Experiments on the synthesis of substances related to sterols. Part XXII. Synthesis of x-norequilenin methyl ether. *J. Chem. Soc.*, 1994–7.

Koebner, A. & Robinson, R. (1941). Experiments on the synthesis of substances related to the sterols. Part XXXVI (Continuation of Part XXII). *J. Chem. Soc.*, 566–9.

Mejer, S. & Kalinowska, K. (1969). Reduction of (+ −)-14β-gona-1,3,5(10),6,8-pentaene-11,17-dione with lithium aluminium hydride. *Bull. Acad. Polon. Sci., Sér. Sci. Chim.*, **17**, 145–9.

Mladenova-Orlinova, L., Ivanov, C. & Aleksiev, B. B. (1970). Preparation and dehydration of phenanthyl-substituted hydroxypropionic and hydroxybutyroic acids. *Dokl. Bolg. Akad. Nauk.*, **23**, 73–6.

Posner, G. H., Chapdelaine, M. J. & Lenz, C. M. (1979). Short, simple stereocontrolled steroid synthesis: (±)-11-oxoequilenin methyl ether and a new 9,11-*seco*-13-ethyl-steroid. *J. Org. Chem.*, **44**, 3661–5.

Rahman, A. & Perl, C. (1968). Double acylation of aromatic compounds. IV. Total synthesis of Diels' hydrocarbon by succinoylation and acetylation of naphthalene. *Annalen*, **718**, 127–35.

Rahman, A. & Rodriguez, N. M. (1969). Total synthesis of 1,2-cyclopentenophenanthrene. *Chem. Ind. (London)*, **52**, 1870–1.

Rahman, A. & Rodriguez, N. M. (1971). Double acetylation of aromatic carbons. IX. Synthesis of 16,17-dihydro-15*H*-cyclopenta[a]phenanthrene by succinoylation of ethyl 3-(2-naphthyl)propionate. *Chem. Ber.*, **104**, 2651–6.

Rahman, A. & Vuano, B. M. (1971). Diels' hydrocarbon synthesis [from 2-acetyl-9,10-dihydrophenanthren]. *An. Asoc. Quim. Argent.*, **59**, 265–9.

Ribeiro, O., Hadfield, S. T., Clayton, A. F., Vose, C. W. & Coombs, M. M. (1983). Potentially carcinogenic cyclopenta[a]phenanthrenes. Part 11. Synthesis of the 1-methyl-, 1,11-methano, and 7,11-dimethyl derivatives of 15,16-dihydrocyclopenta[a]phenanthren-17-one. *J. Chem. Soc. Perkin Trans. I*, 87–91.

Riegel, B., Siegel, S. & Kritchevsky, D. (1948). The synthesis of 3-alkyl-1,2-cyclopentenophenanthrenes. *J. Am. Chem. Soc.*, **70**, 2950–2.

Robinson, R. (1938). Experiments on the synthesis of substances related to sterols. Part XXI. A new synthesis of ketocyclopentenophenanthrene. *J. Chem. Soc.*, 1390–7.

Robinson, R. & Rydon, H. N. (1939). Experiments on the synthesis of substances related to the sterols. Part XXVII. The synthesis of x-noroestrone. *J. Chem. Soc.*, 1394–405.

Russell, J. C., Bhatt, T. S., Jones, J. R. & Coombs, M. M. (1985). Comparison of the binding of some carcinogenic and non-carcinogenic cyclopenta[a]phenanthrenes to DNA *in vitro* and *in vivo*. *Carcinogenesis*, **6**, 1223–5.

Short, F. W. & Rockwood, G. M. (1969). Synthesis and interconversion of 6-aryl-4-oxohexanoic acids and 5-aryl-2-furan-propionic acids. Anti-inflammatory agents. *J. Heterocyclic Chem.*, **6**, 713–22.

Shotter, R. G., Johnson, K. M. & Williams, H. J. (1973). Polyphosphoric acid catalysed cyclisation of aryl stryryl ketones. *Tetrahedron*, **29**, 2163–6.

Siewinski, A., Dmochowska, J. & Meyer, S. (1969). Microbiol transformations. III. Microbiol reduction of (+)-14β-gona-1,3,5(10),6,8-pentaene-11,17-dione by *Rhodotorula mucilaginosa*. *Bull. Acad. Pol. Sci., Sér. Chim.*, **17**, 151–4.

Woodward, R. B., Inhoffen, H. H., Larsen, H. O. & Menzel, K. H. (1953). Synthesis of 3′,8-dimethyl-1,2-cyclopentenophenanthrene. *Chem. Ber.*, **8b**, 594–601.

4

General chemistry of cyclopenta[a]phenanthrenes

All cyclopenta[a]phenanthrenes contain an aromatic phenanthrene ring system fused to a five-membered ring, and not unexpectedly chemical reactions due to both these structural moieties are observed. In the D-ring ketones the carbon–oxygen dipole induces electron withdrawal from the whole system, and often reactions at the five-membered ring tend to dominate the chemistry of these compounds.

Oxidation of the parent hydrocarbon (1) with chromic acid (Fig. 40) was found to give mainly the 15-ketone (102) (Hoch, 1938; Butenandt *et al.*, 1946; Badger *et al.*, 1952) together with a trace of the expected 6,7-quinone (104) (Badger *et al.*, 1952). The 11-methyl hydrocarbon (83), conveniently prepared by hydrogenolysis of the 11-methyl-17-ketone (26) with Adam's catalyst and palladium on charcoal in acetic acid containing hydrochloric acid, also gave the 11-methyl-15-ketone (334) in 37% yield (Coombs, 1969). By contrast, the five-membered ring in the 17-ketone, 15,16-dihydrocyclopenta[a]phenanthren-17-one (4), resisted further attack; oxidation with chromic acid in acetic acid led to a nearly quantitative yield of the bright yellow 6,7-quinone (335) (15,16-dihydro-cyclopenta[a]phenanthrene-6,7,17-trione). Similar oxidation of the 11-methyl-17-ketone (26) gave the corresponding 11-methyl-6,7,17-trione (336) in 51% yield, together with unchanged starting material and small amounts of three other oxidation products. Butenandt *et al.* (1946) obtained the 6,7-quinone (104) from the parent hydrocarbon (1) indirectly by first treating it with osmium tetroxide to give the *cis*-6,7-diol (103) in good yield; this was then further oxidized to the quinone with chromic acid. Coombs found that the 17-ketones (4) and (26) also reacted smoothly with osmium tetroxide in pyridine to furnish the keto-diols (337) and (338) which could be further oxidized with chromic acid to the quinones in high yield. The keto-diols were dehydrated when they were

62   *General chemistry*

heated with 2.5-M sulphuric acid; the unsubstituted keto-diol (337) gave mainly the phenol 15,16-dihydro-6-hydroxycyclopenta[a]phenanthren-17-one (339) with a small amount of a second phenol, probably the 7-hydroxy isomer; this 6-phenol (339) was identical with the sample obtained from total synthesis (see Fig. 36). The 11-methyl keto-diol (338) was less readily dehydrated, and gave only the 6-phenol (340). Oxidation of the two 17-ketones with cerium (IV) ammonium nitrate in aqueous acetic acid at ambient temperature, conditions reported to oxidize the methyl group in 1-methyloestrone methyl ether to a formyl group in 90% yield (Laing and Sykes, 1968), led to mixtures containing the 6,7,17-triones and several other unidentified oxidation products in low to moderate yield.

Oxidation of the parent hydrocarbon (1) with lead tetraacetate gave the 15-acetoxy compound (333) (Badger *et al.*, 1952). Similar oxidation of the two ketones (4) and (26) took a different course, leading to the 16-

Fig. 40

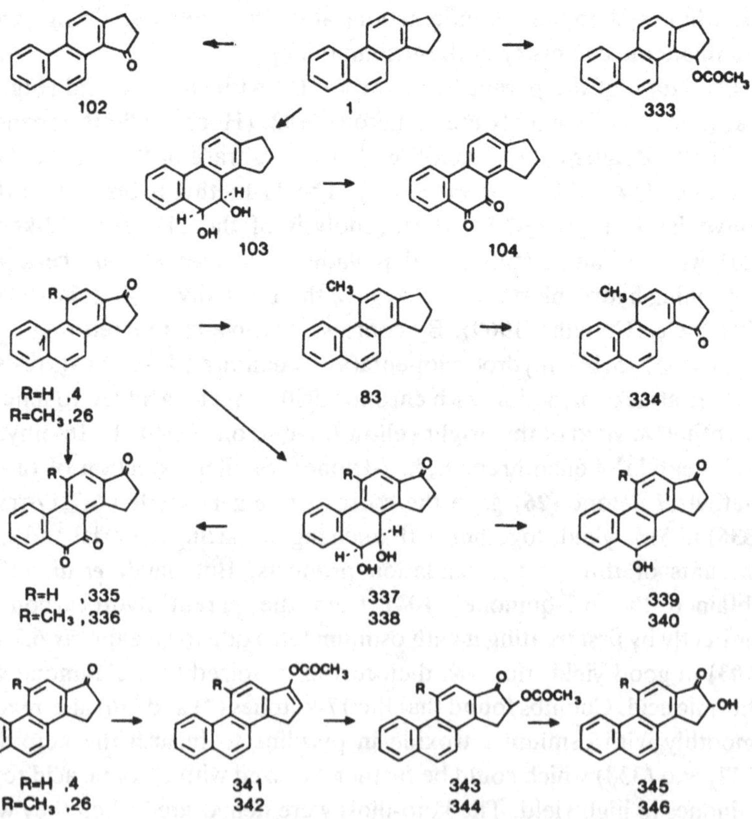

acetoxy derivatives, but better yields of the latter were obtained by similar oxidation of the enol acetates (**341**) and (**342**). These were readily prepared in high yield from the ketones with isopropenyl acetate, catalysed with *p*-toluene sulphonic acid. Oxidation with lead tetraacetate in a mixture and acetic acid and acetic anhydride with irradiation with visible light from a tungsten filament lamp then afforded the 17-keto-16-acetates (**343**) and (**344**) in excellent yield. Based on infrared evidence the initial oxidation products appeared to be the 16,17,17-triacetates, but these gave the 17-keto-16-acetates on recrystallization of the crude reaction products. The 17-ketone-16-ols (**345**) and (**346**) were readily obtained by acid hydrolysis; alkali caused decomposition.

Friedel–Crafts acylation of 16,17-dihydro-15*H*-cyclopenta[a]-phenanthrene (**1**) (Dannenberg *et al.*, 1965) in nitrobenzene with acetyl chloride in the presence of aluminium chloride led to substitution at C-12 (Fig. 41). The 12-acetyl compound (**347**), obtained in 38% yield, was converted via Beckmann rearrangement of its oxime into the 12-amide (**348**) and thence into 12-amino-16,17-dihydro-15*H*-cyclopenta[a]-phenanthrene (**349**). This amide (**348**) was synthesized independently from Robinson's 12-ketone (**96**); the oxime (**350**) of this ketone was acetylated, then heated with acetic anhydride and acetyl chloride (Semmler–Wolff aromatization) to give the 6,7-dihydro-12-diacetylamino compound (**351**) in 60% yield. Treatment with potassium hydroxide followed by dehydrogenation with platinum on charcoal at 300°C furnished the same amide. Friedel–Crafts acylation of the naphthyl

Fig. 41

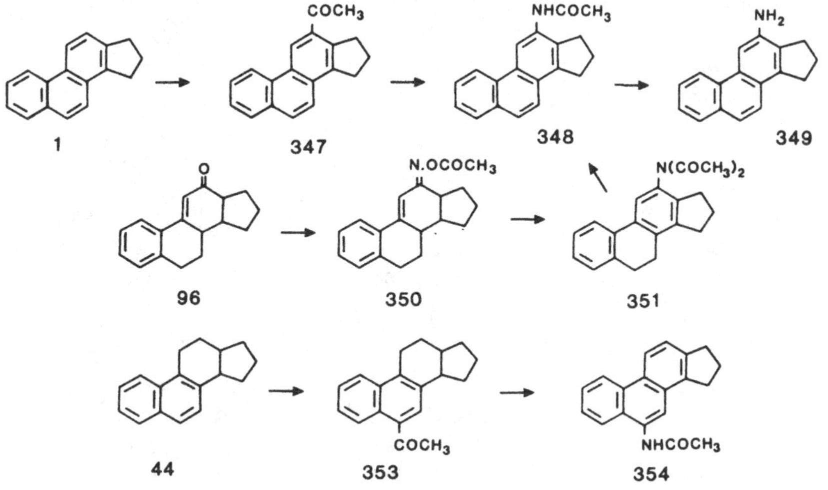

compound   (44)   (11,12,13,14,16,17-hexahydro-15*H*-cyclopenta[a]-
phenanthrene), on the other hand, occurred at C-6 to give the 6-acetyl
derivative (353), which was dehydrogenated and converted into the
6-amide (354) as before. Electrophilic bromination of the 17-ketones (4)
and (26) with bromine in chloroform or acetic acid, even in the absence of
light or in the presence of silver nitrate and acid (Derbyshire and Waters,
1950), conditions known to favour aryl bromination, did not lead to aryl
substitution, but gave instead the 15-bromo (318) and (355) and 15,15-
dibromo derivatives (356) and (357) (Fig. 42) by attack at the benzylic
position in the five-membered ring (Coombs *et al.*, 1973). With a large
excess of bromine addition occurred at the 6,7-position of (4) to form the
6,7-dihydro-6,7,15,15-tetrabromide (360), which on being heated lost
hydrogen bromide to yield 15,16-dihydro-6(or 7),15,15-tribromo-
cyclopenta[a]phenanthren-17-one (361) (Coombs, unpublished work).
At no point did electrophilic bromination of the aromatic phenanthrene
ring system occur, emphasizing the overriding effect of the carbonyl
group at C-17 on the reactivity of the aromatic ring system. Free-radical

Fig. 42

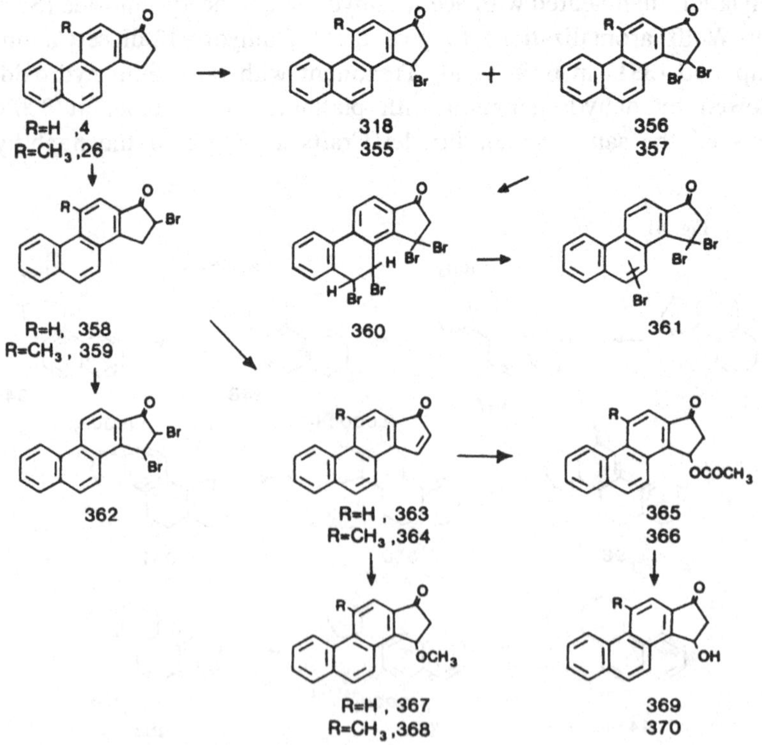

bromination of the ketones (**4**) and (**26**) with N-bromosuccinimide in carbon tetrachloride during irradiation with visible light furnished the 16-bromo-17-ketones (**358**) and (**359**) in high yield. Similar bromination of the 15-bromo-17-ketone led to 15,16-dibromo-15,16-dihydrocyclopenta[a]phenanthren-17-one (**362**), different from the dibromide obtained by direct bromination.

Dehydrobromination of 16-bromo-15,16-dihydrocyclopenta[a]phenanthren-17-one (**358**) with triethylamine in tetrahydrofuran gave bright orange crystals of the fully unsaturated ketone, cyclopenta[a]phenanthren-17-one (**363**). Debromination occurred readily, being complete in a few minutes at room temperature, and could be followed conveniently by ultraviolet spectroscopy. The purification of this compound was complicated by the ease with which it gave rise to insoluble material on attempted recrystallization. In this respect it resembled the analogous compound indenone which is known to undergo spontaneous polymerization (Marvel and Hinmann, 1954). 11-Methylcyclopenta[a]phenanthren-17-one (**364**), obtained from 16-bromo-15,16-dihydro-11-methylcyclopenta[a]phenanthren-17-one (**359**) by the same method (Coombs *et al.*, 1975), appeared to be somewhat more stable. Again by analogy with indenone (Lacey and Smith, 1971) acid-catalysed hydration of the 15(16)-double bond in the enone (**363**) using aqueous sulphuric acid in tetrahydrofuran, followed by acetylation, yielded the 15-acetoxy-17-ketone (**365**) from which the secondary alcohol (**369**) was obtained by acid hydrolysis. Hydration of the corresponding double bond in the 11-methyl homologue (**364**) proceeded more slowly, and recourse was made to sulphuric acid-catalysed addition of acetic acid which occurred much faster; the 11-methyl-15-acetoxy-17-ketone (**366**) was isolated directly by crystallization in 40% yield. As before the alcohol (**370**) was prepared by acid hydrolysis, alkali being detrimental. The 15-methoxy-17-ketones (**367**) and (**368**) were similarly made by acid-catalysed addition of methanol to the double bond (Bhatt *et al.*, 1982).

In an effort to direct electrophilic bromination of these ketones to the aromatic phenanthrene rings, bromination in the presence of thallium triacetate (McKillop *et al.*, 1972) was investigated (Coombs *et al.*, 1973). Under these conditions (Fig. 43) with the parent, unsubstituted ketone 15,16-dihydrocyclopenta[a]phenanthren-17-one (**4**), the main product was a compound $C_{19}H_{14}O_3$ devoid of bromine; this was identified as the 15-acetoxy-17-ketone (**365**) already prepared as described above. It was not formed when either the 17-ketone (**4**) or its 15-bromo derivative (**318**) was treated with thallium triacetate in the absence of bromine, the best yield of the 15-acetate being secured when one equivalent of bromine was

added to the original ketone and thallium triacetate in carbon
tetrachloride at ambient temperature. A bromo derivative of thallium
therefore appears to be involved, and it was proposed that esterification
by it of the 17-enol to form the thallic ester (371) was followed by attack at
C-15 by acetate, giving (318) as shown. This mechanism is similar to that
proposed previously for the formation of 10β-trifluoroacetoxy-19-noran-
drosta-1,4-diene-3,17-dione (373) by the action of thallium trifluoroacetate on oestrone via the phenolic thallic ester (372) (Coombs and
Jones, 1972). The proposed intermediate (371) involves bond rearrangement in the five-membered ring to a quinoid structure; this has been
observed in other reactions involving substitution in ring-D. Thus
attempted nucleophilic replacement of bromine in the 15-bromo-17-
ketone (318) by acetate led smoothly not to the expected 15-acetate, but
to the 16-acetoxy-17-ketone (343) identical with the specimen prepared
by lead tetraacetate oxidation (Coombs *et al.*, 1973). Also attempted
demethylation of the 15-methoxy-17-ketone (367) with boron tribromide
gave instead the 16-bromo-17-ketone (Coombs, unpublished work). In
both these reactions quinoid intermediates (374) and (375), arising from
nucleophilic attack at C-16 in the enol accompanied by bond migration,
account reasonably for these unexpected results.

Reduction of the 16-hydroxy-17-ketones (345) and (346) with sodium
borohydride (Fig. 44) readily furnished the 16,17-*trans*-diols (376) and

Fig. 43

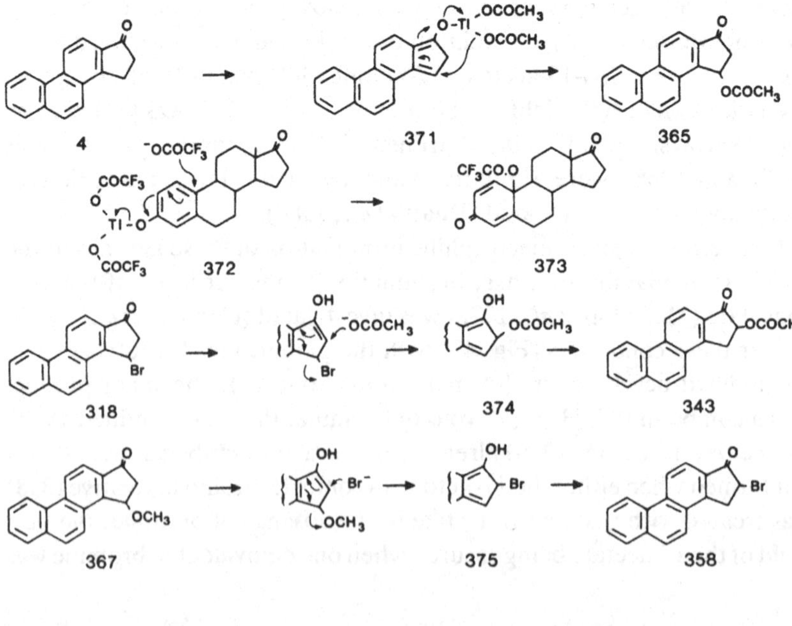

(377), whilst addition of osmium tetroxide to the D-ring double bond in 15*H*-cyclopenta[a]phenanthrene (3) and its 11-methyl homologue (150) gave the 16,17-*cis*-diols (378) and (379). In a similar way oxidation of 17*H*-cyclopenta[a]phenanthrene (2) with osmium tetroxide led to the 15,16-*cis*-diol (382) (Coombs and Hall, 1973). On acid-catalysed dehydration all these diols gave rise to the previously unknown 16-ketones (380) and (381), analogous to the unconjugated ketone similarly formed on dehydration of indan-1,2-diol (Brooks and Young, 1956). These ketones are easily distinguished from their 15- and 17-isomers by their ultraviolet absorption spectra which are similar to those of the hydrocarbons, and by their infrared carbonyl stretching frequencies at 1750 cm⁻¹ as opposed to those of the conjugated ketones at 1690 cm⁻¹. Presumably formation of 16-ketones occurs with gain in energy due to relief of strain in ring-D outweighing that which would have been gained by conjugation of the carbonyl group at either C-15 or C-17. Synthesis of partially hydrogenated 16-ketocyclopenta[a]phenanthrenes have been reported in two papers summarized in Fig. 44. Wilds (1942) brominated

Fig. 44

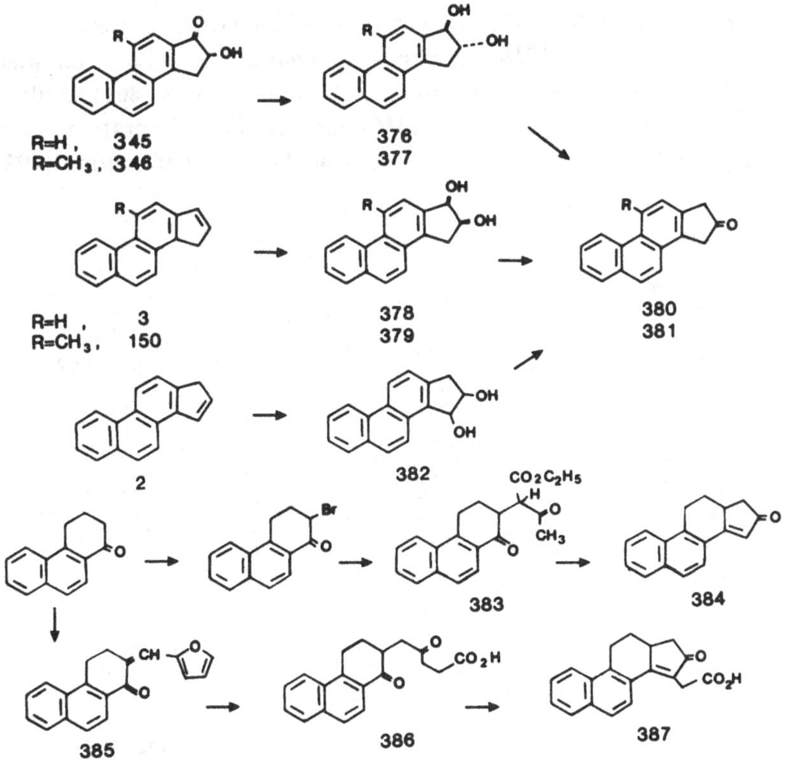

1,2,3,4-tetrahydrophenanthren-1-one and condensed the 2-bromo-1-ketone with sodioacetoacetic ester to form the diketone (**383**). Treatment of the latter with dilute potassium hydroxide led to cyclization with the formation of 11,12,13,17-tetrahydro-16*H*-cyclopenta[a]phenanthren-16-one (**384**) in high yield. On Clemmensen reduction followed by dehydrogenation with palladium on charcoal it was converted into the known hydrocarbon (**1**). In the second report (Turner, 1949) the same tricyclic ketone was transformed almost quantitatively into its furfurylidene derivative (**385**), which with hot acid yielded the diketo acid (**386**) by a reaction analogous to that reinvestigated by Robinson and described previously. Treatment of this diketone with dilute alkali caused ring closure to the 16-ketone (**387**) which had ultraviolet absorption very similar to that described by Wilds (1942) for (**384**).

Grignard reactions with the 17-ketone (**4**) (Fig. 45) yielded 17-methyl- and 17-isopropyl-15*H*-cyclopenta[a]phenanthrenes (**133**) and (**388**) which on treatment with osmium tetroxide yielded the corresponding 16,17-*cis*-diols (**389**) and (**400**) (Dannenberg *et al.*, 1960). Oxidation of the methyl-diol (**389**) with periodate cleaved ring-D to form the phenanthrene ketoaldehyde, whereas oxidation of this diol or of the precursor hydrocarbon (**133**) with chromic acid led to the corresponding ketoacid; 15-methyl-17*H*-cyclopenta[a]phenanthrene (**128**) likewise gave the isomeric ketoacid on similar oxidation. The diol (**401**) resulted from ozonolysis of the 17-methyl-15*H*-hydrocarbon. Dehydration of the 17-methyl-16,17-*cis*-diol (**389**) afforded the 17-methyl-16-ketone (**402**)

Fig. 45

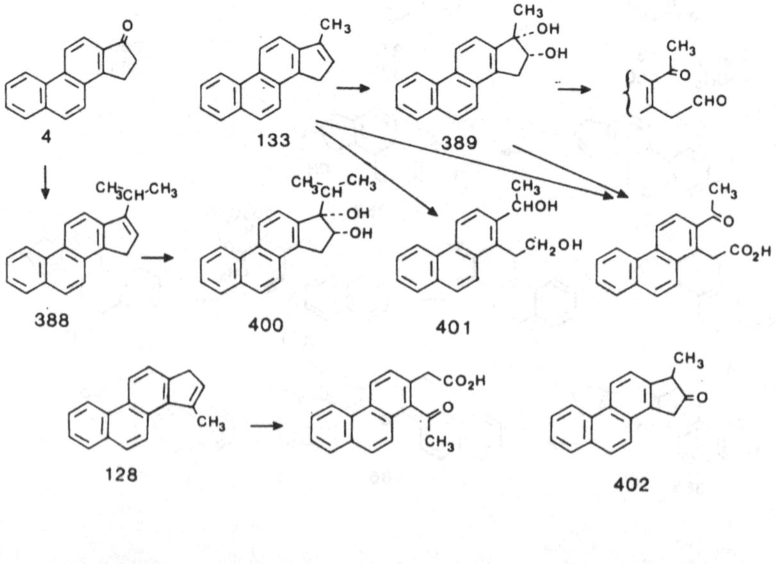

closely similar in properties to the parent 16-ketone (**380**). The 17-ketones also react normally in the Reformatsky reaction as first shown by Robinson and Slater (1941) who condensed the readily available 11-methoxy- and 3,11-dimethoxy-17-ketones with ethyl bromoacetate in the presence of zinc to give the unsaturated esters (**403**) and (**404**) or their $\Delta^{16(17)}$ isomers (Fig. 46). In the course of the synthesis of cholanthrenes Dannenberg (1950) prepared the unsubstituted ester (**405**) and, by employing ethyl 2-bromopropionate, also the 20-methyl homologue (**406**) (Dannenberg and Dannenberg-von Dresler, 1964). The double bonds in these two esters were reduced by catalytic hydrogenation and the side chains in the products (**407**) and (**408**) were extended by means of the Arndt–Eistert reaction to (**409**) and (**410**) before cyclization at C-12 and after further transformations to furnish the cholanthrenes (**411**) and (**412**). For the synthesis of the isomeric ring system 16,17-benzo-15*H*-cyclopenta[a]phenanthrene [indeno(2′,3′:1,2)phenanthrene] (**416**), derivatives of which have been isolated as minor products during

Fig. 46

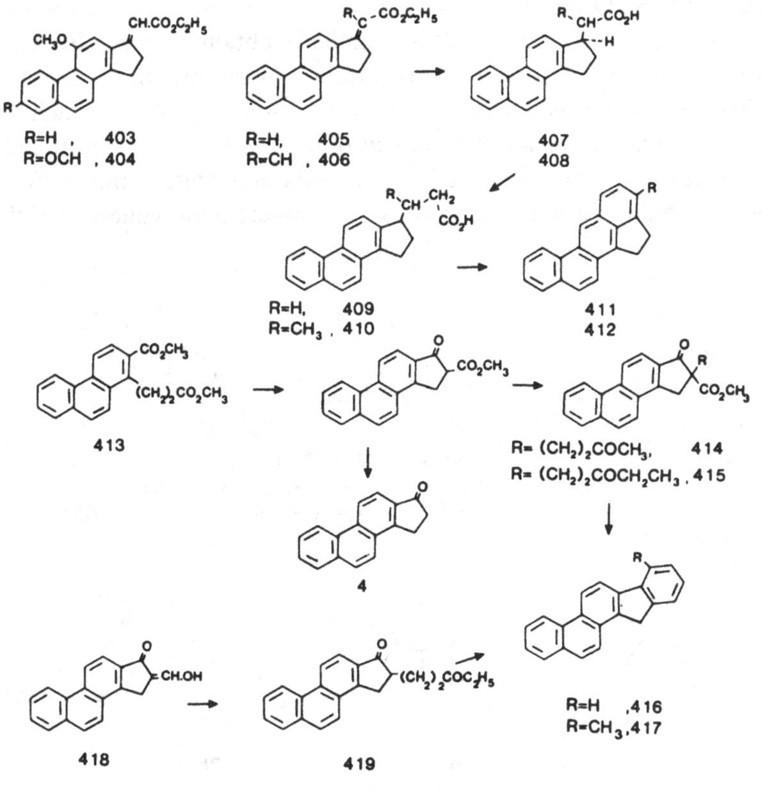

dehydrogenation of various sterols (Ruzicka and Goldberg, 1937), Nasipuri and Roy (1961) prepared the sodium salt of methyl 15,16-dihydro-17-oxo-cyclopenta[a]phenanthrene-16-carboxylate by Dieckmann cyclization of the phenanthrene-1,2-diester (**413**). Acid hydrolysis of the 16-carboxylate led to 15,16-dihydrocyclopenta[a]phenanthren-17-one (**4**), mp 200–201°C, whilst condensation with the Mannich base 4-piperidinobutan-2-one methiodide or with 1-chloropentan-3-one gave the diketo-esters (**414**) and (**415**), converted in several steps to the desired pentacyclic hydrocarbons (**416**) and (**417**). This ring system was also obtained (Buchta and Kraetzer, 196s) via Michael addition of ethyl vinyl ketone to the 16-hydroxymethylene-17-ketone (**418**) to form 15,16-dihydro-16-(3-oxopentyl)cyclopenta[a]phenanthren-17-one (**419**) which was cyclized and aromatized as before.

The 17-methylene group in cyclopenta[a]phenanthrenes, situated between two double bonds, is acidic. Thus the parent 17*H*- hydrocarbon (**2**) (Fig. 47) condensed readily with benzaldehyde and with *p*-dimethylaminobenzaldehyde in the presence of sodium hydroxide to yield the yellow 17-benzylidine compounds (**420**) and (**421**); hydrogenation of (**420**) gave the 17-benzyl derivatives (**423**) (Coombs, 1966). The yellow isopropylidene derivative (**422**) was similarly obtained by condensation with acetone in the presence of piperidine; in the presence of sodium hydroxide there was isolated a colourless isomer (**424**) in which the terminal double bond had rotated out of conjugation with the aromatic ring system, thereby presumably relieving the steric interaction between the side chain and hydrogen at C-12. Complete hydrogenation of this

Fig. 47

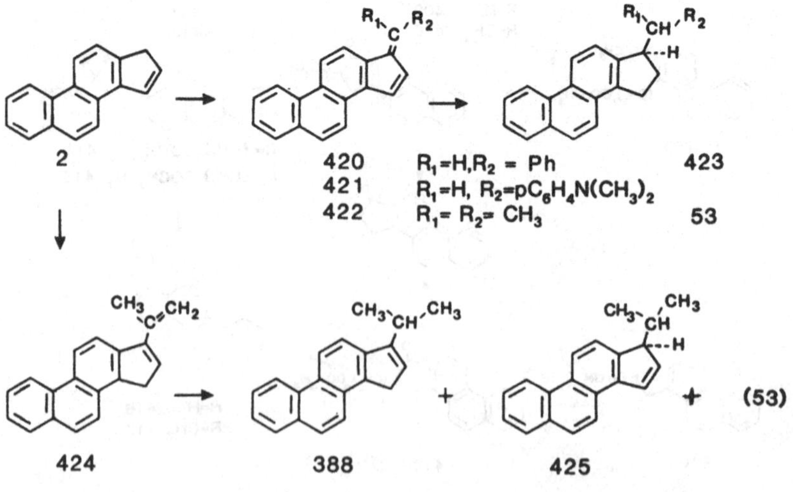

diene readily gave 15,16-dihydro-17-isopropyl-17H-cyclopenta[a]-phenanthrene (**53**), but when hydrogenation was interrupted after two atom-equivalents had been absorbed, the starting material was recovered along with the fully reduced hydrocarbon (**53**) and both the 17-isopropyl-16(17)-ene (**388**) and its 15(16)-isomer (**425**), demonstrating that isomerization of the double bond in the five-membered ring from C-16(17) to C-15(16) had occurred in the course of the reduction. Partial reduction of the aromatic system in 17-ketocyclopenta[a]phenanthrenes cannot be conveniently accomplished by direct catalytic hydrogenation because the benzylic carbonyl group is eliminated comparatively readily (Robinson and Rydon, 1939). For example, reduction of the easily accessible 3,11-dimethoxy-17-ketone (**426**) in acetic acid over Adam's catalyst at 70°C gave 11,12,13,14,16,17-hexahydro-15H-11-hydroxy-3-methoxy-cyclopenta[a]phenanthrene (**427**) among other products. In order to preserve the 17-carbonyl function, present in oestrogens and many C_{19} steroids, Robinson first opened the five-membered D-ring prior to hydrogenation as depicted in Fig. 48. The 16-hydroxymethylene derivative (**429**) was obtained by condensation of the dimethoxy-17-ketone with ethyl formate in pyridine, catalysed by sodium ethoxide; other methods gave more or less of the dimer (**428**). Conversion to the nitrile (**430**) was brought about with hydroxylamine in acetic acid, and without purification it was hydrolysed to the di-acid (**431**) with hot aqueous alcoholic potassium hydroxide. This di-acid was esterified and reduced catalytically as before; three partially hydrogenated products (**432-434**) were isolated from the reduction-product mixture. Re-formation of the D-ring was achieved by heating the lead salts of these di-acids *in vacuo*. In this way di-acid (**432**) gave 3,11-dimethoxy-6,7,15,16-tetrahydrocyclopenta[a]phenanthren-17-one (**332**) whilst 18-noroestrone methyl ether, 6,7,8,9,11,12,13,14,15,16-decahydro-3-methoxycyclopenta[a]phenanthren-17-one (**22**) of unknown stereochemistry was obtained from the di-acid (**434**); the isomeric di-acid (**433**) resisted cyclization by this method. Two years later Robinson and Slater (1941) approached this problem from a different angle. Starting with the readily available 12-ketones (**96**) and (**437**), reduction by the Pondorff procedure gave the corresponding alcohols (**438**) and (**439**), dehydration of which with potassium hydrogen sulphate yielded the required 9(11),12(13)-dienes (**440**) and (**441**) together with the products of their further dehydrogenation, the 6,7,16,17-tetrahydro-15H-cyclopenta[a]phenanthrenes (**442**) and (**443**). The latter were the only products obtained when oxidation of the dienes to the corresponding 17-ketones with selenium dioxide was attempted. More recently Jacob *et al.*

(1971) found that reduction of the 12-ketone (**96**) with lithium aluminium hydride gave, in addition to the diene (**440**) and triene (**442**) reported by Robinson, also the isomeric 11,12,13,14,16,17-hexahydro-15*H*-hydrocarbon (**44**) as well as the alcohol containing only one aromatic A-ring (**444**). Robinson and Slater also found that the Reformatsky product (**405**) already described, on vigorous reduction (with Raney nickel at 200–220°C under 65 atm. pressure) was hydrogenated to the 18-noroestrogen derivative (**445**) with elimination of the 11-methoxy group.

In a recent study (Elvidge *et al.*, 1985) the relative rates of proton exchange at C-16 in a series of 17-ketocyclopenta[a]phenanthrenes were measured. These compounds were labelled at C-16 specifically by acid-

Fig. 48

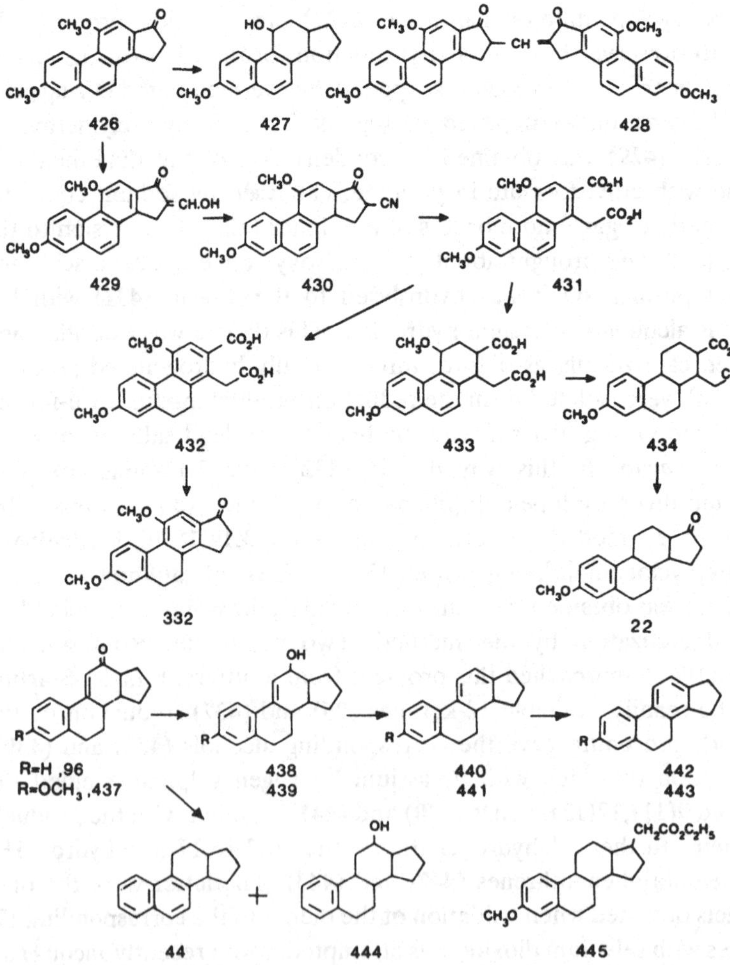

catalysed or hydroxide-catalysed exchange with tritiated water, and the position of the label in the product was checked by tritium nmr (δ 2.70–2.86 in deuterated chloroform). Hydroxide-catalysed detritiation in 9:1 (v/v) water–dioxane was followed by measuring the radioactivity remaining in aliquots of the substrate at fixed time intervals; the results are shown in Table 4. The rate constants for the unsubstituted 17-ketone (4) and its 1-methyl homologue (302) were essentially the same, but as expected methyl groups elsewhere in the molecule decreased this rate, the effect being greater the nearer the methyl group was to C-16. The rate for the 12-methyl isomer (130) was the lowest for the monomethyl compounds and was decreased further by introduction of a second methyl group at C-11 (131). The 7-methyl-17-ketone (230) was, however, anomalous because the rate was markedly increased, and this was true also of the other two 7-methyl derivatives (309) and (447). The 7-methyl group also had an effect on H-15 because in its nmr spectrum these protons were deshielded 0.42–0.46 ppm compared with the other isomers (see Table 4). These effects of 7-methyl substitution can be attributed to the strain it introduces into these molecules. This was indicated by the unexpected difficulties encountered in the synthesis of both the 7-methyl- and 7,11-dimethyl-17-ketones, and is fully confirmed by the results of X-ray crystallography discussed in Chapter 8.

Table 4. *Hydroxide-catalysed second order rate constants ($k_{OH^-}^T$) at 298.2°K for detritiation of various [16-^{3}H]-15,16-dihydrocyclopenta[a]-phenanthren-17-ones, and their nmr H-15 resonance signals (δ) measured in ppm from tetramethylsilane*

Compound	$10^2 k_{OH^-}^T$ mol^{-1} s^{-1}	H-15 (δ)
unsubstituted-17-ketone (4)	1.83±0.14	3.28
1-methyl-17-ketone (302)	1.85±0.05	3.25
3-methyl-17-ketone (304)	1.42±0.02	3.25
4-methyl-17-ketone (305)	1.47±0.19	3.26
6-methyl-17-ketone (306)	1.15±0.14	3.27
7-methyl-17-ketone (230)	3.17±0.08	3.70
11-methyl-17-ketone (26)	1.47±0.06	3.24
12-methyl-17-ketone (130)	0.67±0.07	3.28
11,12-dimethyl-17-ketone (131)	0.30±0.05	3.22
7,11-dimethyl-17-ketone (309)	2.45±0.19	3.63
11-hydroxy-17-ketone (206)	0.23±0.02	—
11-methoxy-17-ketone (132)	2.06±0.06	3.22
7-methyl-11-methoxy-17-ketone (447)	2.50±0.17	3.58
11-ethyl-17-ketone (211)	1.58±0.03	—
1,11-methano-17-ketone (310)	0.87±0.07	3.25

4.1   References

Badger, G. M., Carruthers, W. & Cook, C. W. (1952). New derivatives of 1,2-cyclopentenophenanthrene. *J. Chem. Soc.*, 4996–5000.

Bhatt, T. S., Hadfield, S. T. & Coombs, M. M. (1982). Carcinogenicity and mutagenicity of some alkoxy cyclopenta[a]phenanthren-17-ones: effect of obstructing the bay region. *Carcinogenesis*, **3**, 677–80.

Brooks, C. W. J. & Young, L. (1956). Biochemical studies of toxic agents. 9. The metabolic conversion of indene into *cis*- and *trans*- indane-1:2-diol. *Biochem. J.*, **63**, 264–9.

Buchta, E. & Kraetzer, H. (1962). Polycyclic compounds. X. 5-methyl-naphtho[2′,1′:1,2]fluorene. *Ber.*, **95**, 1820–5.

Butenandt, A., Dannenberg, H. & von Dresler, D. (1946). Methylhomolage des 1,2-cyclopentenophenanthrens, III. Mitteilung: synthese des 9,10-dimethyl-1,2-cyclopentenophenanthrens. *Z. Naturforsch.*, **1**, 222–6.

Coombs, M. M. (1966). Potentially carcinogenic cyclopenta[a]phenanthrenes. Part II. Derivatives containing further unsaturation in ring-D. *J. Chem. Soc. (C)*, 963–8.

Coombs, M. M. (1969). Potentially carcinogenic cyclopenta[a]phenanthrenes. Part III. Oxidation studies. *J. Chem. Soc. (C)*, 2484–8.

Coombs, M. M. & Hall, M. (1973). Potentially carcinogenic cyclopenta[a]phenanthrenes. Part VII. Ring-D diols and related compounds. *J. Chem. Soc. Perkin Trans. I*, 1255–8.

Coombs, M. M., Hall, M., Siddle, V. A. & Vose, C. W. (1975). Potentially carcinogenic cyclopenta[a]phenanthrenes. Part X. Oxygenated derivatives of the carcinogen 15,16-dihydro-11-methylcyclopenta[a]thren-17-one of metabolic interest. *J. Chem. Soc. Perkin Trans. I*, 265–70.

Coombs, M. M., Hall, M. & Vose, C. W. (1973). Potentially carcinogenic cyclopenta[a]phenanthrenes. Part VIII. Bromination of 17-ketones. *J. Chem. Soc. Perkin Trans. I*, 2236–40.

Coombs, M. M. & Jones, M. B. (1972). Oxidation of oestrone with thallium trifluoroacetate. *Chem. Ind. (London)*, 169.

Dannenberg. H. (1950). Attempts to synthesise 'Steranthrene'. I. 5-propyl-3-methylcholanthrene. *Annalen*, **568**, 100–16.

Dannenberg, H. & Dannenberg-von Dresler, D. (1964). Relation between steroids and carcinogenic compounds. IV. Cholanthrene-5-acetic and 5-propionic acids, their synthesis and carcinogenic action. *Z. Naturforsch.*, **19B**, 801–6.

Dannenberg, H., Dannenberg-von Dresler, D. & Neumann, H.-G. (1960). Dehydrierung von Steroiden. III. 1:2-cyclopentenphenanthrene. *Annalen*, **636**, 74–87.

Dannenberg, H., Sonnenbichler, J. & Gross, H. J. (1965). 3-Amino and 9-acetamido-1,2-cyclopentenophenanthrene. *Annalen*, **684**, 200–9.

Derbyshire, D. H. & Waters, W. A. (1950). The significance of the bromine cation in aromatic substitution. Part II. Preparative applicability. *J. Chem. Soc.*, 575–7.

Elvidge, J. A., Jones, J. R., Russell, J. C., Wiseman, A. & Coombs, M. M. (1985). A kinetic investigation of the hydroxide-catalysed detritiation of various [16-³H]-15,16-dihydrocyclopenta[a]phenanthren-17-ones and related compounds. *J. Chem. Soc. Perkin Trans. II*, 563–5.

Hoch, J. (1938). Substances with female hormone effect. The synthesis of two oxo-1,2-cyclopentenophenanthrenes. *C. R. Hebd. Séances Acad. Sci.*, **207**, 921–3.

Jacob, G., Cagniant, D. & Cagniant, P. (1971). Recherches dans le domaine du dihydro-16,17-15*H*-cyclopenta[a]phenanthrene. *C. R. Hebd. Séances Acad. Sci., Sér. C*, **272**, 650–2.

Lacey, P. H. & Smith, D. C. C. (1971). A convenient preparation of indenone. *J. Chem. Soc. (C)*, 41–3.

Laing, S. B. & Sykes, P. J. (1968). Synthetic steroids. Part IX. A new route to 19-nor-steroids. *J. Chem. Soc.*, 2915–18.

Marvel, C. S. & Hinmann, C. W. (1954). The synthesis of indone and some related compounds. *J. Am. Chem. Soc.*, **76**, 5435–7.

McKillop, A., Bromley, D. & Taylor, E. C. (1972). Thallium in organic synthesis. XXV. Electrophilic aromatic bromination using bromine and thallium (III) acetate. *J. Org. Chem.*, **37**, 88–92.

Nasipuri, D. & Roy, D. N. (1961). Polycyclic systems. Part IX. A new synthesis of indeno (2',3':1,2)phenanthrene. *J. Chem. Soc.*, 3361–6.

Robinson, R. & Rydon, H. N. (1939). Experiments on the synthesis of substances related to the sterols. Part XXVII. The synthesis of x-noroestrone. *J. Chem. Soc.*, 1394–1405.

Robinson, R. & Slater, S. N. (1941). Experiments on the synthesis of substances related to the sterols. Part XXIX. *J. Chem. Soc.*, 376–85.

Ruzicka, L. & Goldberg, M. W. (1937). Polyterpene und polyterpenoide CXVII. Zur kenntnis der bedingungen und des mechanisms des dehydrierung der homologen sterine und des cholsaur. *Helv. Chim. Acta*, **20**, 1245–53.

Turner, D. L. (1949). Some aryl-substituted cyclopentenones; a new synthesis of the cyclopentenophenanthrene structure. *J. Am. Chem. Soc.*, **71**, 612–15.

Wilds, A. C. (1942). The synthesis of 2'-ketodihydro-1,2-cyclopentenophenanthrene and derivatives of phenanthro[1,2-b]furan. *J. Am. Chem. Soc.*, **64**, 1421–9.

5

Physical and spectral properties of cyclopenta[a]phenanthrenes

Some 350 individual cyclopenta[a]phenanthrenes have so far been reported in the chemical literature, and at least some physical characteristics of the majority of these have been described. In the earlier papers often only the melting point of the compound and possibly those of certain readily prepared derivatives were given. In somewhat later reports it is usual also to find ultraviolet absorption data, while in papers published during the last 25 years infrared, nuclear magnetic resonance, and mass spectra are frequently encountered. In this chapter melting points and spectroscopic data are summarized for the great majority of these cyclopenta[a]phenanthrenes, and this is followed by a separate section on the mass spectrometry of a few of these compounds. Consideration of structural data derived from X-ray crystallographic studies appears in a separate chapter.

5.1   Melting points and spectral data

In the compilation which follows cyclopenta[a]phenanthrenes have been listed by molecular formula according to the convention adopted by Chemical Abstracts. The molecular formula is followed by the serial (**arabic**) number, when one has been assigned to it in the text, tables and figures, and by the complete chemical name. The Chemical Abstracts Registry Number [enclosed in square brackets] is also quoted when this is available. The compilation ends with a reverse index, relating serial number to molecular formula to assist location of individual compounds referred to elsewhere in the book. Melting points are quoted in degrees Centigrade, and ultraviolet spectra as λ_{max} ($\log_{10}\varepsilon$) where ε is the molecular absorption coefficient, usually measured in ethanolic solution. Infrared absorption wavelengths (μm), especially of the strong aromatic bands in the 11–14 μm region, are tabulated to provide an additional means of identification; measurements are for Nujol mulls unless otherwise specified. Nuclear magnetic (proton) resonance chemical shifts (δ) measured in parts per million (ppm) relative to tetramethylsilane in deuterated chloroform are also quoted where available.

The ultraviolet absorption spectra of 16,17-dihydro-15H-cyclopenta[a]phenanthrene hydrocarbons were discussed by Dannenberg and Steidle (1954) who pointed out that these compounds, like simple phenanthrenes, possess four groups of absorption bands, shown in Fig. 49 for Diels' hydrocarbon. The most intensive band with a maximum around 260 nm ($\log_{10}\varepsilon$ 4.7–4.8) was designated the β-group, that with the shortest wavelength around 220 nm ($\log_{10}\varepsilon$ 4.5) the β'-group, the three maxima between 280 and 310 nm ($\log_{10}\varepsilon$ 4.0–4.2) the p-group, and the three weak maxima between 320 and 360 nm ($\log_{10}\varepsilon$ 2.5–3.2) the α-group in accordance with the notation originated by Clar (1952). As expected addition of one or even two methyl groups to the five-membered ring has little effect on the chromophore, whereas substitution of one methyl group in the phenanthrene ring system causes a bathochromic shift of the β-band of up to 7 nm, depending upon the position of substitution. Substitution of a second methyl group causes a further shift in the same direction of 4–11 nm, from the parent hydrocarbon. By contrast the p- and α-band groups do not undergo this red shift to the same extent.

Fig. 49. Ultraviolet spectra recorded in ethanol of Diels' hydrocarbon (**7**) showing the β', β, p and α bands, and of 15,16-dihydrocyclopenta[a]phenanthren-17-one (**4**) and its borohydride reduction product, the 17-ol.

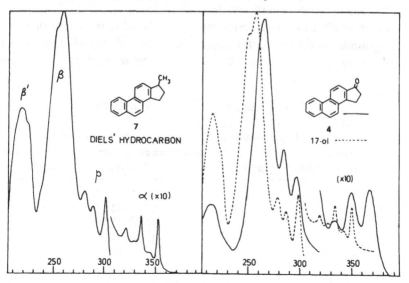

Wavelength (nm)

Conjugation of a double bond at C-15 or C-17 in the five-membered ring also causes a bathochromic shift of the β-band (10.0–14.5 nm); the 17H-hydrocarbons are readily distinguished by the presence of an additional absorption band at 239 nm absent in their 15H-isomers (Coombs, 1966b). Conjugation of an exocyclic carbon–carbon double bond at C-17 results in a similar shift of the β-band, but conjugation of a carbonyl oxygen at this position has less effect. Thus 15,16-dihydrocyclopenta[a]-phenanthren-17-one (4) absorbs at 265 nm; however, the α-bands are shifted 10–15 nm in the same direction (compared with the 16,17-dihydro hydrocarbon) whereas the p-bands are not and one of these (λ_{max} ~280 nm) is lost (see Fig. 49). Aryl methyl substitution is accompanied by the usual red shift in these 17-ketones. Surprisingly, conjugation of a carbonyl group at C-15 to give the isomeric ketone (102) causes a blue shift of the β-band to 251.5 nm, and introduction of a C-15(16) double bond into the 17-ketone to yield cyclopenta[a]phenanthren-17-one (363) is also accompanied by a similar blue shift to 253 nm. In this compound the three maxima constituting the p-group are not greatly displaced, but the three weak α maxima are replaced by one broad maximum at 380–390 nm which imparts a yellow colour to this ketone and its 11-methyl homologue (364). The ultraviolet spectra of all these ketones become very similar to those of the corresponding hydrocarbons after mild reduction *in situ* with sodium borohydride to the secondary alcohol as shown in Fig. 49. The spectra of the various tetrahydro, hexahydro, etc., hydrocarbons are generally similar to those of the analogous phenanthrene derivatives.

Little needs to be said about the infrared and nmr spectra of these compounds. In the former the conjugated carbonyl group in the 15- and 17-ketones absorbs at about 5.92 μm as expected and slightly lower in the

Table 5. *Wavelength ranges associated with different aryl substitution patterns in 16,17-dihydro-15H-cyclopenta[a]phenanthrenes in carbon disulphide solution*

Ring substitution pattern	Wavelength range (μm)
1,2	13.26–13.44
1,2,3	12.67–12.77
	13.27–13.29
1,2,4	12.03–12.05
1,2,3,4	12.20–12.35
1,2,3,4,5	11.42–11.62

D-ring bromo ketones, but at 5.71 μm in the unconjugated 16-ketone (**380**). The strong out-of-plane deformation bands in the 11.0–14.0 μm region are characteristic of each structure and give information regarding the substitution patterns. Dannenberg *et al.* (1953) discussed these absorption bands in the spectra of 16 variously substituted mono- and di-methyl derivatives of 16,17-dihydro-15*H*-cyclopenta[a]phenanthrene measured in both the solid state (potassium bromide discs) and in solution in carbon disulphide. With few exceptions bands occurred within the wavelength ranges shown in Table 5 for the various ring-substitution patterns for spectra obtained in solution.

In the nmr spectra of the 15,16-dihydro-17-ketones the aromatic protons resonate between δ 7.3 and 7.8, but the bay-region protons at C-1 and C-11 are deshielded by about 1 ppm. The C-15 methylene group resonates as a multiplet at δ 3.24–3.28 for the unsubstituted 17-ketone (**4**) and all its isomeric arylmethyl derivatives with the exception of the 7-methyl compound (δ 3.70), disclosing steric compression in this region of the molecule confirmed by X-ray crystallographic studies (Chapter 8).

5.2   Mass spectrometry of cyclopenta[a]phenanthrenes

The use of mass spectrometry for the determination of molecular weights of organic compounds including cyclopenta[a]phenanthrenes is commonplace, and it has recently led to the identification of several hydrocarbons of this series from a number of natural sources. Generally no difficulty is experienced with relatively simple aromatic compounds because often the molecular ion is also the most abundant ion in the spectrum. The technique is particularly valuable for the study of metabolites, usually obtainable only in very limited quantities. However, *trans*-1,2-dihydrodiols which commonly occur as metabolites derived from aromatic compounds often give problems because they undergo facile dehydration, so that the M$^+$-18 ion is abundant and the molecular ion is weak or non-existent.

As a preliminary to employing mass spectrometric fragmentation patterns to assist in the elucidation of the structures of unknown metabolites of the carcinogen 15,16-dihydro-11-methylcyclopen-ta[a]phenanthren-17-one (**26**) and related compounds, the mass spec-trometry of several assorted synthetic compounds shown in Fig. 50 was studied in detail (Vose and Coombs, 1977). Table 6 shows the ions of abundance greater than 2% of the base peak produced from these compounds under comparable conditions (AEI MS-902 mass spec-trometer with an ionizing potential of 70 eV; samples inserted directly into the source). The first four compounds, the parent 17-ketone (**4**), its

Table 6. *Compound (see Fig. 50) and ionic abundance*

Loss (in mass units) from the molecular ion	(4)	(26)	(215)	(339)	(343)	(365)	(446)	(341)	Tentative assignment
+1	19	21	20	20	5	5	4	9	
0	100	100	100	100	15	28	18	46	molecular ion M^+
−1	8	4	9	5					
−2	7		7	4					
−15	4	4							M^+-CH_3
−28	27	4	10	8					M^+-CO
−29	59	9	32	18					M^+-CHO
−30	42	5	6	4					M^+-CH_2O
−31	4		8						M^+-CH_2OH
−42	10	5				18		100	M^+-CH_2CO
−43		36							M^+-CH_3-CO
−44		29							M^+-CH_3-CHO
−45		4							
−56	16	2	10	6					
−57		12	8	8					
−58				5	25				
−59					25	25			
−60		3		15	100	39	27		M^+-CH_3CO_2H

m/z						Assignment
−69	5					
−70					26	M⁺-CH₂CO-CO
−71		2			46	M⁺-CH₂CO-CHO
−72			7		20	M⁺-CH₂CO-CH₂O
−73						
−83		3				
−85	2	6				
−87	5	7	5			
−88			16	100	12	M⁺-CO-CH₃CO₂H
−98					6	
−101				24		
−102				100	100	M⁺-CH₃CO₂H-CH₂CO
−114			6			
−115			5			
−117					19	M⁺-CH₃CO₂H-CH₂CO-CH₃
−129					18	M⁺-CH₃CO₂H-CH₂CO-CO
−130					10	M⁺-CH₃CO₂H-CH₂CO-CO
−145					15	M⁺-CH₃CO₂H-CH₂CO-CH₃-CO
−146					20	M⁺-CH₃CO₂H-CH₂CO-CH₃-CHO
−159					9	
−173					3	

11-methyl (**26**) and 11-hydroxymethyl (**215**) derivatives, and the 6-phenol (**339**) have the molecular ion as the base peak, behaviour characteristic of aromatic compounds. All show M$^+$-28 ions arising from loss of the carbonyl group, and other ions which follow from the general degradative pathways proposed in Fig. 51. This is similar to the scheme reported by

Fig. 50. Synthetic cyclopenta[a]phenanthrenes studied by mass spectrometry (Vose and Coombs, 1977).

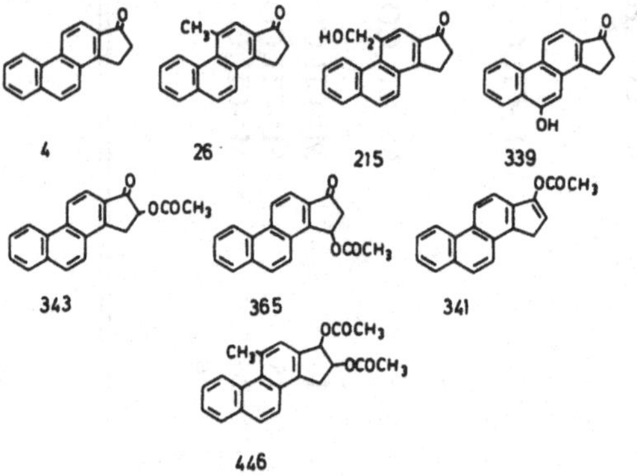

Fig. 51. Proposed origin of ions formed by fragmentation of ring-D in 15,16-dihydrocyclopenta[a]phenanthren-17-ones, and the loss of ketene involving a concerted six-membered hydrogen shift.

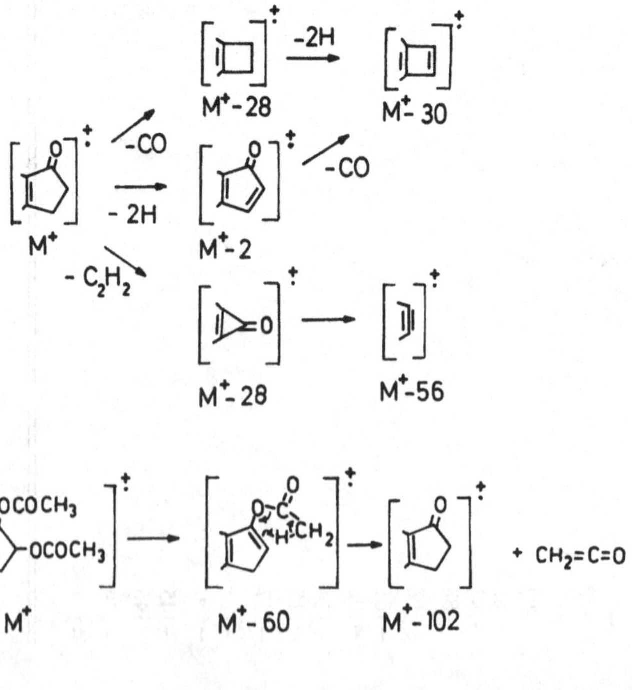

Bowie (1966) for the related ketone indan-1-one. The 11-methyl and 11-hydroxymethyl ketones yield in addition weak ions at M$^+$-15 and M$^+$-31, respectively, indicating the loss of these substitutents from the molecular ion. By contrast the molecular ion is of low abundance with the other four cyclopenta[a]phenanthrenes. The M$^+$-60 ion arising from the loss of acetic acid from the molecular ion is the base peak in the spectrum of the 16-acetoxy-17-ketone (343), with a less-abundant ion at M$^+$-88 due to further loss of CO; the reverse is true for the isomeric 15-acetoxy-17-ketone (365). The ion at M$^+$-42 in the spectrum of the latter is absent in that of its 16-isomer and a metastable ion (m* at 212.2) confirms that this ion arises by one-step loss of ketene from the molecular ion, probably by loss of the 17-carbonyl and 16-methylene groups. The ion at M$^+$-42 constitutes the base peak in the spectrum of the enol acetate (341); again it is shown to arise by one-step loss of ketene from the molecular ion by the presence of a metastable ion m* 196.5. This may occur via a concerted six-membered shift as shown in Fig. 51, leading to the molecular ion of the 17-ketone which then undergoes further fragmentation as already described. The enol acetate (341) is homologous with the M$^+$-60 ion in the spectrum of the diacetate (446), and in this compound the base peak arises by loss of 42 mass units from the molecular ion, so that this rearrangement is probably general for compounds and ions of this series possessing or capable of forming an enol acetate structure.

The use of mass spectrometry in the identification of various metabolites is described in the chapter on the metabolism of cyclopenta[a]phenanthrenes. However, a rather unusual use of this technique is described here because it illustrates the power of this method to help solve otherwise intractable problems. After metabolic activation the carcinogen (26) binds covalently to DNA if it is added to the incubation mixture. As will be described later, reaction occurs mainly (~80%) with the guanine moieties to the extent of about one base in 10^4 bases in the DNA. From separate considerations it was thought that this reaction occurred between the exocyclic amino group in the deoxyguanine bases and a 3,4-dihydrodihydroxy-1,2-epoxide derived from the carcinogen to yield an adduct of the type shown as the ion of m/z 447 in Fig. 52. When DNA treated in this way was submitted to pyrolysis electron-impact mass spectrometry without further derivatization (Wiebers *et al.*, 1981), in addition to the usual ion products derived from the four common DNA component bases (adenosine, guanine, cytosine, and thymine) other peaks of low abundance (about one-hundredth of the peak heights of the normal components) were seen. It was readily possible, in view of the previous studies, to fit these into the postulated fragmentation scheme shown in which the numbers represent the masses of the ions observed. The structures proposed for the molecular ion and two fragment ions are also displayed in this figure. The most abundant ion m/z 368 was selected for further scrutiny by mass-analysed ion kinetic-energy spectrometry (MIKES), a technique which allows the further fragmentation of a single ion to be followed in detail. Ideally the molecular ion would be selected for this purpose, but in this case it was of extremely low abundance and it was felt that fragmentations leading to the relatively stable m/z 368 ion were reasonably well understood. Major daughter ions in the MIKE spectrum of this ion are shown in Table 7 and fully substantiate the structures proposed. In particular the ion at m/z 218 demonstrates loss of guanine (150 mass units), whilst the ion at m/z 233 (loss of 135 mass units) indicates that the entity of mass 218 derived from the carcinogen is attached to the NH of the exocyclic N^2-amino group of this purine. This confirmation of the supposed structure of the major DNA adduct is

Fig. 52. Proposed molecular ion (m/z 447) formed from the DNA adduct, and fragmentation pathways leading to the ions m/z 368 and 365.

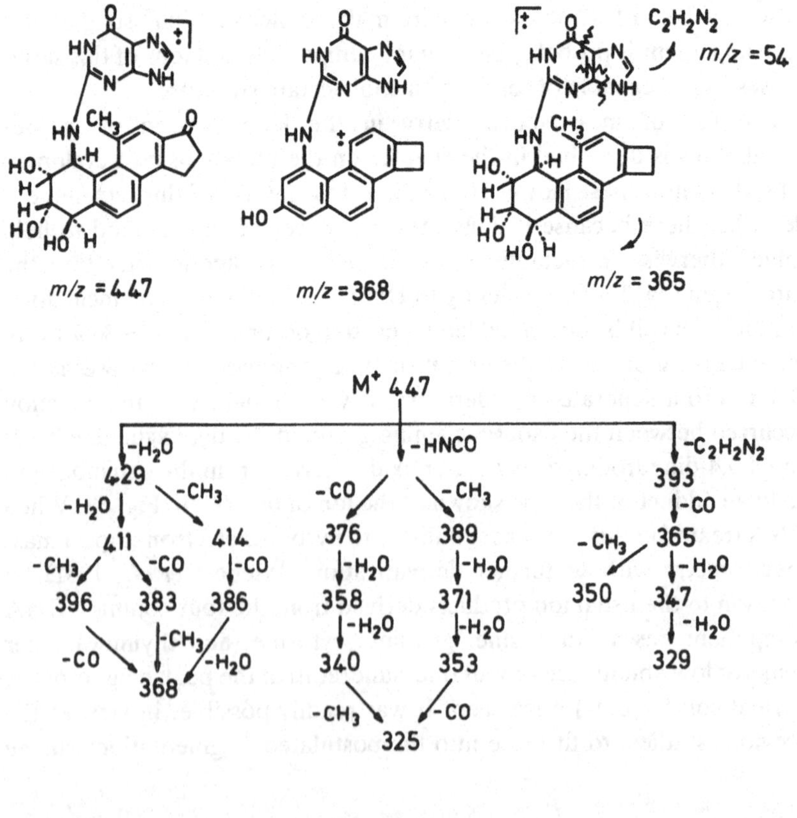

$m/z = 447$ $m/z = 368$ $m/z = 365$

Table 7. *Ions in the MIKE spectrum of the major DNA adduct ion of* m/z *368*

Daughter ion	Relative intensity	Loss of parent ion m/z 368 ($C_{21}H_{14}N_5O_2$)	Composition of daughter ion
354	100.0	14(CH_2)	$C_{20}H_{12}N_5O_2$
351	77.0	17(OH)	$C_{21}H_{13}N_5O$
340	52.3	28(C_2H_4)	$C_{19}H_{10}N_5O_2$
325	38.3	43(HNCO)	$C_{20}H_{13}N_4O$
316	21.7	52(C_4H_4)	$C_{17}H_{10}N_5O_2$
289	31.8	77(C_6H_5)	$C_{15}H_9N_5O_2$
267	25.0	101(C_8H_5)	$C_{13}H_9N_5O_2$
254	32.0	114(C_9H_6)	$C_{12}H_8N_5O_2$
233	31.8	135($C_5H_3N_4O$)	$C_{16}H_{11}NO$
218	57.0	150($C_5H_4N_5O$)	$C_{16}H_{10}O$
206	41.0	162($C_6H_{10}N_5O$)	$C_{15}H_{10}O$
193	33.6	175($C_7H_5N_5O$)	$C_{14}H_9O$
164	28.0	204($C_8H_6N_5O_2$)	$C_{13}H_8$
151	37.0	217($C_9H_7N_5O_2$)	$C_{12}H_7$
127	27.5	241($C_{11}H_7N_5O_2$)	$C_{10}H_7$

important because, owing to the extremely minute amount available, it is doubtful whether the information could have been obtained in any other way.

It has been known for a long time that during selenium dehydrogenation of steroids at elevated temperatures the long sterol side chain at C-17 is lost, although it is retained on quinone dehydrogenation at substantially lower temperatures. It is therefore interesting to observe that in the mass spectra of cyclopenta[a]phenanthrenes bearing a sterol side chain the molecular ion is of very low abundance; the base peak is the ion formed by loss of this side chain (Ludwig *et al.*, 1981).

5.3 Compilation of physical and spectroscopic data for most of the cyclopenta[a]phenanthrenes reported in the chemical literature up to 1985

$C_{17}H_{10}Br_2O$
  (**356**) 15,15-Dibromo-15,16-dihydrocyclopenta[a]phenanthren-17-one
  [50905-49-2] [74495-83-3]
  MW 390;   mp 213–213.5°C
  λ_{max} 279 (4.70), 298 (4.24), 314.5 (4.18), 360 (3.30), 377 (3.27) nm
  ν_{max} 5.85, 12.45, 14.0 μm
  δ 4.69 s (H-16)   (Coombs *et al.*, 1973*a*)
$C_{17}H_{10}Br_2O$
  (**362**) 15,16-Dibromo-15,16-dihydrocyclopenta[a]phenanthren-17-one
  [50905-50-5]

MW 390;   mp 179–180°C

λ_{max} 283 (4.60), 311.5 (4.33), 361 (3.19), 380 (3.18) nm

ν_{max} 5.85, 12.04, 13.10 μm

δ 5.05 (H-15), 6.10 (H-16)   (Coombs *et al.*, 1973*a*)

$C_{17}H_{10}O$ (**363**) Cyclopenta[a]phenanthren-17-one [50905-54-9]

MW 230;   Orange prisms, mp 202–208°C

λ_{max} 253, 286, 298, 310, 382 nm

ν_{max} 5.85, 12.25, 12.80, 13.26 μm   (Coombs and Hall, 1973)

$C_{17}H_{10}O_2$

(**185**) Cyclopenta[a]phenanthren-15,17-dione

MW 246;   mp 240.5–241.5°C   (Fieser *et al.*, 1936)

$C_{17}H_{10}O_3$

(**335**) 6,7,15,16-Tetrahydrocyclopenta[a]phenanthrene-6,7,17-trione

MW 262;   mp 245–247°C

λ_{max} 271–279 (4.03), 331 (3.31), 406 (3.21) nm

ν_{max} 5.84, 5.97, 6.30, 10.45, 11.63, 11.90, 12.90 μm   (Coombs, 1969)

$C_{17}H_{11}BrO$

(**318**) 15-Bromo-15,16-dihydrocyclopenta[a]phenanthren-17-one
[50905-48-1]

MW 311;   mp 196–197°C

λ_{max} 267 (4.78), 286.5 (4.41), 298.5 (4.36), 310 (4.13), 354 (3.32),
372 (3.31) nm

ν_{max} 5.85, 12.26, 13.25 μm

δ 4.83 (J 3,7) (15-H), 4.19 (J 18,7) and 3.68 (J 18,3) (H-16)
                                        (Coombs *et al.*, 1973*a*)

$C_{17}H_{11}BrO$

(**358**) 16-Bromo-15,16-dihydrocyclopenta[a]phenanthren-17-one
[51013-72-0]

MW 311;   Golden laths, mp 175°C (decomp.)

λ_{max} 230.5 (4.28), 273 (4.73), 300.5 (4.27), 335 (3.00), 354 (3.13),
371 (3.13) nm

ν_{max} 5.88, 12.26, 13.25 μm

δ 3.20 (J 18,2) and 3.48 (J 18,6) (H-15), 5.96 (J 6,2) (H-16)
                                        (Coombs *et al.*, 1973*a*)

$C_{17}H_{12}$ (**3**) 15*H*-Cyclopenta[a]phenanthrene [219-07-8]

MW 216;   mp 165–167°C

λ_{max} 220 (4.45), 269 (4.79), 273 (4.81), 292 (4.23), 302 (4.17),
314 (3.96) nm

ν_{max} (CS$_2$) 12.48, 13.40, 14.50 μm   (Coombs, 1966*b*)

$C_{17}H_{12}$ (**2**) 17*H*-Cyclopenta[a]phenanthrene [219-08-9]

MW 216;   mp 164–165°C (Coombs, 1996*b*); 163–164°C (Badger *et al.*, 1952)

λ_{max} 224 (4.41), 239 (4.24), 269 (4.72), 273.5 (4.70), 292 (4.17),
302.5 (4.16), 314.5 (4.04) nm

ν_{max} (CS$_2$) 12.49, 13.25, 13.30, 14.48 μm   (Coombs, 1966*b*)

$C_{17}H_{12}O$ (**102**) 16,17-Dihydrocyclopenta[a]phenanthren-15-one [32425-83-5]

MW 232;   mp 184–186°C (Coombs, 1966*b*); 183–184°C (Bachmann and Kloetzel, 1937); pale yellow needles, mp 183–184°C (Badger *et al.*, 1952)

λ_{max} 216 (4.41), 251.5 (4.58), 288 (4.06), 319 (4.08), 344 (3.65), 362 (3.49) nm

ν_{max} 5.9, 10.32, 10.4, 11.4, 11.76, 11.9, 12.26, 12.92, 13.2, 13.94 μm

(Coombs, 1966*b*)

$C_{17}H_{12}O$ (**380**) 15,17-Dihydrocyclopenta[a]phenanthren-16-one
MW 232;   mp 172–174°C [42123-03-5]

λ_{max} 258 (4.77), 269 (4.21), 278 (4.11), 300 (4.21), 319 (3.14), 335 (3.10), 350 (3.03) nm

ν_{max} 5.88, 11.92, 12.49, 13.10, 13.30 μm   (Coombs and Hall, 1973)

$C_{17}H_{12}O$ (**4**) 15,16-Dihydrocyclopenta[a]phenanthren-17-one [786-66-3]
[74495-81-1] [74495-82-2]
MW 232;   mp 203–204°C (Coombs *et al.*, 1970); 200–201°C
(Nasipuri and Roy, 1961)

λ_{max} 265 (4.89), 284 (4.52), 296 (4.38), 334 (3.24), 350 (3.40), 367 (3.44) nm

ν_{max} 5.92, 11.48, 11.82, 12.40, 12.86, 13.22, 14.18 μm

δ 3.28 (H-15), 2.70 (H-16)   (Coombs, 1966*a*)

$C_{17}H_{12}O_2$

(**396**) 15,16-Dihydro-2-hydroxycyclopenta[a]phenanthren-17-one
[55651-45-1]
MW 248;   mp 340°C (decomp.)

λ_{max} 274.5 (4.74), 366 (3.40), 383 (3.45)

anion λ_{max} 245 (4.59), 296 (4.62)   (Coombs *et al.*, 1975)

$C_{17}H_{12}O_2$

(**23**) 15,16-Dihydro-3-hydroxycyclopenta[a]phenanthren-17-one
MW 248

λ_{max} 278, 291, 324, 367 nm

anion λ_{max} 234, 277, 288, 371 nm   (Coombs, unpublished)

$C_{17}H_{12}O_2$

(**339**) 15,16-Dihydro-6-hydroxycyclopenta[a]phenanthren-17-one
[24684-45-5]
MW 248;   mp 280°C

λ_{max} 270 (4.81), 287 (4.48), 302 (4.28), 361 (3.37), 378 (3.42) nm

anion λ_{max} 291, 350, 439 nm

ν_{max} 3.20, 5.96, 11.54, 11.80, 12.18, 12.26, 13.08 μm   (Coombs, 1969)

$C_{17}H_{12}O_2$

(**206**) 15,16-Dihydro-11-hydroxycyclopenta[a]phenanthren-17-one
[83053-63-8]
MW 248;   mp 310–315°C (Robinson, 1938); 306–310°C (Bhatt *et al.*, 1982)

λ_{max} 261 (4.98), 293 (4.72), 368 (4.05), 387 (4.16) nm

(Bhatt *et al.*, 1982)

$C_{17}H_{12}O_2$

(**369**) 15,16-Dihydro-15-hydroxycyclopenta[a]phenanthren-17-one
[55081-28-2]

MW 248; Isolated as its acetate (**365**), mp 197–198°C (see
$C_{19}H_{14}O_3$)   (Coombs *et al.*, 1973*a*)

$C_{17}H_{12}O_2$

(**345**) 15,16-Dihydro-16-hydroxycyclopenta[a]phenanthren-17-one
[24684-54-6]
MW 248; mp 186–187°C, 197°C (decomp.)
λ_{max} 265 (4.95), 284 (4.49), 296 (4.39), 335 (3.15), 351 (3.32),
369 (3.33) nm
ν_{max} 2.96, 5.92, 12.16, 12.44, 13.30 μm   (Coombs, 1969)

$C_{17}H_{12}O_2$

(**104**) 6,7,16,17-Tetrahydro-15*H*-cyclopenta[a]phenanthrene-6,7-
dione
MW 248; Bright red needles, mp 209–211°C (Badger *et al.*, 1952);
213°C (Butenandt *et al.*, 1946*b*)

$C_{17}H_{13}BrO$

cis-16-Bromo-17-hydroxy-16,17-dihydro-15*H*-cyclopenta[a]-
phenanthrene [50909-53-8]
MW 313
λ_{max} 256.5, 278, 299 nm
ν_{max} 3.01 μm   (Coombs *et al.*, 1973*a*)

$C_{17}H_{14}$ (**176**) 13,14-Dihydro-17*H*-cyclopenta[a]phenanthrene [81396-17-0]
MW 218
ν_{max} 3.22, 12.80, 13.25 μm
δ 2.1–3.4 (m, 3H), 4.0 (m, 1H), 5.7 (m, 3H), 7.0–8.0 (m, 7H)
                                            (Lee-Ruff *et al.*, 1982)

$C_{17}H_{14}$ (**1**) 16,17-Dihydro-15*H*-cyclopenta[a]phenanthrene [482-66-6]
MW 218; mp 133–134°C (Kon, 1933); 134.5–135°C (Cook and
Hewett, 1933); 132–133°C (Butz *et al.*, 1940); 134–135°C (Coombs,
1966*b*)
λ_{max} 216 (4.48), 259 (4.77), 280 (4.16), 288 (4.07), 300 (4.71) nm
ν_{max} (CS_2) 12.32, 13.27 μm (Dannenberg *et al.*, 1953)
ν_{max} 10.62, 11.56, 12.3, 12.95, 13.4, 14.08 μm (Coombs, 1966*b*)
m/z 218 (100%), 219 (19%), 189 (28%), 188 (7%), 163 (6%)
                                            (Chaffee and Jones, 1983)

$C_{17}H_{14}O$ (**38**) 16,17-Dihydro-3-hydroxy-15*H*-cyclopenta[a]phenanthrene
MW 234; mp 184–188.5°C   (Hoffelmer *et al.*, 1964)

$C_{17}H_{14}O$ 16,17-Dihydro-15*H*-cyclopenta[a]phenanthren-15-ol [42123-05-7]
MW 234; mp 166–167°C
acetate, mp 127–128°C   (Badger *et al.*, 1952)

$C_{17}H_{14}O$ 16,17-Dihydro-15*H*-cyclopenta[a]phenanthren-11-ol
MW 234; mp 174–175°C
λ_{max} 228, 246, 279, 303, 349, 366 nm   (Bhatt, unpublished data)

$C_{17}H_{14}O$ 16,17-Dihydro-15*H*-cyclopenta[a]phenanthren-17-ol
MW 234; mp 183–184°C
λ_{max} 259 (4.77), 280 (4.09), 288 (3.98), 300 (4.12) nm
ν_{max} 3.15, 9.55, 11.50, 12.28, 12.92, 13.40, 13.85 μm
                                                     (Coombs, 1966*b*)

$C_{17}H_{14}O$ (**384**) 11,12,13,17-Tetrahydro-16*H*-cyclopenta[a]phenanthren-16-one

MW 234;   mp 185–185.5°C
oxime, mp 247–250°C   (Wilds, 1942)

$C_{17}H_{14}O$ **(179)** 11,12,15,16-Tetrahydro-cyclopenta[a]phenanthren-17-one
MW 234;   Pale yellow scales, mp 210°C (Bardhan, 1936); colourless
rhombohedral prisms, mp 214–216°C (Bachmann *et al.*, 1943); pale
yellow crystals, mp 219–221°C (Johnson and Peterson, 1945); 218–
220°C (Coombs *et al.*, 1970)
λ_{max} 272 (4.61), 282 (4.70), 325 (3.18), 337 (3.21), 367 (2.97) nm
ν_{max} 11.50, 11.94, 12.14, 13.24, 13.85 μm   (Coombs *et al.*, 1970)

$C_{17}H_{14}O$ **(174)** 11,12,13,14-Tetrahydro-17*H*-cyclopenta[a]phenanthren-12-one
[67279-07-6] [80299-44-1]
MW 234;   mp 84–85°C   (Lee-Ruff *et al.*, 1981)

$C_{17}H_{14}O$ 13,14,15,16-Tetrahydrocyclopenta[a]phenanthren-17-one
[7421-33-2] [5836-87-3]
MW 234;   mp 95–96°C
λ_{max} 239 (4.73), 303 (3.88), 316 (4.01), 330 (3.88), 336 (3.86) nm
ν_{max} 5.75 μm   (Coombs, 1966*a*)

$C_{17}H_{14}O_2$
(116) 16,17-Dihydro-1,4-dihydroxy-15*H*-cyclopenta[a]phenanthrene
MW 252;   mp 210°C   (Tamayo and Martin, 1952)

$C_{17}H_{14}O_2$
(382) 16,17-Dihydro-*cis*-15,16-dihydroxy-15*H*-cyclopenta[a]phenanthrene
MW 250 (characterized as its diacetate **(109)** (see $C_{21}H_{18}O_4$)
(Coombs and Hall, 1973)

$C_{17}H_{14}O_2$
(378) 16,17-Dihydro-*cis*-16,17-dihydroxy-15*H*-cyclopenta[a]-
phenanthrene [42122-94-1]
MW 250;   mp 226–228°C
λ_{max} 250.5 (4.71), 257 (4.83), 279 (4.16), 287 (4.06), 299 (4.16),
320 (2.71), 327.5 (2.56), 334.5 (2.87), 343 (2.49), 350 (2.86) nm
ν_{max} 3.05, 12.15, 12.24, 13.33, 13.48 μm   (Coombs and Hall, 1973)

$C_{17}H_{14}O_2$
(376) 16,17-Dihydro-*trans*-16,17-dihydroxy-15*H*-cyclopenta[a]-
phenanthrene [42122-95-2]
MW 250;   mp 277–278°C
λ_{max} 250.5 (4.71), 257 (4.82), 279 (4.16), 287 (4.05), 299 (4.17),
320 (2.65), 327.5 (2.49), 335 (2.84), 343 (2.44), 350 (2.84) nm
ν_{max} 3.08, 12.10, 13.44 μm   (Coombs and Hall, 1973)

$C_{17}H_{14}O_2$
(324) 1,2,3,4,16,17-Hexahydrocyclopenta[a]phenanthrene-1,15-dione
MW 250;   mp 173–175°C   (Rahman and Rodriguez, 1969)

$C_{17}H_{14}O_2$
(±) **(193)** 11,12,13,14,15,16-Hexahydrocyclopenta[a]phenanthrene-
11,17-dione [23462-83-1] [24808-98-8] [67530-16-9]
MW 250;   Colourless needles, mp 115°C (Koebner and Robinson,
1938); 120°C (Coombs, 1965)
λ_{max} 216 (4.61), 248 (4.33), 315 (3.82)
ν_{max} 5.78, 5.98 μm   (Coombs, 1965)

$C_{17}H_{14}O_2$

(+) (**193**) (+)-11,12,13,14,15,16-Hexahydrocyclopenta[a]-
phenanthrene-11,17-dione
MW 250;   mp 138°C, $[\alpha]_D^{20°}$ +266° ($CHCl_3$)
λ_{max} 248 (4.32), 314 (3.80) nm
ν_{max} 5.75, 5.95 μm   (Cagara and Siewinski, 1975)

$C_{17}H_{14}O_2$

(−) (**193**) (−)-11,12,13,14,15,16-Hexahydrocyclopenta[a]-
phenanthrene-11,17-dione
MW 250;   mp 138°C, $[\alpha]_D^{20°}$ −258° ($CHCl_3$)
λ_{max} 248 (4.33), 314 (3.86) nm
ν_{max} 5.75, 5.95 μm   (Cagara and Siewinski, 1975)

$C_{17}H_{14}O_3$

(**337**) 17-Oxo-6,7,15,16-tetrahydrocyclopenta[a]phenanthrene-*cis*-
6,7-diol
MW 266;   mp 232–234°C
λ_{max} 245 (4.02), 309–317 (4.43) nm
ν_{max} 2.86, 2.96, 5.78, 10.31, 11.91, 12.90, 13.51 μm   (Coombs, 1969)

$C_{17}H_{15}N$ (**349**) 12-Amino-16,17-dihydro-15*H*-cyclopenta[a]phenanthrene
[3036-49-5]
MW 233;   mp 250°C
λ_{max} 255.5 (4.64), 314 (3.98), 360 (3.11)
ν_{max} (KBr) 3.03, 3.47–4.41, 10.87, 12.20, 13.25 μm
$C_{17}H_{15}N.HCl$ [2960-80-7]   (Dannenberg et al., 1965)

$C_{17}H_{16}$ (**442**) 6,7,16,17-Tetrahydro-15*H*-cyclopenta[a]phenanthrene
MW 220;   mp 60°C (Jacob et al., 1971); 61–62°C (Robinson and
Slater, 1941)
λ_{max} 272 (4.30) nm
ν_{max} 12.20, 13.07 μm
δ 7 (m), 7.5 (m), 2.1 (m), 2.8 (m)   (Jacob et al., 1971)

$C_{17}H_{16}$ 13,14,16,17-Tetrahydro-15*H*-cyclopenta[a]phenanthrene [7421-32-1]
[5836-83-9]
MW 220;   mp 79–80°C
λ_{max} 239 (4.76), 303 (3.84), 315 (3.91), 337 (3.63) nm
ν_{max} 10.55, 11.54, 12.15, 12.42, 13.25, 13.50, 13.80 μm
                                                             (Coombs, 1966a)

$C_{17}H_{16}O$ (**325**) 1,2,3,4,16,17-Hexahydrocyclopenta[a]phenanthren-15-one
MW 236   (Rahman and Rodriguez, 1969)

$C_{17}H_{16}O$ (**237**) 1,2,3,4,15,16-Hexahydrocyclopenta[a]phenanthren-17-one
MW 236;   mp 145–146°C
λ_{max} 256.5 (3.98), 282 (3.25), 292.5 (3.27), 333.5 (2.86), 348 (2.91) nm
ν_{max} 5.89, 9.55, 11.8, 12.1, 12.5 μm   (Coombs and Bhatt, 1973)

$C_{17}H_{16}O$ (**82**) 11,12,13,14,16,17-Hexahydro-15*H*-cyclopenta[a]phenanthren-11-
one
MW 236;   mp 119–120°C   (Butenandt et al., 1946a)

$C_{17}H_{16}O$ (**205**) 11,12,13,14,15,16-Hexahydrocyclopenta[a]phenanthren-17-one
[786-64-1]
MW 236;   mp 114–114.5°C   (Coombs, 1966a)

$C_{17}H_{16}O$ 12-Hydroxy-11,12,13,14-tetrahydro-17H-cyclopenta[a]phenanthrene
[67279-08-7] [80299-45-2]
MW 236 (Dao *et al.*, 1978)
$C_{17}H_{16}O$ 13,14,16,17-Tetrahydro-15H-cyclopenta[a]phenanthren-17-ol
[788-65-2] [7421-34-3]
MW 236; mp 117–118°C
λ_{max} 239 (4.75), 301.5 (3.85), 315 (3.95), 330 (3.79), 336 (3.69) nm
ν_{max} 3.00, 9.35 μm (Coombs, 1966a)
$C_{17}H_{16}O_2$
(103) 6,7-*cis*-Dihydroxy-6,7,16,17-tetrahydro-15H-cyclopenta[a]-
phenanthrene
MW 252; mp 193°C (Butenandt *et al.*, 1946b)
$C_{17}H_{16}O_2$
(115) 1,4-Dihydroxy-6,7,16,17-tetrahydro-15H-cyclopenta[a]phenan-
threne
MW 252 (Tamayo and Martin, 1952)
$C_{17}H_{16}O_2$
11,12,13,14,15,16-Hexahydro-11-hydroxycyclopenta[a]phenanthren-
17-one [23462-85-3] [23462-84-2]
(Mejer and Kalinowska, 1969)
$C_{17}H_{16}O_2$
11,12,13,14,15,16-Hexahydro-11α-hydroxycyclopenta[a]phenanthren-
17-one [23462-84-2]
MW 252; mp 115°C
λ_{max} 229 (4.91), 278 (3.78) nm
ν_{max} (Nujol) 2.93, 5.75 μm
ν_{max} (CCl$_4$) 2.77 μm (Mejer and Kalinowska, 1969)
$C_{17}H_{16}O_2$
11,12,13,14,15,16-Hexahydro-11β-hydroxycyclopenta[a]phenanthren-
17-one [23462-85-3]
MW 252; mp 201°C
λ_{max} 230 (4.96), 278 (3.84) nm
ν_{max} (Nujol) 2.88, 5.78 μm
ν_{max} (CCl$_4$) 2.77 μm (Mejer and Kalinowska, 1969)
$C_{17}H_{16}O_2$
11,12,13,14,16,17-Hexahydro-17α-hydroxy-15H-cyclopenta[a]-
phenanthren-11-one [23462-86-4]
MW 252; mp 119°C
λ_{max} 243 (4.35), 310 (3.88)
ν_{max} (Nujol) 2.93, 6.02 μm
ν_{max} (CCl$_4$) 2.76 μm (Mejer and Kalinowska, 1969)
$C_{17}H_{16}O_2$
11,12,13,14,16,17-Hexahydro-17β-hydroxy-15H-cyclopenta[a]-
phenanthren-11-one [23462-87-5]
MW 252; mp 132°C
λ_{max} 243 (4.35), 310 (3.93) nm
ν_{max} (Nujol) 2.93, 6.02 μm
ν_{max} (CCl$_4$) 2.76 μm (Mejer and Kalinowska, 1969)

$C_{17}H_{16}O_2$

(+)11,12,13,14,16,17-Hexahydro-17β-hydroxy-15H-cyclopenta[a]-
phenanthren-11-one [23462-88-6]
MW 252;   mp 111–112°C, $[\alpha]_D^{20°}$ −13° $(CHCl_3)$
Spectra as for (±) compound   (Mejer and Kalinowska, 1969)

$C_{17}H_{16}O_2$

(114) 1,4,5,6,9,10,16,17-Octahydro-15H-cyclopenta[a]phenanthrene-
1,4-dione
MW 252   (Tamayo and Martin, 1952)

$C_{17}H_{18}$ (326) 1,2,3,4,16,17-Hexahydro-15H-cyclopenta[a]phenanthrene
MW 222;   mp 94–96°C   (Rahman and Rodriguez, 1969)

$C_{17}H_{18}$ (440) 6,7,8,14,16,17-Hexahydro-15H-cyclopenta[a]phenanthrene
MW 222;   mp 79°C (Robinson & Slater, 1941); 78°C (Jacob et al.,
1971)
λ_{max} 230 (3.78), 242 (3.75), 250 (3.66), 321 (4.09), 335 (4.15),
352 (3.97) nm
ν_{max} 13.25 μm
δ 8(m), 7.4(m), 6.76(d), 6.15(d), 3.2(m), 2.2(m) (Jacob et al., 1971)

$C_{17}H_{18}$ (44) 11,12,13,14,16,17-Hexahydro-15H-cyclopenta[a]phenanthrene
[31301-56-1]
MW 222;   mp 91–92°C (Coombs, 1966a); 85–87°C (Buchta and
Ziemer, 1956)
λ_{max} 230 (4.28), 275 (3.63), 285 (3.76), 292 (3.54) nm
(Coombs, 1966a)

$C_{17}H_{18}O$ (96) 6,7,8,12,13,14,16,17-Octahydro-15H-cyclopenta[a]phenanthren-
12-one
MW 238;   mp 171°C (Robinson and Slater, 1941); 173°C (Jacob et
al., 1971); 169–170°C (Hawthorne and Robinson, 1936)
λ_{max} 295 (4.20) nm
ν_{max} 5.99 μm
δ 7.7(m), 7.2(s), 6.5(s), 1.8(m)   (Jacob et al., 1971)

$C_{17}H_{18}O_2$

11α,17α-Dihydroxy-11,12,13,14,16,17-hexahydro-15H-cyclopenta[a]-
phenanthrene [23462-89-7]
MW 254;   mp 164°C
λ_{max} 229 (5.12), 279 (3.86) nm
ν_{max} (CCl_4) 2.77 and 290 μm   (Mejer and Kalinowska, 1969)

$C_{17}H_{18}O_2$

11β,17α-Dihydroxy-11,12,13,14,16,17-hexahydro-15H-cyclopenta[a]-
phenanthrene [23462-92-2]
MW 254;   mp 192°C
λ_{max} 229 (5.11), 279 (3.81) nm
ν_{max} (CCl_4) 2.77 μm   (Mejer and Kalinowska, 1969)

$C_{17}H_{18}O_2$

(±)11,17β-Dihydroxy-11,12,13,14,16,17-hexahydro-15H-
cyclopenta[a]phenanthrene
MW 254;   mp 115°C [23462-90-0]

λ_{max} 229 (5.03), 278 (3.79) nm
ν_{max} (CCl$_4$) 2.77 μm   (Mejer and Kalinowska, 1969)

C$_{17}$H$_{18}$O$_2$
(+)11,17β-Dihydroxy-11,12,13,14,16,17-hexahydro-15*H*-cyclopenta[a]phenanthrene [23462-91-1]
MW 254;   mp 170–175°C, [α]$_D^{20°}$ +63° (EtOH)
λ_{max} 299 (5.08), 279 (3.87) nm
ν_{max} (CHCl$_3$) 2.77 μm   (Mejer and Kalinowska, 1969)

C$_{17}$H$_{18}$O$_2$
(**233**) 1,2,3,4,11,12,13,14,15,16-Decahydrocyclopenta[a]-phenanthrene-11,17-dione
MW 254;   mp 111–113°C
λ_{max} 200 (4.25), 257 (3.91), 308 (3.33) nm
ν_{max} 5.75, 5.95, 10.1, 10.7, 11.9 μm   (Coombs and Bhatt, 1973)

C$_{17}$H$_{20}$O (**438**) 12-Hydroxy-6,7,8,12,13,14,16,17-octahydro-15*H*-cyclopenta[a]-phenanthrene
MW 240;   mp 131–132°C   (Robinson and Slater, 1941)

C$_{17}$H$_{22}$O (**444**) 6,7,8,9,11,12,13,14,16,17-Decahydro-12-hydroxy-15*H*-cyclopenta[a]phenanthrene
MW 242;   mp 165°C
λ_{max} 265 (2.71) nm
ν_{max} 2.97, 13.70 μm
δ 7.2(m), 1.5(s), 3.2(m)   (Jacob *et al.*, 1971)

C$_{18}$H$_{12}$Br$_2$O
(**357**) 15,15-Dibromo-15,16-dihydro-11-methyl-cyclopenta[a]-phenanthren-17-one [50905-51-6] [74495-85-5]
MW 234;   Orange crystals, mp 206–207°C
λ_{max} 267.5 (4.68), 302.5 (4.32), 315 (4.12), 369 (3.29), 384 (3.31) nm
ν_{max} 5.84, 12.15, 13.44, 13.93, 14.12 μm
δ 4.69 (H-16)   (Coombs *et al.*, 1973*a*)

C$_{18}$H$_{12}$O (**310**)15,16-Dihydro-1,11-methanocyclopenta[a]phenanthren-17-one
MW 244;   mp 195°C
λ_{max} 266.5 (4.77), 277 (4.76), 303 (3.34), 348 (3.03), 365.5 (2.86) nm
ν_{max} 5.94, 6.12, 7.14, 7.74, 12.20, 12.42 μm
δ2.8 (H-16), 3.25 (H-15), 4.2 (bridge CH$_2$)   (Ribeiro *et al.*, 1983)

C$_{18}$H$_{12}$O (**364**) 11-Methylcyclopenta[a]phenanthren-17-one
MW 244 [55651-29-1]
λ_{max} 256, 288, 298, 312, 389 nm   (Coombs *et al.*, 1975)

C$_{18}$H$_{12}$O$_2$
(**148**) 17*H*-Cyclopenta[a]phenanthrene-17-carboxylic acid
MW 260;   mp 250–270°C   (Süss, 1953)

C$_{18}$H$_{12}$O$_2$
(**418**) 15,16-Dihydro-16-formylcyclopenta[a]phenanthren-17-one
MW 260;   mp 197–198°C   (Buchta and Kraetzer, 1962)

C$_{18}$H$_{12}$O$_3$
(**336**) 11-Methyl-6,7,15,16-tetrahydrocyclopenta[a]phenanthrene-6,7,17-trione

MW 276; mp 230°C
λ_{max} 263 (4.15), 345 (3.44), 410 (2.94) nm
ν_{max} 5.80, 6.00, 6.24, 10.30, 11.91, 12.08, 13.70, 13.86 μm
(Coombs, 1969)

$C_{18}H_{13}BrO$

(355) 15-Bromo-15,16-dihydro-11-methylcyclopenta[a]phenanthren-17-one [50905-52-7]
MW 325; mp 211.5–212°C
λ_{max} 267.5 (4.68), 290 (4.37), 303 (4.29), 363 (3.31), 381 (3.35) nm
ν_{max} 5.88, 12.20, 13.18, 13.85, 14.29 μm
δ 4.85 (J 7,3) (H-15), 3.72 (J 18,3) and 4.23 (J 18,7) (H-16)
(Coombs *et al.*, 1973a)

$C_{18}H_{13}BrO$

(359) 16-Bromo-15,16-dihydro-11-methylcyclopenta[a]phenanthren-17-one [55651-28-0]
λ_{max} 275.4, 359, 377 nm
ν_{max} 5.81, 11.49, 12.09, 12.50, 12.99, 13.19, 14.81 μm
δ 5.94 (J 2,6) (H-16), 3.49 (J 6,20) and 3.30 (J 2,20) (H-15)
(Coombs *et al.*, 1975)

$C_{18}H_{13}ClO_2$

(322) 7-Chloro-15,16-dihydro-6-methoxycyclopenta[a]phenanthren-17-one
MW 296.5; mp 220°C   (Badger *et al.*, 1952)

$C_{18}H_{14}$ (143) 15,16-Dihydro-17-methylenecyclopenta[a]phenanthrene
[5837-17-2]
MW 230; mp 217–218°C
λ_{max} 215 (4.22), 273.5 (4.69), 287 (4.44), 299 (4.34), 307 (4.09),
333 (3.08), 349 (3.28), 367 (3.34) nm
ν_{max} 3.25, 6.18, 10.62, 11.6, 12.04, 12.42, 13.42, 13.9 μm
δ 5.56 and 5.13 (olefinic protons), 3.25 and 3.05 (methylene protons)
(Coombs, 1966b)

$C_{18}H_{14}$ (150) 11-Methyl-15H-cyclopenta[a]phenanthrene [42122-99-6]
MW 230; mp 87–89°C
λ_{max} 221.5 (4.47), 267 (4.65), 274 (4.65), 294 (4.08), 306 (4.08),
317 (2.83), 348 (2.85), 364 (2.74) nm
ν_{max} 12.27, 13.32, 14.27 μm   (Coombs and Hall, 1973)

$C_{18}H_{14}$ (128) 15-Methyl-17H-cyclopenta[a]phenanthrene
MW 230; mp 135°C
λ_{max} 221 (4.68), 241 (4.45), 267.5 (4.60), 293 (4.02), 305 (4.17),
317.5 (4.15), 344 (3.08), 361 (2.99) nm
ν_{max} (KBr) 12.29, 12.40, 13.24, 13.41 μm   (Dannenberg *et al.*, 1960)

$C_{18}H_{14}$ (133) 17-Methyl-15H-cyclopenta[a]phenanthrene [3353-08-0]
MW 230; Cream needles, mp 209–212°C
λ_{max} 223 (4.30), 270 (4.70), 276 (4.73), 293 (4.14), 316 (3.74),
331 (2.71), 348 (2.69), 366 (2.46) nm
ν_{max} 11.0, 11.55, 12.0, 12.3, 12.8, 13.4, 13.82 μm   (Coombs, 1966b)

$C_{18}H_{14}O$ (302) 15,16-Dihydro-1-methylcyclopenta[a]phenanthren-17-one
[85616-38-2]

MW 246; mp 189–190°C

λ_{max} 266 (4.84), 288 (4.53), 303 (4.30), 359 (3.77), 375 (3.77) nm

ν_{max} 5.92, 12.09, 12.99 μm

δ 2.73 (H-16), 3.08 (methyl), 3.38 (H-15)   (Ribeiro *et al.*, 1983)

$C_{18}H_{14}O$ **(303)** 15,16-Dihydro-2-methylcyclopenta[a]phenanthren-17-one
[27343-46-0]

MW 246; mp 221–222°C

λ_{max} 267 (5.05), 284 (4.22), 298 (4.12), 336 (3.11), 352 (3.34),
370 (3.27) nm

ν_{max} 5.85, 11.72, 11.90, 12.10, 12.50, 12.95, 14.08 μm

(Coombs *et al.*, 1970)

$C_{18}H_{14}O$ **(304)** 15,16-Dihydro-3-methylcyclopenta[a]phenanthren-17-one
[27363-65-1]

MW 246; mp 203–204°C

λ_{max} 267 (5.02), 285 (4.67), 298 (4.41), 344 (3.28), 366 (3.25) nm

ν_{max} 5.88, 11.10, 11.60, 11.90, 12.36, 13.05, 13.90, 14.10 μm

(Coombs *et al.*, 1970)

$C_{18}H_{14}O$ **(305)** 15,16-Dihydro-4-methylcyclopenta[a]phenanthren-17-one
[27343-45-9]

MW 246; mp 265–266°C

λ_{max} 266 (4.98), 284 (4.67), 300 (4.36), 336 (3.06), 352 (3.22),
370 (3.23) nm

ν_{max} 5.92, 11.10, 11.88, 12.05, 12.34, 12.60, 13.85, 14.15 μm

(Coombs *et al.*, 1970)

$C_{18}H_{14}O$ **(306)** 15,16-Dihydro-6-methylcyclopenta[a]phenanthren-17-one
[27343-44-8]

MW 246; mp 210.5–212°C

λ_{max} 266 (5.06), 284 (4.69), 298 (4.45), 336 (3.10), 352 (3.32),
370 (3.33) nm

ν_{max} 5.86, 11.44, 12.12, 13.00, 14.25 μm   (Coombs *et al.*, 1970)

$C_{18}H_{14}O$ **(230)** 15,16-Dihydro-7-methylcyclopenta[a]phenanthren-17-one
[30835-65-5]

MW 246; mp 198–199°C

λ_{max} 268 (4.79), 286 (4.42), 301 (4.28), 343 (3.23), 360 (3.41),
378 (3.42) nm

ν_{max} 5.91, 11.3, 11.98, 12.92, 13.34 μm

δ 2.72 (H-15), 2.92 (methyl), 3.70 (H-16) (Coombs and Jaitly, 1971)

$C_{18}H_{14}O$ **(381)** 15,17-Dihydro-11-methylcyclopenta[a]phenanthren-16-one
[42123-04-6]

MW 246; mp 152.5–153°C

λ_{max} 256.5 (4.77), 282 (4.06), 295 (4.08), 307 (4.16), 324 (2.99),
339 (306), 355 (3.04) nm

ν_{max} 5.75, 12.08, 12.58, 13.46 μm   (Coombs and Hall, 1973)

$C_{18}H_{14}O$ **(26)** 15,16-Dihydro-11-methylcyclopenta[a]phenanthren-17-one
[892-17-1] [74495-84-4] [74524-21-3]

MW 246; mp 171–172°C

λ_{max} 222 (4.11), 264 (4.83), 288 (4.49), 301 (4.32), 342 (3.11),
358 (3.38), 376 (3.43) nm

ν_{max} 5.92, 11.40, 12.28, 13.34, 14.00, 14.52 μm

δ 2.68 (H-16), 3.00 (methyl), 3.23 (H-15)   (Coombs, 1966*b*)

$C_{18}H_{14}O$ (**130**) 15,16-Dihydro-12-methylcyclopenta[a]phenanthren-17-one [789-46-8]

MW 245;   mp 233°C (Coombs, 1966*b*; Riegel *et al.*, 1948)

λ_{max} 219 (4.18), 268 (4.85), 286 (4.42), 299 (4.36), 340 (2.96), 355 (3.22), 373 (3.28) nm

ν_{max} 5.92, 11.36, 12.32, 12.70, 13.20 μm

δ 2.70 (H-16), 2.82 (methyl), 3.28 (H-15)   (Coombs, 1966*b*)

$C_{18}H_{14}O$ (**49**) 16,17-Dihydro-17-methylcyclopenta[a]phenanthren-15-one

MW 246;   mp 138–139°C   (Tatta and Bardhan, 1968)

$C_{18}H_{14}O$ (**402**) 15,17-Dihydro-17-methylcyclopenta[a]phenanthren-16-one [42123-02-4]

MW 246;   mp 231–233°C   (Dannenberg *et al.*, 1960)

$C_{18}H_{14}O$ (**334**) 16,17-Dihydro-11-methylcyclopenta[a]phenanthren-15-one [24684-42-2]

MW 246;   mp 182–183°C

λ_{max} 217 (4.57), 253 (4.63), 284 (4.15), 323 (4.14), 363 (3.41) nm

ν_{max} 5.94, 11.60, 12.22, 13.28, 13.72, 14.02 μm   (Coombs, 1969)

$C_{18}H_{14}O_2$

(**458**) 15,16-Dihydro-4-hydroxy-1-methylcyclopenta[a]phenanthren-17-one

MW 262.0994; found, 262.0992

λ_{max} 270, 305 nm

λ_{max} (anion) 260, sh 284, 325 nm   (Coombs *et al.*, 1985)

$C_{18}H_{14}O_2$

(**340**) 15,16-Dihydro-6-hydroxy-11-methylcyclopenta[a]phenanthren-17-one [24684-47-7]

MW 262;   Golden yellow needles, mp 335°C

λ_{max} 265 (4.76), 289 (4.51), 306 (4.27), 368 (3.37), 384 (3.41) nm

ν_{max} 3.08, 5.95, 11.46, 12.05, 12.86, 13.04, 13.74, 14.50 μm

     (Coombs, 1969)

$C_{18}H_{14}O_2$

(**215**) 15,16-Dihydro-11-hydroxymethylcyclopenta[a]phenanthren-17-one [55651-36-0]

MW 262;   mp 190–192°C

λ_{max} 264.5 (4.85), 285 (4.51), 300 (4.32), 356 (3.29), 372.5 (3.41) nm

m/z 262; (M$^+$, 100%), 234 (M$^+$-CO, 20%), 235 (M$^+$-CHO, 45%), 233 (M$^+$-CH$_2$OH, 18%)   (Coombs *et al.*, 1975)

$C_{18}H_{14}O_2$

15,16-Dihydro-11-hydroxy-7-methylcyclopenta[a]phenanthren-17-one [30835-60-0]

MW 262;   mp 335–340°C

  acetate, mp 243–244°C

λ_{max} 230.5 (4.24), 267 (4.79), 295.5 (4.38), 360 (3.47), 378 (3.77), 398 (3.86) nm   (Coombs and Jaitly, 1971)

$C_{18}H_{14}O_2$

(**370**) 15,16-Dihydro-15-hydroxy-11-methylcyclopenta[a]phenanthren-17-one [55651-31-5]

MW 262
λ_{max} 265 (4.84), 300 (4.53), 356 (3.29), 374 (3.21) nm
(Coombs *et al.*, 1975)

$C_{18}H_{14}O_2$

(**346**) 15,16-Dihydro-16-hydroxy-11-methylcyclopenta[a]phenanthren-17-one [24684-56-8]
MW 262; mp 205–207°C
λ_{max} 264 (4.88), 288 (4.52), 301 (4.35), 345 (3.14), 361 (3.36), 379 (3.39) nm
ν_{max} 3.00, 5.92, 11.44, 11.62, 12.06, 12.28, 12.55, 12.80, 13.56, 14.10 μm
(Coombs, 1969)

$C_{18}H_{14}O_2$

(**307**) 15,16-Dihydro-2-methoxycyclopenta[a]phenanthren-17-one [55651-43-9]
MW 262; mp 180–180.5°C
λ_{max} 271 (4.81), 360 (3.45), 377 (3.51) nm
ν_{max} 5.87–5.95, 9.59, 10.47, 12.14, 12.66, 13.16, 13.89 μm
(Coombs *et al.*, 1975)

$C_{18}H_{14}O_2$

(**24**) 15,16-Dihydro-3-methoxycyclopenta[a]phenanthren-17-one
MW 262; mp 209 and 230°C
λ_{max} 218–220 (4.21), 269 (4.78), 277 (4.83), 319 (4.22), 347 (3.62), 366 (3.28) nm
ν_{max} 5.92, 11.42, 12.38, 13.04 μm
(Coombs, 1966*b*)

$C_{18}H_{14}O_2$

(**308**) 15,16-Dihydro-6-methoxycyclopenta[a]phenanthren-17-one [24684-46-6]
MW 262; mp 196–197°C
λ_{max} 270 (4.98), 287 (4.69), 302 (4.37), 361 (3.36), 378 (3.33) nm
ν_{max} 5.90, 11.86, 12.24, 12.76, 13.04, 13.78, 14.12 μm
(Coombs *et al.*, 1970)

$C_{18}H_{14}O_2$

(**132**) 15,16-Dihydro-11-methoxycyclopenta[a]phenanthrene-17-one [5836-85-1]
MW 262; mp 179°C (Robinson, 1938); 184°C (Coombs, 1966*b*)
λ_{max} 214 (4.21), 261 (4.86), 292 (4.42), 303 (4.29), 346 (3.42), 363 (3.72), 381 (3.82) nm
ν_{max} 5.88, 11.30, 12.30, 13.32 μm
(Coombs, 1966*b*)

$C_{18}H_{14}O_2$

(**367**) 15,16-Dihydro-15-methoxycyclopenta[a]phenanthren-17-one [83053-56-9]
MW 262; mp 155°C
λ_{max} 268, 297, 352, 369 nm
(Bhatt *et al.*, 1982)

$C_{18}H_{14}O_3$

(**465**) 15,16-Dihydro-2,15-dihydroxycyclopenta[a]phenanthren-17-one [55081-26-0]
MW 278; Yellow solid, mp 278°C
λ_{max} 276; anion 250, 300 nm
(Coombs and Crawley, 1974)

98   *Physical and spectral properties*

$C_{18}H_{14}O_3$
15,16-Dihydro-11-hydroxy-3-methoxycyclopenta[a]phenanthren-17-
one
MW 278;   mp 293–299°C   (Robinson, 1938)

$C_{18}H_{14}O_4$
(463) 8,9-Epoxy-2,15-dihydroxy-11-methyl-8,9-secogona-
1,3,5,7,9,11,13-heptaen-17-one
MW 294;   mp 280–282°C
λ_{max} 278 (4.55); anion 255 (4.50), 299 (4.50) nm
                              (Coombs and Crawley, 1974)

$C_{18}H_{15}NO$
16,17-Dihydro-17-methyl-15H-cyclopenta[a]phenanthren-15-one,
oxime [17981-86-1]
MW 261;   mp 169–171°C   (Tatta and Bardhan, 1968)

$C_{18}H_{16}$ (107) 16,17-Dihydro-1-methyl-15H-cyclopenta[a]phenanthrene
[63020-74-6]
MW 232;   mp 75–76°C (Butenandt *et al.*, 1950)
λ_{max} 256 (4.80), 285 (4.05), 297 (4.03), 306 (4.11), 323 (2.68),
339 (2.69), 355 (2.54) nm (Dannenberg and Steidle, 1954)
ν_{max} (CS$_2$) 12.22, 12.77, 13.28 μm   (Dannenberg *et al.*, 1953)

$C_{18}H_{16}$ (98) 16,17-Dihydro-2-methyl-15H-cyclopenta[a]phenanthrene
[3988-20-3]
MW 232;   mp 106–107°C (Butenandt *et al.*, 1946c)
λ_{max} 261 (4.81), 282 (4.16), 291 (4.07), 303 (4.16), 323 (2.85),
338 (3.08), 354 (3.10) nm (Dannenberg and Steidle, 1954)
ν_{max} (CS$_2$) 12.03, 12.20 μm   (Dannenberg *et al.*, 1953)

$C_{18}H_{16}$ (70) 16,17-Dihydro-3-methyl-15H-cyclopenta[a]phenanthrene
MW 232;   mp 132°C   (Kon and Woolman, 1939)

$C_{18}H_{16}$ (100) 16,17-Dihydro-4-methyl-15H-cyclopenta[a]phenanthrene
[63020-75-7]
MW 232;   mp 151–152°C (Butenandt *et al.*, 1949a)
λ_{max} 255 (4.69), 263 (4.78), 283.5 (4.14), 294.5 (4.12), 306.5 (4.22),
324 (2.80), 339 (2.85), 355 (2.73) nm (Dannenberg and Steidle,
1954)
ν_{max} (CS$_2$) 12.33, 12.72, 13.29 μm   (Dannenberg *et al.*, 1953)

$C_{18}H_{16}$ (67) 16,17-Dihydro-6-methyl-15H-cyclopenta[a]phenanthrene
[63020-26-8]
MW 232;   mp 109–110°C (Gamble and Kon, 1935); 98–101°C
(Butenandt and Suranyi, 1942)
λ_{max} 262 (4.80), 282 (4.16), 290 (4.06), 303.5 (4.09), 322 (2.83),
337 (2.92), 354 (2.87) nm (Dannenberg and Steidle, 1954)
ν_{max} (CS$_2$) 11.52, 12.26, 13.27 μm   (Dannenberg *et al.*, 1953)

$C_{18}H_{16}$ (94) 16,17-Dihydro-7-methyl-15H-cyclopenta[a]phenanthrene
[63020-76-8]
MW 232;   mp 106–108°C (Butenandt *et al.*, 1949a)
λ_{max} 261 (4.77), 281 (4.24), 291 (4.06), 304 (4.08), 323.5 (2.91),
339 (3.15), 355 (3.19) nm (Dannenberg and Steidle, 1954)
ν_{max} 11.42, 12.22, 13.44 μm   (Dannenberg *et al.*, 1953)

$C_{18}H_{16}$ (**83**) 16,17-Dihydro-11-methyl-15H-cyclopenta[a]phenanthrene
[24684-41-1]
MW 232;   mp 80–81°C (Butenandt *et al.*, 1946*a*); 81–82°C (Coombs, 1969)
λ_{max} 256 (4.81), 285 (4.05), 297 (4.03), 306 (4.10), 323.5 (2.91), 340 (3.05), 356 (3.07) nm (Dannenberg and Steidle, 1954)
ν_{max} (CS$_2$) 11.58, 12.28, 13.43 μm   (Dannenberg *et al.*, 1953)

$C_{18}H_{16}$ (**97**) 16,17-Dihydro-12-methyl-15H-cyclopenta[a]phenanthrene
[63020-73-5]
MW 232;   mp 86–87°C (Butenandt *et al.*, 1946*a*); 85–86°C (Riegel *et al.*, 1948)
λ_{max} 261 (4.79), 282 (4.16), 291 (4.05), 303 (4.15), 321 (2.70), 337 (2.70), 353 (2.56) nm (Dannenberg and Steidle, 1954)
ν_{max} (CS$_2$) 11.53, 12.27, 13.39 μm (Dannenberg *et al.*, 1953)
Trinitro deriv., mp 196–197°C   (Riegel *et al.*, 1948)

$C_{18}H_{16}$ (**45**) 16,17-Dihydro-15-methyl-15H-cyclopenta[a]phenanthrene
MW 232;   mp 76–77°C (Ruzicka *et al.*, 1933)
Trinitrobenzene deriv., mp 143–144°C

$C_{18}H_{16}$ (**46**) 16,17-Dihydro-16-methyl-15H-cyclopenta[a]phenanthrene
MW 232;   mp 106–107°C; bp 160–170°C/0.3 mm (Ruzicka *et al.*, 1933)
Trinitrobenzene deriv., mp 140–141°C

$C_{18}H_{16}$ (**7**) Diels' hydrocarbon [549-38-2]
16,17-Dihydro-17-methyl-15H-cyclopenta[a]phenanthrene
MW 232;   mp 125–126°C (Diels and Gadke, 1927; Diels and Rickert, 1935; Bergmann and Hillemann, 1933); 126–127°C (Riegel *et al.*, 1942); 125.5–126°C (Tatta and Bardhan, 1968); 126.5–127.5°C (Coombs, 1966*b*)
λ_{max} 259 (4.80), 280 (4.14), 288.5 (4.04), 300.5 (4.11), 321 (2.74), 336 (2.94), 351.5 (2.33) nm (Dannenberg and Steidle, 1954)
ν_{max} 11.6, 12.06, 12.36, 13.06, 13.4, 13.9 μm
(Coombs, 1966*b*)

$C_{18}H_{16}O$ (**11**) 16,17-Dihydro-3-methoxy-15H-cyclopenta[a]phenanthrene
MW 248;   mp 76–77°C (Cook and Girard, 1934)
Orange picrate, mp 135–136.5°C
Trinitrobenzene deriv., mp 160–161°C

$C_{18}H_{16}O$ (**59**) 16,17-Dihydro-4-methoxy-15H-cyclopenta[a]phenanthrene
MW 248;   mp 153°C
picrate, mp 160°C   (Kon and Ruzicka, 1935)

$C_{18}H_{16}O$ (**61**) 16,17-Dihydro-6-methoxy-15H-cyclopenta[a]phenanthrene
MW 248;   mp 129°C   (Kon and Ruzicka, 1935)

$C_{18}H_{16}O$ 16,17-Dihydro-11-methoxy-15H-cyclopenta[a]phenanthrene
MW 248;   mp 106–107°C
λ_{max} 229, 248, 254, 278, 300, 332, 348, 364 nm
(Bhatt, unpublished data)

$C_{16}H_{16}O$ (**448**) 16,17-Dihydro-11-methyl-15H-cyclopenta[a]phenanthren-17-ol
[40951-13-1]
MW 248;   mp 140–141°C

λ_{max} 227 (4.22), 255 (4.78), 281 (4.02), 293 (4.02), 304.5 (4.10), 323 (2.79), 338.5 (2.96), 354 (2.98) nm

ν_{max} 3.08, 12.12, 12.24, 13.33 μm   (Coombs and Hall, 1973)

$C_{18}H_{16}O$ 1-Methyl-11,12,15,16-tetrahydrocyclopenta[a]phenanthren-17-one [85616-49-5]

MW 248;   mp 138–140°C

λ_{max} 276 (4.55), 286 (4.62), 330 (4.09), 343 (4.11), 376 (3.87) nm

ν_{max} 5.94, 6.06 μm   (Ribeiro *et al.*, 1983)

$C_{18}H_{16}O$ 2-Methyl-11,12,15,16-tetrahydrocyclopenta[a]phenanthren-17-one [27343-51-7]

MW 248;   mp 139–140°C

λ_{max} 272.5 (4.56), 283 (4.68), 327 (3.29), 338 (3.31), 370 (2.94) nm

ν_{max} 10.25, 11.80, 12.10 μm   (Coombs *et al.*, 1970)

$C_{18}H_{16}O$ 3-Methyl-11,12,15,16-tetrahydrocyclopenta[a]phenanthren-17-one [27343-51-7]

MW 248;   mp 222–223°C

λ_{max} 272 (4.61), 283 (4.70), 327 (3.25), 340 (3.31), 368 (3.12) nm

ν_{max} 11.16, 12.24, 12.98, 13.78, 14.10 μm   (Coombs *et al.*, 1970)

$C_{18}H_{16}O$ (**257**) 4-Methyl-11,12,15,16-tetrahydrocyclopenta[a]phenanthren-17-one [27343-34-6]

MW 248;   mp 237.5–241.3°C (Woodward *et al.*, 1953); 245–246°C (Coombs *et al.*, 1970)

λ_{max} 276 (4.50), 288 (4.59), 327 (3.07), 242 (3.11), 372 (2.89) nm

ν_{max} 12.20, 12.44, 13.18 μm   (Coombs *et al.*, 1970)

$C_{18}H_{16}O$ 6-Methyl-11,12,15,16-tetrahydrocyclopenta[a]phenanthren-17-one [27343-49-3]

MW 248;   mp 180.5–181.5°C

λ_{max} 276 (4.50), 287 (4.65), 327 (3.06), 342 (3.12), 375 (2.99) nm

ν_{max} 11.42, 12.15, 13.10 μm   (Coombs *et al.*, 1970)

$C_{18}H_{16}O$ (**252**) 11-Methyl-11,12,15,16-tetrahydrocyclopenta[a]phenanthren-17-one [27343-48-2]

MW 248;   mp 177–178°C

λ_{max} 271 (4.58), 282 (4.68), 327 (3.14), 341 (3.19), 368 (3.00) nm

ν_{max} 11.52, 12.10, 12.28, 13.26 μm   (Coombs *et al.*, 1970)

$C_{18}H_{16}O$ (**249**) 12-Methyl-11,12,15,16-tetrahydrocyclopenta[a]phenanthren-17-one

MW 248;   mp 156.5–157°C   (Riegel *et al.*, 1948)

$C_{16}H_{16}O_2$

2-Methoxy-11,12,15,16-tetrahydrocyclopenta[a]phenanthren-17-one [55651-42-8]

MW 264;   mp 154–154.5°.C

λ_{max} 273.5 (4.39), 284 (4.44), 328 (4.30) nm   (Coombs *et al.*, 1975)

$C_{18}H_{16}O_2$

(**66**) 3-Methoxy-11,12,15,16-tetrahydrocyclopenta[a]phenanthren-17-one

MW 264;   mp 210–211°C (Chuang *et al.*, 1939)

Colourless plates, mp 211–212°C   (Bachmann and Holman, 1951)

$C_{18}H_{16}O_2$

6-Methoxy-11,12,15,16-tetrahydrocyclopenta[a]phenanthren-17-one [27343-47-1]

MW 264; mp 175–176°C

λ_{max} 280 (4.53), 290 (4.64), 327 (2.92), 342 (2.94), 375 (2.99) nm

ν_{max} 11.70, 12.20, 13.15 μm   (Coombs *et al.*, 1970)

$C_{18}H_{16}O_2$

(379) 16,17-Dihydro-*cis*-16,17-dihydroxy-11-methyl-15*H*-cyclopenta[a]phenanthrene [42123-00-2]

MW 264; mp 181–182°C

λ_{max} 227 (4.19), 255 (4.83), 281 (4.07), 292.5 (4.03), 305 (4.11), 323.5 (2.80), 338.5 (2.96), 354 (2.94) nm

ν_{max} 3.02, 9.11, 12.20, 13.46 μm   (Coombs and Hall, 1973)

$C_{18}H_{16}O_2$

(377) 16,17-Dihydro-*trans*-16,17-dihydroxy-11-methyl-15*H*-cyclopenta[a]phenanthrene

MW 264; mp 224–226°C [42123-09-1]

λ_{max} 227 (4.22), 256 (4.85), 281 (4.07), 292.5 (4.04), 305 (4.13), 323 (2.82), 338.5 (2.97), 354 (2.98) nm

ν_{max} 3.05, 9.36, 12.12, 13.42 μm   (Coombs and Hall, 1973)

$C_{18}H_{16}O_2$

(389) 16,17-Dihydro-*cis*-16,17-dihydroxy-17-methyl-15*H*-cyclopenta[a]phenanthrene [42202-82-4]

MW 264; mp 171–172°C

λ_{max} 215 (4.56), 251 (4.73), 257.5 (4.84), 279 (4.18), 287.5 (4.08), 299 (4.19), 320 (2.65), 334 (2.84), 351 (2.82) nm

ν_{max} (KBr) 2.94, 8.56, 8.63, 8.95, 9.30, 12.15, 13.30 μm

(Dannenberg *et al.*, 1960)

$C_{18}H_{16}O_3$

(194) 11,12,13,14,15,16-Hexahydro-3-methoxycyclopenta[a]phenanthrene-11,17-dione

MW 250; mp 126–127°C   (Koebner and Robinson, 1938)

$C_{18}H_{16}O_3$

(338) 11-Methyl-17-oxo-6,7,15,16-tetrahydrocyclopenta[a]phenanthrene-*cis*-6,7-diol

MW 280; mp 244–245°C

λ_{max} 232 (4.13), 308–314 (4.22) nm

ν_{max} 2.90, 3.05, 5.96, 10.20, 10.38, 11.14, 12.04, 12.78, 13.10, 13.40, 13.80, 14.46 μm   (Coombs, 1969)

$C_{18}H_{16}O_3$

(457) 3α,4β-Dihydroxy-11-methyl-3,4,15,16-tetrahydrocyclopenta[a]phenanthren-17-one

MW 280 (see Chap. 7 for spectral data) (Coombs *et al.*, 1979; 1980)

$C_{18}H_{16}O_3$

(459) 1α,2β-Dihydroxy-11-methyl-1,2,15,16-tetrahydrocyclopenta[a]phenanthren-17-one

MW 280 (see Chap. 7 for spectral data) (Coombs *et al.*, 1979; 1980)

$C_{18}H_{16}O_4$

(454) 11-Methyl-1,2,15,16-tetrahydro-1α,2β,15-trihydroxycyclopenta[a]phenanthren-17-one

MW 296 (see Chap. 7 for spectral data)

(Coombs and Crawley, 1974; Coombs *et al.*, 1980)

$C_{18}H_{16}O_4$

(456) 11-Methyl-3,4,15,16-tetrahydro-3α,4β,16-trihydroxy-
cyclopenta[a]phenanthren-17-one
MW 296 (see Chap. 7 for spectral data)   (Coombs *et al.*, 1980)

$C_{18}H_{16}O_4$

(455) 11-Methyl-3,4,15,16-tetrahydro-3α,4β,15-trihydroxy-
cyclopenta[a]phenanthren-17-one
MW 296 (see Chap. 7 for spectral data)   (Coombs *et al.*, 1980)

$C_{18}H_{16}O_5$

(460) 8,9-Epoxy-1α,2β,15-trihydroxy-11-methyl-8,9-secogona-
3,5,7,9,11,13-hexaen-17-one
MW 312;   mp 120°C (decomp.), $[\alpha]_D^{26°}$ −214° (*c.* 0.134, EtOH)
λ_{max} 267 (4.57), 320 (4.03), 332 (4.04), 352 (3.67), 370 (3.61) nm
v_{max} 2.94–3.16, 5.91, 6.23, 9.62, 9.95 μm
δ H-1, 5.85 ($J_{1,2}$ 2); H-2, 4.36 ($J_{1,2}$ 2, $J_{2,3}$ 6); H-3, 6.30 ($J_{2,3}$ 6, $J_{3,4}$ 9);
H-4, 6.85 ($J_{3,4}$ 9); H-6, 7.52 ($J_{6,7}$ 9); H-7, 8.48 ($J_{6,7}$ 9); H-12, 7.52;
H-15, 5.76 ($J_{15,16}$ 2, $J_{15,16}$ 6); H-16, 3.19 ($J_{15,16}$ 6, $J_{16,16}$ 19); H-16,
2.60 ($J_{15,16}$ 2, $J_{16,16}$ 19); 11-CH$_3$, 3.22   (Coombs and Crawley, 1974)

$C_{18}H_{18}O$ (443) 3-Methoxy-6,7,16,17-tetrahydro-15H-cyclopenta[a]phenan-
threne
MW 250;   mp 101–102°C   (Robinson and Slater, 1941)

$C_{18}H_{18}O$ (238) 1,2,3,4,15,16-Hexahydro-11-methylcyclopenta[a]phenanthren-
17-one
MW 250;   mp 150–152°C
λ_{max} 223 (4.23), 261 (4.77), 287 (3.97), 297.5 (4.02), 308 (3.87),
344 (3.69), 354 (3.74) nm
v_{max} 5.95, 11.5, 12.45 μm
m/z 250.13574 (M⁺), 235, 222, 207, 194, 179
(Coombs and Bhatt, 1973)

$C_{18}H_{18}O$ (86) 11,12,13,14,16,17-Hexahydro-12-methyl-15H-cyclopenta[a]-
phenanthren-11-one
MW 250
12β-methyl, mp 85–86°C
12α-methyl, mp 117–118°C   (Butenandt *et al.*, 1946a)

$C_{18}H_{18}O_4$

(462) 1,2,3,4,15,16-Hexahydro-1α,2β,15-trihydroxy-11-
methylcyclopenta[a]phenanthren-17-one
MW 298;   mp 225–227°C
λ_{max} 260 (4.70), 285 (3.89), 295 (3.94), 342 (3.46), 354 (3.49) nm
(Coombs and Crawley, 1974)

$C_{18}H_{20}O$ (441) 6,7,8,14,16,17-Hexahydro-3-methoxy-15H-cyclopenta[a]-
phenanthrene
MW 252;   mp 82–85°C   (Robinson and Slater, 1941)

$C_{18}H_{20}O_2$

(427) 11,12,13,14,16,17-Hexahydro-11-hydroxy-3-methoxy-15H-
cyclopenta[a]phenanthrene
MW 268;   mp 141–142°C   (Robinson and Rydon, 1939)

$C_{18}H_{20}O_2$

(437) 3-Methoxy-6,7,8,12,13,14,16,17-octahydro-15*H*-cyclopenta[a]-
phenanthren-12-one
MW 268;   mp 192°C   (Robinson and Slater, 1941)

$C_{18}H_{20}O_2$

3-Methoxy-6,7,8,12,13,14,15,16-octahydrocyclopenta[a]phenanthren-
15-one
MW 268;   mp 142°C   (Nazarov *et al.*, 1953)

$C_{18}H_{20}O_2$

3-Methoxy-6,7,8,12,13,14,15,16-octahydrocyclopenta[a]phenanthren-
17-one
MW 268;   bp 210–215°C/0.5 mm   (Nazarov *et al.*, 1953)

$C_{18}H_{22}O$ (313) 6,7,8,9,11,12,13,14,15,16-Decahydro-1-methylcyclopenta[a]-
phenanthren-17-one
MW 254;   mp 85–88°C   (Coombs and Vose, 1974)

$C_{18}H_{22}O$ (93) 1,2,3,4,11,12,13,14,16,17-Decahydro-7-methyl-15*H*-
cyclopenta[a]phenanthren-11-one
MW 254;   mp 102–103°C (Butenandt *et al.*, 1949a)
λ_{max} 261, 311 nm

$C_{18}H_{22}O_2$

(22) 6,7,8,9,11,12,13,14,15,16-Decahydro-3-methoxycyclopenta[a]-
phenanthren-17-one
MW 270
    mp 13β, 149–150°C; 13α, 120–121°C (Loke *et al.*, 1958)
    mp 13β, 161–163°C; 13α, 121–122°C (Johns, 1958)
    mp 13β, 163–164°C; 13α, 120–122°C   (Coombs and Vose, 1974)

$C_{18}H_{22}O_2$

(439) 12-Hydroxy-3-methoxy-6,7,8,12,13,14,16,17-octahydro-15*H*-
cyclopenta[a]phenanthrene
MW 270;   mp 157–161°C   (Robinson and Slater, 1941)

$C_{18}H_{22}O_2$

3-Methoxy-6,7,8,9,11,12,13,14,15,16-decahydrocyclopenta[a]-
phenanthren-15-one
MW 270;   two isomers, mp 160–160.3°C and 116–117°C
                                        (Nazarov *et al.*, 1953)

$C_{19}H_{14}O_2$

(341) 17-Acetoxy-15*H*-cyclopenta[a]phenanthrene [24684-52-4]
MW 274;   mp 210–211°C
λ_{max} 222 (4.48), 269 (4.91), 273 (4.92), 291 (4.28), 312 (3.89),
329 (2.91), 345 (2.83), 363 (2.66) nm
ν_{max} 5.72, 8.24, 11.00, 12.02, 12.28, 12.85, 13.34, 13.88 μm
                                        (Coombs, 1969)

$C_{19}H_{14}O_3$

(397) 2-Acetoxy-15,16-dihydrocyclopenta[a]phenanthren-17-one
[55651-44-0]
MW 290;   mp 248–249°C
λ_{max} 265.5 (5.84), 282.5 (4.46), 296 (4.36), 352 (3.37), 369 (3.39) nm

ν_{max} 5.70 (acetate), 5.90 (aryl CO), 9.85, 10.75 μm
δ 3.44 (15-H$_2$), 2.83 (16-H$_2$), 2.39 (acetate Me)

(Coombs *et al.*, 1975)

$C_{19}H_{14}O_3$

(80) 11-Acetoxy-15,16-dihydrocyclopenta[a]phenanthren-17-one
[24684-58-0]
MW 290;   mp 207°C   (Robinson, 1938)

$C_{19}H_{14}O_3$

(343) 16-Acetoxy-15,16-dihydrocyclopenta[a]phenanthren-17-one
[24684-53-5]
MW 290;   mp 178°C
λ_{max} 266 (4.92), 284 (4.50), 297 (4.39), 352 (3.31), 370 (3.32) nm
ν_{max} 5.70, 8.16, 5.81, 12.14, 12.40, 12.92, 13.16 μm (Coombs, 1969)
δ 3.25 (J 4,17) and 4.3 (J 7.5,17) (H-15), 5.63 (J 4,7.5)

(Coombs *et al.*, 1973a)

$C_{19}H_{14}O_3$

(365) 15-Acetoxy-15,16-dihydrocyclopenta[a]phenanthren-17-one
[50905-55-0]
MW 290;   mp 197–198°C
λ_{max} 269 (4.76), 297 (4.26), 330 (3.10), 349 (3.09), 366 (3.07) nm
ν_{max} 5.74, 5.84, 9.78, 11.69, 12.19, 13.20 μm

(Coombs *et al.*, 1973a)

$C_{19}H_{14}O_4$

(186) 1,6-Dimethoxy-cyclopenta[a]phenanthrene-15,17-dione
MW 306;   Deep yellow needles, mp 281–283°C

(Fieser and Hershberg, 1936)

$C_{19}H_{16}$ **(135)** 11,17-Dimethyl-15H-cyclopenta[a]phenanthrene [5831-10-7]
MW 244;   mp 149–150°C
λ_{max} 222 (4.32), 270 (4.70), 276.5 (4.81), 295 (4.13), 306 (4.13),
317 (3.69), 350 (2.93), 368 (2.83) nm
ν_{max} 10.90, 11.52, 12.20, 13.06, 13.32, 13.86 μm   (Coombs, 1966b)

$C_{19}H_{16}$ **(136)** 12,17-Dimethyl-15H-cyclopenta[a]phenanthrene [5831-09-4]
MW 244;   mp 161–162°C
λ_{max} 222.5 (4.38), 272 (4.81), 276 (4.81), 290 (4.27), 318 (3.88),
349 (2.71), 367 (2.43) nm
ν_{max} 10.96, 11.44, 12.28, 12.34, 13.15, 13.34 μm   (Coombs, 1966b)

$C_{19}H_{16}O$ **(347)** 12-Acetyl-16,17-dihydro-15H-cyclopenta[a]phenanthrene
[2960-75-0]
MW 260;   mp 128°C
λ_{max} 242 (4.50), 262 (4.66), 290.5 (4.03), 320.5 (4.16), 350 (3.50),
369 (3.43) nm
ν_{max} 5.99, 11.45, 12.20, 13.30 μm
δ (CCl$_4$) 2.68 (3H, methyl), 2.0–3.5 (6H), 7.4–7.9 (5H, aromatic),
8.4–8.9 (2H, aromatic)   (Dannenberg *et al.*, 1965)

$C_{19}H_{16}O$ **(309)** 15,16-Dihydro-7,11-dimethylcyclopenta[a]phenanthren-17-one
[85616-56-4]
MW 260;   mp 208–210°C
λ_{max} 275 (4.76), 293 (4.48), 307 (4.29), 368 (3.46), 389 (3.51) nm
ν_{max} 5.96 μm

δ 2.65 (H-16), 2.82 and 2.98 (methyls), 3.63 (H-15)

(Ribeiro *et al.*, 1983)

$C_{19}H_{16}O$ (**131**) 15,16-Dihydro-11,12-dimethylcyclopenta[a]phenanthren-17-one [894-52-0]

MW 260; mp 149–150°C

λ_{max} 218 (4.09), 264 (4.88), 292 (4.45), 304 (4.32), 349 (3.05), 366 (3.34), 383 (3.40) nm

ν_{max} 5.94, 11.40, 12.38, 13.26, 14.00 μm

δ 2.70 (H-16), 2.75 (methyls), 3.17 (H-15)   (Coombs, 1966*a*)

$C_{19}H_{16}O$ (**211**) 15,16-Dihydro-11-ethylcyclopenta[a]phenanthren-17-one [42028-27-3]

MW 260; mp 129–130°C

λ_{max} 264.5 (4.91), 289 (4.47), 302 (4.33), 360 (3.51), 378 (3.54) nm

ν_{max} 5.88, 12.38, 13.36, 13.90, 14.54 μm   (Coombs *et al.*, 1973*b*)

$C_{19}H_{16}O$ (**253**) 15,16-Dihydro-12-ethylcyclopenta[a]phenanthren-17-one

MW 260; mp 206.5–207°C   (Riegel *et al.*, 1948)

$C_{19}H_{16}O$ (**50**) 16,17-Dihydro-17-ethylcyclopenta[a]phenanthren-15-one

MW 260; mp 110–111.2°C (Riegel *et al.*, 1943)

Oxime, mp 169–170.8°C

$C_{19}H_{16}O$ (**134**) 3-Methoxy-17-methyl-15*H*-cyclopenta[a]phenanthrene

MW 260; mp 204–205°C

λ_{max} 223 (4.28), 273 (4.84), 294 (4.22), 304 (4.16), 318 (4.10), 338 (2.92), 355 (3.04), 374 (3.03) nm

ν_{max} 10.94, 11.64, 12.22, 13.10, 13.82 μm   (Coombs, 1966*b*)

$C_{19}H_{16}O$ (**138**) 11-Methoxy-17-methyl-15*H*-cyclopenta[a]phenanthrene [5831-12-9]

MW 260; mp 159–160°C

λ_{max} 221 (4.37), 272 (4.70), 280 (4.74), 287 (4.63), 324 (3.69), 339 (3.29), 356 (3.49), 374 (3.57) nm

ν_{max} 10.92, 11.95, 12.10, 12.20, 12.55, 13.10, 13.35, 13.90 μm

(Coombs, 1966*b*)

$C_{19}H_{16}O_2$

(**333**) 15-Acetoxy-16,17-dihydro-15*H*-cyclopenta[a]phenanthrene

MW 276; mp 127–128°C   (Badger *et al.*, 1952)

$C_{19}H_{16}O_2$

(**390**) 15,16-Dihydro-11-ethoxycyclopenta[a]phenanthren-17-one [83053-57-0]

MW 276; mp 191–193°C

λ_{max} 261 (4.91), 291 (4.54), 362 (3.98), 381 (4.00) nm (Bhatt *et al.*, 1982)

$C_{19}H_{16}O_2$

(**311**) 15,16-Dihydro-4-methoxy-1-methylcyclopenta[a]phenanthren-17-one

MW 276; mp 199–200°C

λ_{max} 262, 302, 366, 384 nm

δ 2.80 (H-16), 3.07 (methyl), 3.40 (H-15), 4.03 (O-methyl)

(Coombs *et al.*, 1985)

$C_{19}H_{16}O_2$

(**468**) 15,16-Dihydro-6-methoxy-11-methylcyclopenta[a]phenanthren-17-one [24684-49-9]

106   *Physical and spectral properties*

MW 276;   mp 203–205°C
v_{max} 5.86, 12.26, 13.18, 13.78 µm   (Coombs, 1969)
$C_{19}H_{16}O_2$
(**447**) 15,16-Dihydro-11-methoxy-7-methylcyclopenta[a]phenanthren-
17-one [30835-61-1]
MW 276;   mp 215–216°C
λ_{max} 267 (4.81), 293.5 (4.37), 321 (3.92), 355 (3.44), 373 (3.74),
393 (3.81) nm   (Coombs and Jaitly, 1971)
$C_{19}H_{16}O_2$
(**368**) 15,16-Dihydro-15-methoxy-11-methylcyclopenta[a]-
phenanthren-17-one [83053-62-7]
MW 276;   mp 158°C
λ_{max} 265, 299.5, 355, 373 nm   (Bhatt *et al.*, 1982)
$C_{19}H_{16}O_2$
(**407**) 17-(16,17-Dihydro-15*H*-cyclopenta[a]phenanthryl)-acetic acid
MW 276;   mp 164–166°C
λ_{max} 215 (4.56), 259 (4.74), 280 (4.19), 288 (4.10), 300 (4.10),
320 (2.65), 327.5 (2.47), 333 (2.83), 342.5 (2.41), 351 (2.83) nm
v_{max} 3.32, 3.75, 3.85, 5.87, 12.35, 13.37 µm
                    (Dannenberg and Dannenberg-von Dresler, 1964)
$C_{19}H_{16}O_3$
(**111**) 8,12,13,14,16,17-Hexahydro-15*H*-cyclopenta[a]phenanthrene-
13,14-dicarboxylic acid anhydride
MW 292;   mp 172–173°C   (Sen Gupta and Bhattacharyya, 1954)
$C_{19}H_{16}O_3$
(**112**) 11,12,13,14,16,17-Hexahydro-15*H*-cyclopenta[a]phenanthrene-
13,14-dicarboxylic acid anhydride
MW 292;   Flakes, mp 183°C   (Sen Gupta and Bhattacharyya, 1954)
$C_{19}H_{16}O_3$
(**426**) 15,16-Dihydro-3,11-dimethoxycyclopenta[a]phenanthren-
17-one
MW 292;   mp 200–201°C   (Robinson, 1938)
$C_{19}H_{16}O_3$
(**387**) 15-(16-Oxo-11,12,13,17-tetrahydro-16*H*-cyclopenta[a]-
phenanthryl)-acetic acid
MW 292;   mp 221–223°C   (Turner, 1949)
$C_{19}H_{17}Cl$
(**172**) 3-Chloro-15,17-dihydro-17,17-dimethylcyclopenta[a]-
phenanthrene [13914-44-8]
MW 280.5;   mp 134°C
λ_{max} 220 (4.66), 224 (4.67), 255 (4.78), 261 (4.84), 283 (4.24),
292 (4.18), 304 (4.26), 323 (2.99), 331 (2.74), 338 (3.24), 347 (2.75),
355 (3.31) nm
v_{max} (KBr) 11.10, 11.62, 11.94, 12.09 µm
                    (Dannenberg and Hebenbrock, 1966)
$C_{19}H_{17}NO$
(**354**) 6-Acetamido-16,17-dihydro-15*H*-cyclopenta[a]phenanthrene
[2960-73-8]

MW 275; mp 273°C
λ_{max} 262 (4.68), 291 (3.97), 304 (4.02), 338 (2.96), 350 (2.81) nm
ν_{max} 3.09, 6.05, 6.51, 11.55, 12.35, 13.25 μm
(Dannenberg et al., 1965)

$C_{19}H_{17}NO$

(**348**) 12-Acetamido-16,17-dihydro-15H-cyclopenta[a]phenanthrene
[2960-79-4]
MW 275; mp 248°C
λ_{max} 222.5 (4.48), 242.5 (4.49), 262.5 (4.81), 303 (4.17), 312 (4.03) nm
ν_{max} 3.05, 6.01, 6.46, 11.52, 12.26, 13.45 μm
δ 2.0–3.5, 7.3–8.0 (5H, aromatic), 8.0–8.6 (2H, aromatic),
8.1 (singlet)   (Dannenberg et al., 1965)

$C_{19}H_{18}$ (**99**) 16,17-Dihydro-2,12-dimethyl-15H-cyclopenta[a]phenanthrene
[3974-81-0]
MW 246; mp 136–137°C (Butenandt et al., 1946c)
λ_{max} 264 (4.71), 284 (4.10), 292 (3.98), 305 (4.08), 322 (2.75),
339 (2.87), 355 (2.84) nm (Dannenberg and Steidle, 1954)
ν_{max} (CS$_2$) 11.60, 12.05 μm   (Dannenberg et al., 1953)

$C_{19}H_{18}$ (**71**) 16,17-Dihydro-3,17-dimethyl-15H-cyclopenta[a]phenanthrene
MW 246; mp 139–140°C   (Kon and Woolman, 1939)

$C_{19}H_{18}$ (**101**) 16,17-Dihydro-4,12-dimethyl-15H-cyclopenta[a]phenanthrene
[63020-70-2]
MW 246; mp 106–107°C (Butenandt et al., 1949b)
λ_{max} 250 (4.59), 264 (4.70), 286 (4.03), 296.5 (4.02), 308.5 (4.13),
339.5 (2.63), 356 (2.24) nm (Dannenberg and Steidle, 1954)
ν_{max} (CS$_2$) 11.62, 12.35, 13.27 μm   (Dannenberg et al., 1953)

$C_{19}H_{18}$ (**110**) 16,17-Dihydro-4,17-dimethyl-15H-cyclopenta[a]phenanthrene
[63020-71-3]
MW 246; mp 130–131°C (Inhoffen et al., 1949); 134.5–136°C
(Woodward et al., 1953)
λ_{max} 216 (4.58), 255 (4.72), 262.5 (4.80), 283 (4.18), 293 (4.16),
306 (4.27), 322.5 (2.77), 338 (2.84), 254 (2.73) nm (Dannenberg and
Neumann, 1961a)
ν_{max} (CS$_2$) 12.34, 12.67 μm   (Dannenberg et al., 1953)

$C_{19}H_{18}$ (**68**) 16,17-Dihydro-6,17-dimethyl-15H-cyclopenta[a]phenanthrene
MW 246; mp 80°C (Gamble and Kon, 1935); 78–78.5°C
(Butenandt and Suranyi, 1942)
λ_{max} 271 (4.82), 282 (4.18), 290 (4.06), 303.5 (4.10), 323 (2.75),
337 (2.88), 354 (2.84) nm (Dannenberg and Steidle, 1954)
ν_{max} (CS$_2$) 11.47, 12.22, 13.27 μm   (Dannenberg et al., 1953)

$C_{19}H_{18}$ (**105**) 16,17-Dihydro-6,7-dimethyl-15H-cyclopenta[a]phenanthrene
[63020-72-4]
MW 246; mp 98–99°C (Butenandt et al., 1946a)
λ_{max} 263.5 (4.78), 286 (4.15), 296.5 (4.04), 307 (3.95), 327 (2.86),
342 (3.02), 358 (3.12) nm (Dannenberg and Steidle, 1954)
ν_{max} (CS$_2$) 12.25, 13.00, 13.31 μm   (Dannenberg et al., 1953)

$C_{19}H_{18}$ (**87**) 16,17-Dihydro-11,12-dimethyl-15H-cyclopenta[a]phenanthrene
[63020-69-9]   MW 246; mp 105–106°C (Butenandt et al., 1946a)

λ_{max} 261 (4.73), 288 (3.96), 300 (3.98), 311 (4.01), 343 (2.83), 360 (2.72) nm   (Dannenberg and Steidle, 1954)

ν_{max} 12.32, 13.37 μm   (Dannenberg *et al.*, 1953)

$C_{19}H_{18}$ (**139**) 16,17-Dihydro-11,17-dimethyl-15*H*-cyclopenta[a]phenanthrene [5831-16-3]

MW 246;   mp 65°C

λ_{max} 219 (4.45), 227 (4.19), 257 (4.80), 294 (4.02), 306 (4.07), 324 (2.85), 339 (3.00), 355 (3.03) nm

ν_{max} 11.40, 12.02, 12.24, 13.28, 13.40, 13.94, 14.60 μm

(Coombs, 1966*b*)

$C_{19}H_{18}$ (**140**) 16,17-Dihydro-12,17-dimethyl-15*H*-cyclopenta[a]phenanthrene [5831-15-2]

MW 246;   mp 56–57°C

λ_{max} 217 (4.63), 261 (4.83), 290 (4.06), 303 (4.13), 321 (2.57), 337 (2.64), 353 (2.41) nm

ν_{max} 11.50, 12.22, 13.42 μm   (Coombs, 1966*b*)

$C_{19}H_{18}$ (**255**) 16,17 Dihydro-12-ethyl-15*H*-cyclopenta[a]phenanthrene [7478-25-3]

MW 246;   mp 64.5–65°C   (Riegel *et al.*, 1948)

$C_{19}H_{18}$ (**52**) 16,17-Dihydro-17-ethyl-15*H*-cyclopenta[a]phenanthrene [17290-34-5]

MW 246;   Irregular platelets, mp 85–86°C (Riegel *et al.*, 1943); 78–79°C (Schontube and Janak, 1968)

Picrate, mp 94.8–96.4°C

$C_{19}H_{18}O$ (**58**) 16,17-Dihydro-3-methoxy-15-methyl-15*H*-cyclopenta[a]phenanthrene

MW 262;   mp 97.5–98°C   (Cohen *et al.*, 1935)

$C_{19}H_{18}O$ 12,12-Dimethyl-11,12,15,16-tetrahydrocyclopenta[a]phenanthren-17-one [5837-18-3]

MW 262;   mp 186–187°C

λ_{max} 219 (4.87), 241 (4.11), 251 (4.16), 262 (4.57), 270 (4.89), 281 (5.00), 324 (4.48), 336 (4.51), 362 (4.25) nm

ν_{max} 5.90, 10.10, 12.30, 12.78, 13.22 μm

δ 1.32 (6H,s,two geminal methyls), 314 (2H,s,C-11 methylene), 2.90 (2H,m,C-15 methylene), 2.7 (2H,m,C-16 methylene)

(Coombs, 1966*a*)

$C_{19}H_{18}O$ (**57**) 16,17-Dihydro-3-methoxy-16-methyl-15*H*-cyclopenta[a]phenanthrene

MW 262;   mp 136.5–137.5°C   (Cohen *et al.*, 1935)

$C_{19}H_{18}O$ (**17**) 16,17-Dihydro-3-methoxy-17-methyl-15*H*-cyclopenta[a]phenanthrene

MW 262;   mp 147.5–148.5°C (Cohen *et al.*, 1935); 149–150°C (Coombs, 1966*b*)

λ_{max} 212 (4.42), 225 (4.30), 236 (4.36), 261 (4.82), 282 (4.20), 291 (4.12), 302 (3.95), 326 (2.83), 341 (3.16), 358 (3.28) nm

ν_{max} 11.64, 12.28, 12.45, 13.80 μm   (Coombs, 1966*b*)

$C_{19}H_{18}O$ (**62**) 16,17-Dihydro-6-methoxy-17-methyl-15*H*-cyclopenta[a]phenanthrene

MW 262; mp 111°C   (Kon and Ruzicka, 1935)

$C_{19}H_{18}O$ **(142)** 16,17-Dihydro-11-methoxy-17-methyl-15*H*-cyclopenta[a]-
phenanthrene
MW 262; Viscous syrup, bp 80°C/10^{-3} mm
λ_{max} 218–220 (4.42), 228 (4.45), 246.5 (4.60), 252.5 (4.59), 276 (4.44),
298 (3.95), 330 (3.25), 345 (3.55), 362 (3.65) nm
ν_{max} 11.92, 12.26, 12.56, 13.30, 13.96 μm   (Coombs, 1966*b*)

$C_{19}H_{18}O$ 7,11-Dimethyl-11,12,15,16-tetrahydrocyclopenta[a]phenanthren-17-
one [85616-55-3]
MW 262; mp 145–146°C
λ_{max} 265 (4.47), 274 (4.75), 285 (4.84), 335 (4.39) nm
ν_{max} 5.94, 6.13, 6.20 μm
δ 1.06 (3H,d,J 7 Hz, CH*Me*), 2.68 (3H,s,aryl methyl)
                                              (Ribeiro *et al.*, 1983)

$C_{19}H_{18}O$ **(250)** 12-Ethyl-11,12,15,16-tetrahydrocyclopenta[a]phenanthren-
17-one
MW 262; mp 102–103°C   (Riegel *et al.*, 1948)

$C_{19}H_{18}O_3$
(332) 3,11-Dimethoxy-6,7,15,16-tetrahydrocyclopenta[a]phenanthren-
17-one
MW 294; mp 143°C (Robinson and Rydon, 1939); 142–143°C
(Corey and Estreicher, 1981)
    dinitrophenylhydrazone, mp 242–243°C
                                              (Robinson and Rydon, 1939)

$C_{19}H_{18}O_3$
(235) 11-Acetoxy-1,2,3,4,15,16-hexahydrocyclopenta[a]phenanthren-
17-one
MW 294; mp 207–208°C
λ_{max} 222 (4.27), 257.5 (4.84), 286 (4.00), 296 (4.04), 307 (3.91),
340 (3.72), 352 (3.81) nm
ν_{max} 5.69, 5.89, 8.30, 9.60, 10.50, 12.40 μm
                                              (Coombs and Bhatt, 1973)

$C_{19}H_{18}O_3$
(201) 17,17-Ethylenedioxy-11,12,13,14,15,16-hexahydrocyclopen-
ta[a]phenanthren-11-one
MW 294; mp 98°C
λ_{max} 216.5, 244, 310 nm
ν_{max} 6.05 μm   (Coombs, 1965)

$C_{19}H_{18}O_3$
(85) 12-Carbomethyoxy-11,12,13,14,16,17-hexahydro-15*H*-cyclopen-
ta[a]phenanthren-11-one
MW 294; mp 149–150°C   (Butenandt *et al.*, 1946*a*)

$C_{19}H_{20}O$ **(353)** 6-Acetyl-11,12,13,14,16,17-hexahydro-15*H*-cyclopenta[a]-
phenanthrene [2960-76-1]
MW 264; mp 73°C
λ_{max} 228 (4.64), 312 (3.84), 333 (3.78) nm
ν_{max} 5.96, 11.30, 13.08 μm
δ 2.73, 3.24, 7.1–7.9, 8.65   (Dannenberg *et al.*, 1965)

$C_{19}H_{20}O_3$

(199) 17,17-Dimethoxy-8,9,11,12,13,14-hexahydrocyclopenta[a]-
phenanthren-11-one
MW 296
ν_{max} 5.85 μm
δ 6.9–7.3 (4H,m), 5.8–6.3 (4H,m), 3.17 (3H,s), 3.09 (3H,s),
2.3–3.5 (6H,m)
m/z 296 (M$^+$), 264 (M$^+$-MeOH), 262 (M$^+$-MeOH-H$_2$)
(Jung and Hudspeth, 1978)

$C_{19}H_{22}$ (48) 11,12,13,14,16,17-Hexahydro-14,17-dimethyl-15H-cyclopenta[a]-
phenanthrene
MW 250; bp 160°C/0.4 mm, n_D 1.60681   (Harper *et al.*, 1934)

$C_{19}H_{22}O$ (56) 11,12,13,14,16,17-Hexahydro-3-methoxy-14-methyl-15H-
cyclopenta[a]phenanthrene
MW 266;   Thick yellowish gum which refused to crystallize
Nitrobenzene derivative scarlet needles, mp 110–110.5°C
(Cohen *et al.*, 1935)

$C_{19}H_{22}O$ (63) 11,12,13,14,16,17-Hexahydro-3-methoxy-17-methyl-15H-
cyclopenta[a]phenanthrene
MW 266;   mp 73–77°C   (Hoffsomner *et al.*, 1966)

$C_{19}H_{24}O$ (16) 3-Methoxy-17-methyl-6,7,8,9,11,12,14,15-octahydro-16H-
cyclopenta[a]phenanthrene
MW 268;   mp 141–146°C   (Cohen *et al.*, 1935)

$C_{19}H_{24}O_3$

(200) 17,17-Dimethoxy-6,7,8,9,11,12,13,14,16,17-decahydro-15H-
cyclopenta[a]phenanthren-11-one
MW 300
δ 3.95 (2H,d,J$_{8,9}$ 10 Hz)   (Jung and Hudspeth, 1978)

$C_{20}H_{15}NO_3$

(430) 15,16-Dihydro-3,11-dimethoxy-16-cyanocyclopenta[a]-
phenanthren-17-one
MW 317   (Robinson and Rydon, 1939)

$C_{20}H_{16}$ (422) 17-Isopropylidenecyclopenta[a]phenanthrene [5830-65-9]
MW 256:   Bright yellow leaflets, mp 188–189°C
λ_{max} 214 (4.44), 228 (4.50), 270 (4.63), 302 (4.67), 310 (4.77),
347 (3.61), 366 (3.50) nm
ν_{max} 6.10, 11.66, 12.00, 12.14, 12.50, 13.20 μm   (Coombs, 1966b)

$C_{20}H_{16}$ (424) 17-(2-Propenyl)-15H-cyclopenta[a]phenanthrene [5837-12-7]
MW 256:   Colourless needles, mp 255°C
λ_{max} 223 (4.40), 271 (4.74), 276 (4.75), 295 (4.30), 3.16 (3.40) nm
ν_{max} 10.20, 10.90, 12.08, 12.38, 12.86, 13.48, 14.60 μm
(Coombs, 1966b)

$C_{20}H_{16}O_2$

(342) 17-Acetoxy-11-methyl-15H-cyclopenta[a]phenanthrene
MW 288   (Coombs, 1969)

$C_{20}H_{16}O_3$

(469) 6-Acetoxy-15,16-dihydro-11-methylcyclopenta[a]phenanthren-
17-one [24684-48-8]

MW 304;   mp 225–227°C   (Coombs, 1969)

$C_{20}H_{16}O_3$

(227) 11-Acetoxy-15,16-dihydro-7-methylcyclopenta[a]phenanthren-17-one

MW 304; mp 243–244°C

δ 2.92 (3H,s,aryl methyl), 2.49 (3H,s,acetate), 2.80 (2H,m, C-16 methylene), 3.76 (2H,m,C-15 methylene)

(Coombs and Jaitly, 1971)

$C_{20}H_{16}O_3$

(72) 11-Acetoxy-15,16-dihydro-3-methylcyclopenta[a]phenanthren-17-one

MW 304;   mp 224°C   (Kon and Woolman, 1939)

$C_{20}H_{16}O_3$

(366) 15-Acetoxy-15,16-dihydro-11-methylcyclopenta[a]phenanthren-17-one [55651-30-4]

MW 304;   mp 209–210°C

λ_{max} 266 (4.81), 301 (4.30), 356 (3.11), 374 (3.19) nm

(Coombs *et al.*, 1975)

$C_{20}H_{16}O_3$

(344) 16-Acetoxy-15,16-dihydro-11-methylcyclopenta[a]phenanthren-17-one [24684-55-7]

MW 304;   mp 156–157°C

λ_{max} 263 (4.87), 288 (4.52), 301 (4.35), 342 (3.12), 357 (3.37), 375 (3.42) nm

ν_{max} 5.72, 5.81, 8.10, 12.02, 12.14, 12.90, 13.18, 13.30, 13.96 μm

(Coombs, 1969)

$C_{20}H_{16}O_3$

11-Acetoxymethyl-15,16-dihydrocyclopenta[a]phenanthren-17-one [55651-35-9]

MW 304;   mp 175–176°C

λ_{max} 265 (4.88), 285 (4.50), 300.5 (4.36), 356 (3.32), 373 (3.44) nm

δ (CD_3SOCD_3), 2.08 (s,acetate), 2.82 (m,16-H_2), 3.12 (m,15-H_2), 5.32 (s,11-CH_2)

m/z 304 (M^+, 100%), 245 (M^+-CH_3CO_2, 20%), 231 (M^+-$CH_2CO_2CH_3$, 30%)   (Coombs *et al.*, 1975)

$C_{20}H_{16}O_4$

(190) 11-Acetoxy-15,16-dihydro-3-methoxycyclopenta[a]phenanthren-17-one

MW 320;   mp 241–242°C   (Robinson and Rydon, 1939)

$C_{20}H_{16}O_4$

(429) 15,16-Dihydro-3,11-dimethoxy-16-formylcyclopenta[a]-phenanthren-17-one

MW 320;   mp 195°C (decomp.)   (Robinson and Rydon, 1939)

$C_{20}H_{18}$ 17-Ethyl-17-methylcyclopenta[a]phenanthrene

MW 258;   mp 117°C, $[\alpha]_D^{23°}$ −63.8° (ethanol)

λ_{max} 221 (4.78), 242 (4.51), 265.5 (4.63), 295 (4.01), 307 (4.16), 319 (4.15), 345 (3.03), 361 (2.62) nm

(Dannenberg and Neumann, 1961*b*)

$C_{20}H_{18}$　(**388**) 17-Isopropyl-15*H*-cyclopenta[a]phenanthrene
MW 258;　mp 153°C (Coombs, 1966*b*); 154–156°C (Dannenberg *et al.*, 1960)
λ_{max} 224 (4.31), 271 (4.70), 275 (4.71), 316 (4.02) nm
ν_{max} 10.26, 10.90, 11.50, 12.22, 12.90, 13.34, 13.66 μm
(Coombs, 1966*b*)

$C_{20}H_{18}$　(**425**) 17-Isopropyl-17*H*-cyclopenta[a]phenanthrene [5830-63-7]
MW 258;　mp 106–107°C
λ_{max} 221 (4.66), 240 (4.33), 269 (4.65), 274 (4.60), 292.5 (4.07), 303 (4.08), 317 (3.95) nm
ν_{max} 10.30, 10.52, 10.76, 10.90, 11.50, 12.30, 13.00, 13.26, 13.65, 14.00 μm
(Coombs, 1966*b*)

$C_{20}H_{18}$　(**137**) 11,12,17-Trimethyl-15*H*-cyclopenta[a]phenanthrene [5831-11-8]
MW 258;　mp 126–126.5°C
λ_{max} 219 (4.35), 280 (4.93), 311 (4.14), 355 (2.78) nm
ν_{max} 10.90, 12.30, 13.18, 13.34, 13.64, 14.90 μm　(Coombs, 1966*b*)

$C_{20}H_{18}O$　(**254**) 15,16-Dihydro-12-isopropylcyclopenta[a]phenanthren-17-one
MW 274;　mp 183.5–184°C　　　　　　(Riegel *et al.*, 1948)

$C_{20}H_{18}O$　(**73**) 3,17-Dimethyl-11-methoxy-15*H*-cyclopenta[a]phenanthrene [5831-18-5]
MW 274;　mp 130–131°C　　　　　　(Kon and Woolman, 1939)

$C_{20}H_{18}O$　(**51**) 16,17-Dihydro-17-isopropylcyclopenta[a]phenanthren-15-one
MW 274;　mp 143.6–144.4°C (Riegel *et al.*, 1943)
oxime, mp 205–211°C

$C_{20}H_{18}O$　(**165**) 3-Hydroxy-1,17,17-trimethylcyclopenta[a]phenanthrene
[isolated as its acetate $C_{22}H_{20}O_2$:
MW 316;　mp 121–122°C
λ_{max} 263, 297, 310, 322
ν_{max} 5.65, 8.13 μm
δ 1.42 (s,17-gem-diMe), 2.38 (s,3-OAc), 3.15 (s,1-Me), 6.75 (d,J 6, 16-H), 7.2–8.8 (m, olefinic and Ar H)
m/z 316 (44%, M$^+$), 275 (23%), 274 (100%, M$^+$-CH$_2$CO), 259 (29%), 244 (15%), 215 (15%)]　　　(Brown and Turner, 1971)

$C_{20}H_{18}O_2$
(**391**) 15,16-Dihydro-11-*n*-propoxycyclopenta[a]phenanthren-17-one [83053-58-1]
MW 290;　mp 181–182°C
λ_{max} 262.5 (4.92), 292 (4.66), 363 (4.05), 382 (4.12) nm
(Bhatt *et al.*, 1982)

$C_{20}H_{18}O_2$
(**392**) 15,16-Dihydro-11-isopropoxycyclopenta[a]phenanthren-17-one [83053-59-2]
MW 290;　mp 172–173°C
λ_{max} 261 (4.78), 292 (4.41), 364 (4.01), 384 (4.05) nm
(Bhatt *et al.*, 1982)

$C_{20}H_{18}O_2$
(**408**) 17-(16,17-Dihydro-15*H*-cyclopenta[a]phenanthyl)-2-propionic acid

MW 290;   mp 235–240°C

λ_{max} 256 nm   (Dannenberg, 1950)

$C_{20}H_{18}O_2$

(409) 17-(16,17-Dihydro-15*H*-cyclopenta[a]phenanthyl)-3-propionic acid

MW 290;   mp 187–190°C

λ_{max} 215 (4.54), 259 (4.80), 280 (4.18), 288 (4.08), 300 (4.06), 320 (278), 327.5 (2.58), 335 (2.94), 342.5 (2.50), 350 (2.88) nm

ν_{max} 3.00, 3.80–3.85, 5.78, 13.20, 13.24 μm

                        (Dannenberg and Dannenberg-von Dressler, 1964)

$C_{20}H_{18}O_4$

(84) 11,12,13,14,16,17-Hexahydro-12-methoxyoxalyl-15*H*-cyclopenta[a]phenanthren-11-one

MW 322;   mp 157–158°C   (Butenandt *et al.*, 1946*a*)

$C_{20}H_{18}O_4$

(216) 17,17-Ethylenedioxy-12-formyl-11,12,13,14,15,16-hexahydrocyclopenta[a]phenanthren-11-one

MW 322;   Large yellow prisms, mp 144–145°C

λ_{max} 218 (4.54), 254.5 (4.13), 362 (3.87) nm

ν_{max} 6.24, 6.30 μm   (Coombs, 1966*a*)

$C_{20}H_{20}$ (36) 15,16-Dihydro-17-ethyl-17-methylcyclopenta[a]phenanthrene [3750-94-5] [81943-50-2]

MW 260;   mp 94–96°C, $[\alpha]_D$ −28° (Bharucha *et al.*, 1962); 97–98.5°C, $[\alpha]_D$ −28.5° (Chinn and Mihina, 1965)

λ_{max} 216 (4.50), 220 (4.46), 253 (4.69), 280 (4.15), 287 (4.05), 300 (4.14), 319 (2.73), 326 (2.53), 334 (2.96), 340 (2.47), 350 (3.00) nm

ν_{max} (CS$_2$) 11.63, 12.28, 13.37, 13.96 μm   (Bharucha *et al.*, 1962)

$C_{20}H_{20}$ (467) 16,17-Dihydro-17-*n*-propyl-15*H*-cyclopenta[a]phenanthrene

MW 260;   mp 88–89°C

ν_{max} (CS$_2$) 12.33, 13.39 μm   (Dannenberg *et al.*, 1953)

$C_{20}H_{20}$ (256) 16,17-Dihydro-12-isopropyl-15*H*-cyclopenta[a]phenanthrene

MW 260;   mp 88.5–89°C   (Riegel *et al.*, 1948)

$C_{20}H_{20}$ (53) 16,17-Dihydro-17-isopropyl-15*H*-cyclopenta[a]phenanthrene [5830-64-8]

MW 260;   Thin plates, mp 97.6–98.4°C (Riegel *et al.*, 1943); 85°, 93°C (Coombs, 1966*b*)

Picrate, mp 108–113°C   (Riegel *et al.*, 1943)

$C_{20}H_{20}$ (69) 16,17-Dihydro-6,17,17-trimethyl-15*H*-cyclopenta[a]phenanthrene [63642-51-3]

MW 260;   mp 96–97°C (Butenandt and Suranyi, 1942)

λ_{max} 262 (4.82), 282 (4.18), 290 (4.06), 303.5 (4.10), 323 (2.76), 337 (2.87), 354 (2.80) nm (Dannenberg and Steidle, 1954)

ν_{max} (CS$_2$) 11.47, 12.22, 13.26 μm   (Dannenberg *et al.*, 1953)

$C_{20}H_{20}$ (141) 16,17-Dihydro-11,12,17-trimethyl-15*H*-cyclopenta[a]phenanthrene [5831-17-4]

MW 260;   mp 75–77°C

114   *Physical and spectral properties*

λ_{max} 218 (4.33), 224.9 (4.26), 261 (4.71), 287 (3.98), 301 (3.97),
312 (4.01), 343 (3.17), 360 (3.07) nm
ν_{max} 11.50, 12.12, 12.56, 13.30, 13.86 μm   (Coombs, 1966b)
$C_{20}H_{20}O$ (74) 16,17-Dihydro-3,17-dimethyl-11-methoxy-15H-cyclopenta[a]-
phenanthrene
MW 276; mp 83–84°C   (Kon and Woolman, 1939)
$C_{20}H_{20}O$ (162) 15,16-Dihydro-3-hydroxy-1,17,17-trimethylcyclopenta[a]-
phenanthrene
MW 276; mp 142–144°C
λ_{max} 263 (4.83), 285 (4.09), 295 (4.01), 306 (3.94), 344 (3.11),
362 (3.11) nm
ν_{max} 3.01, 6.17, 10.00, 11.56, 12.27 μm   (Brown and Turner, 1971)
$C_{20}H_{20}O$ (14)
15,16-Dihydro-17,17-dimethyl-3-methoxycyclopenta[a]phenanthrene
MW 276; mp 166–167°C   (Cohen *et al.*, 1935)
$C_{20}H_{20}O$ (126) 16,17-Dihydro-11-hydroxy-17-isopropyl-15H-cyclopenta[a]-
phenanthrene
MW 276; mp 162°C   (Birch and Robinson, 1944)
$C_{20}H_{20}O$ (251) 12-Isopropyl-11,12,15,16-tetrahydrocyclopenta[a]phenanthren-
17-one
MW 276; mp 115–116°C   (Riegel *et al.*, 1948)
$C_{20}H_{20}O_2$
(400) 16,17-Dihydro-*cis*-16,17-dihydroxy-17-isopropyl-15H-
cyclopenta[a]phenanthrene
MW 292; mp 183°C
λ_{max} 215 (4.56), 251 (4.75), 258 (4.87), 279 (4.21), 287 (4.10),
299 (4.21), 320 (2.67), 334 (2.86), 350 (2.85) nm
ν_{max} 2.99, 9.22, 8.70, 12.30, 13.33 μm   (Dannenberg *et al.*, 1960)
$C_{20}H_{20}O_3$
(209) 17,17-Ethylenedioxy-11,12,13,14,15,16-hexahydro-12-
methylcyclopenta[a]phenanthren-11-one
MW 308; mp 123–124°C
λ_{max} 217 (4.61), 240 (4.32), 310 (3.81) nm
ν_{max} 6.00 μm   (Coombs, 1966a)
$C_{20}H_{20}O_4$
(202) 17,17-Ethylenedioxy-11,12,13,14,15,16-hexahydro-3-methoxy-
cyclopenta[a]phenanthren-11-one
MW 324; mp 114°C
λ_{max} 221 (4.65), 246 (4.49), 310 (3.76) nm
ν_{max} 6.00 μm   (Coombs, 1966a)
$C_{20}H_{22}O_4$
(213) 17,17-Ethylenedioxy-11,12,13,14,15,16-hexahydro-11-hydroxy-
11-hydroxymethylcyclopenta[a]phenanthrene
MW 326; needles, mp 168–170.5°C
λ_{max} 230.5 (4.92), 272.5 (3.74), 282 (3.76), 291 (3.62) nm
δ 3.85 (1H,d, J 11.5, $H_A CH_B OH$), 4.33 (1H,d, J 11.5, $H_B CH_A OH$),
3.96 (4H,s,$OCH_2 CH_2 O$)

m/z 326.1511 (M⁺, 35%), 380 (M⁺-H₂O, 20%), 295
(M⁺-CH₂OH, 100%), 99 (acetal ion, 89%)   (Coombs *et al.*, 1975)

$C_{20}H_{24}O$ **(164)** 3-Hydroxy-11,12,13,14,15,16-hexahydro-1,17,17-
trimethylcyclopenta[a]phenanthrene
MW 280; mp 158–160°C
λ_{max} 263, 283, 294, 307 nm
ν_{max} 3.13 μm
δ 0.90 (s, methyl), 1.10 (s, methyl), 2.88 (s, 1-methyl), 6.80–
7.75 (4H, aromatic)   (Brown and Turner, 1971)

$C_{20}H_{24}O$ **(123)** 17-Isopropyl-6,7,8,9,11,14,16,17-octahydro-15*H*-cyclopenta[a]-
phenanthren-11-one
MW 280; bp 193–195°C/0.08 nm   (Birch and Robinson, 1944)

$C_{20}H_{26}O$ **(13)** 17,17-Dimethyl-3-methoxy-6,7,8,9,11,12,15,16-octahydrocyclo-
penta[a]phenanthrene
MW 282; mp 58–60°C   (Cohen *et al.*, 1935)

$C_{20}H_{28}O$ 6,7,8,9,11,12,13,14,15,16-Decahydro-17α-ethyl-17-methylcyclopen-
ta[a]phenanthren-3-ol
MW 284; mp 152–153.5°C, $[\alpha]_{D}$ −17°
λ_{max} 279.5, 286 nm
ν_{max} (KBr) 3.07, 6.22, 6.32 μm   (Chinn and Mihina, 1965)

$C_{21}H_{14}$ **(416)** 16,17-Benzo-15*H*-cyclopenta[a]phenanthrene
MW 266; mp 331–332°C
      (Nasipuri and Roy, 1961; Ruzicka and Goldberg, 1937)

$C_{21}H_{18}O_{2}$
(405) Ethyl 17-(cyclopenta[a]phenanthrylidene)-acetate
MW 302; mp 183–184°C
λ_{max} 215 (4.34), 274 (4.68), 285 (4.63), 299 (4.67), 314–324 (4.53),
355 (3.85), 373 (3.80) nm
ν_{max} (KBr) 5.88, 6.13, 8.5–8.7, 9.63, 9.74, 11.65, 12.12, 12.43, 12.89,
13.28 μm   (Dannenberg *et al.*, 1964)

$C_{21}H_{18}O_{4}$
(109) *cis*-15,16-Diacetoxy-16,17-dihydro-15*H*-cyclopenta[a]-
phenanthrene [42122-92-9]
MW 334; mp 189–191°C
λ_{max} 223 (4.29), 255 (4.76), 279 (4.13), 287.5 (4.06), 299.5 (4.11),
319 (2.58), 325.5 (2.49), 334 (2.59), 340 (2.35), 350 (2.23) nm
ν_{max} 5.90, 12.26, 13.25 μm   (Coombs and Hall, 1973)

$C_{21}H_{18}O_{4}$
cis-16,17-Diacetoxy-16,17-dihydro-15*H*-cyclopenta[a]phenanthrene
[42122-93-0]
MW 344; mp 173–175°C
λ_{max} 249.5 (4.74), 256.5 (4.87), 278.5 (4.20), 286 (4.09), 298 (4.18),
319.5 (2.63), 327.5 (2.48), 333.5 (2.82), 343 (2.43), 350 (2.82) nm
ν_{max} 5.75, 12.24, 13.26 μm
δ H$_{A}$-15, 3.42 (J 16,5); H$_{B}$-15, 3.70 (J 16,7); H-16, 4.28 m;
H-17, 6.42 d (J 6)   (Coombs and Hall, 1973)

$C_{21}H_{20}$ 1,17-Dimethyl-17-ethylcyclopenta[a]phenanthrene

MW 272;   mp 123–124°C, $[\alpha]_D^{23°}$ −56.2 (alcohol)
λ_{max} 224 (4.70), 244 (4.40), 266 (4.64), 297.5 (4.01), 309 (4.32), 322 (4.23), 347 (2.91), 364 (2.63) nm

(Dannenberg and Neumann, 1961b)

$C_{21}H_{20}O$ (212) 11-*n*-Butyl-15,16-dihydrocyclopenta[a]phenanthren-17-one [63642-51-3]
MW 288;   mp 113–114°C
λ_{max} 264.5 (4.90), 289.5 (4.45), 302 (4.32), 360 (3.41), 377 (3.46) nm
ν_{max} 5.90, 11.44, 12.72, 13.40, 14.08 μm   (Coombs *et al.*, 1973b)

$C_{21}H_{20}O_2$
(393) 11-*n*-Butoxy-15,16-dihydrocyclopenta[a]phenanthren-17-one [83053-60-5]
MW 304;   mp 156–157°C
λ_{max} 261.5 (4.87), 292 (4.44), 363.5 (3.76), 382 (3.82) nm

(Bhatt *et al.*, 1982)

$C_{21}H_{20}O_2$
(410) 17-(16,17-Dihydro-15*H*-cyclopenta[a]phenanthryl)-3-butyric acid
MW 304;   mp 157–159°C
λ_{max} 257 (4.79) nm   (Dannenberg, 1950)

$C_{21}H_{20}O_6$
(118) 1,2,3,4,5,6,7,11,12,13,16,17-Dodecahydro-15*H*-cyclopenta[a]phenanthrene-6,7,11,12-tetracarboxylic-acid-6,7,11,12-dianhydride
MW 368;   mp 249–251°C
λ_{max} 255.5 (4.28) nm   (Butz *et al.*, 1940)

$C_{21}H_{21}NO_2$
(351) 12-Diacetylamino-6,7,16,17-tetrahydro-15*H*-cyclopenta[a]phenanthrene
MW 319;   mp 151°C
λ_{max} 211 (4.77), 273 (4.31), 284 (4.18), 301 (3.55) nm
ν_{max} 5.85, 13.03 μm
δ 2.3 (10 aliphatic), 7.15–7.35 (5 aromatic)

(Dannenberg *et al.*, 1965)

$C_{21}H_{21}O_5P$
(228) 15,16-Dihydro-17-oxocyclopenta[a]phenanthren-11-ol diethylphosphate [30835-59-7]
λ_{max} 262 (4.83), 288.5 (4.48), 302 (4.32), 340 (3.27), 357 (3.52), 375 (3.59) nm
ν_{max} 5.90, 7.9, 9.8 μm   (Coombs and Jaitly, 1971)

$C_{21}H_{22}$ (76) 15,16-Dihydro-4,17-dimethyl-17-ethylcyclopenta[a]phenanthrene
MW 274;   mp 145–147°C   (Brown and Kupchan, 1962)

$C_{21}H_{22}$ (37) 16,17-Dihydro-15-isopropyl-4-methyl-15*H*-cyclopenta[a]phenanthrene [72814-88-1] [77327-08-3]
MW 272   (Laflamme and Hites, 1979)

$C_{21}H_{22}O$ (127) 16,17-Dihydro-17-isopropyl-3-methoxy-15*H*-cyclopenta[a]phenanthrene
MW 290;   mp 129°C   (Birch and Robinson, 1944)

$C_{21}H_{22}O_3$

(210) 17,17-Ethylenedioxy-12,12-dimethyl-11,12,13,14,15,16-hexa-
hydrocyclopenta[a]phenanthren-11-one
MW 322; mp 167°C
λ_{max} 217 (4.35), 244 (4.14), 306 (3.59) nm
ν_{max} 5.95 μm   (Coombs, 1966a)

$C_{21}H_{22}O_4$

(203) 11,11:17,17-Bis(ethylenedioxy)-11,12,13,14,15,16-
hexahydrocyclopenta[a]phenanthrene
MW 338; mp 170°C   (Coombs, 1966a)

$C_{21}H_{26}$ (125) 6,7,8,14,16,17-Hexahydro-17-isopropyl-11-methyl-15*H*-
cyclopenta[a]phenanthrene
MW 278; Colourless oil, bp 190°C/0.1 mm
                                          (Birch and Robinson, 1944)

$C_{21}H_{26}O_2$

(124) 17-Isopropyl-3-methoxy-6,7,8,9,11,14,16,17-octahydro-15*H*-
cyclopenta[a]phenanthren-11-one
MW 310; Yellow glass, bp 128–134°C/0.15 mm
                                          (Birch and Robinson, 1944)

$C_{22}H_{18}O_5$

(466) 2,15-Diacetoxy-15,16-dihydrocyclopenta[a]phenanthren-17-one
[55081-27-1]
MW 362
λ_{max} 267 nm
ν_{max} 5.76, 5.81, 5.88 μm   (Coombs and Crawley, 1974)

$C_{22}H_{18}O_6$

(464) 2,15-Diacetoxy-8,9-epoxy-11-methyl-8,9-secogona-
1,3,5,7,9,11,13-heptaen-17-one
MW 378; mp 208–210°C
λ_{max} 267, 298sh, 356, 374 nm
ν_{max} 5.68, 5.76, 5.83 μm   (Coombs and Crawley, 1974)

$C_{22}H_{20}O_2$

(406) Ethyl 17-(cyclopenta[a]phenanthrylidene)-2-propionate
MW 316; mp 92–93°C   (Dannenberg, 1950)

$C_{22}H_{20}O_2$

(419) 15,16-Dihydro-16-(3-oxopentyl)cyclopenta[a]phenanthren-
17-one
MW 316; mp 165–166°C   (Buchta and Kraetzer, 1962)

$C_{22}H_{20}O_3$

(403) Ethyl 17-(11-methoxycyclopenta[a]phenanthrylidene)-acetate
MW 332; mp 144°C   (Robinson and Slater, 1941)

$C_{22}H_{20}O_4$

(446) 16,17-Dihydro-11-methyl-15*H*-cyclopenta[a]phenanthrene-*cis*-
16,17-diacetate [42123-07-9]
MW 348; mp 192.5–193°C
λ_{max} 226 (4.15), 254.5 (4.88), 281 (4.11), 292 (4.06), 303.5 (4.14),
323.5 (2.81), 338.5 (2.97), 354 (2.98) nm
ν_{max} 5.75, 7.97, 8.08, 12.23 μm

δ H-15, 3.35 (J 16,4); H-15, 3.64 (J 16,6); H-16, 5.69;
H-17, d 6.39 (J 6)   (Coombs and Hall, 1973)

$C_{22}H_{20}O_4$

16,17-Dihydro-11-methyl-15H-cyclopenta[a]phenanthrene-*trans*-
16,17-diacetate [42123-08-0] [63780-58-5]
MW 348;   mp 156–157°C
λ_{max} 224 (4.14), 254 (4.88), 280.5 (4.09), 292 (4.05), 304 (4.15),
323 (2.80), 338 (2.97), 354 (2.97) nm
ν_{max} 5.79, 7.95, 8.07 μm
δ H$_A$-15, 3.16 (J 17,4); H$_B$-15, 3.90 (J 17,8); H-16, 5.58;
H-17, d 6.42 (J 4)   (Coombs and Hall, 1973)

$C_{22}H_{22}O_2$

(**394**) 15,16-Dihydro-11-*n*-pentoxycyclopenta[a]phenanthren-17-one
[83053-61-6]
MW 318;   mp 138–138.5°C
λ_{max} 262 (4.88), 293 (4.52), 363 (4.09), 382 (4.13) nm
                                            (Bhatt *et al.*, 1982)

$C_{22}H_{22}O_4$

(**214**) 11-Acetoxymethyl-17,17-ethylenedioxy-13,14,15,16-
tetrahydrocyclopenta[a]phenanthrene
MW 350
λ_{max} 237.5 (4.81), 303 (3.88), 315 (3.87), 336 (3.59) nm
                                            (Coombs *et al.*, 1975)

$C_{22}H_{23}O_5P$

(**229**) 15,16-Dihydro-7-methyl-17-oxocyclopenta[a]phenanthren-11-ol
diethylphosphate [30835-64-4]
MW 397;   Brown crystals, mp 140–142°C
λ_{max} 266, 291, 305, 350, 368, 396 nm
ν_{max} 5.88, 7.82, 9.70 μm   (Coombs and Jaitly, 1971)

$C_{22}H_{24}$ (**39**) 16,17-Dihydro-17-isopentyl-15H-cyclopenta[a]phenanthrene
[21549-34-8]
MW 288;   mp 115°C   (Wilk and Taupp, 1969)

$C_{22}H_{24}O_5$

(**204**) 11,11:17,17-Bis(ethylenedioxy)-11,12,13,14,15,16-hexahydro-3-
methoxycyclopenta[a]phenanthrene
MW 368;   mp 174°C   (Coombs, 1966*a*)

$C_{22}H_{30}O_3$

(**445**) Ethyl 17-(6,7,8,9,11,12,13,14,16,17-decahydro-3-methoxy-15H-
cyclopenta[a]phenanthryl)acetate
MW 342;   bp 208–215°C/0.4 mm   (Robinson and Slater, 1941)

$C_{23}H_{16}O$ (**328**) 15,16-Dihydro-15-phenylcyclopenta[a]phenanthren-17-one
[50558-60-6]
MW 308;   White needles, mp 222°C
ν_{max} 5.87, 12.05 μm
δ 1.25–3.10 (13H, aromatic), 5.05 (q,CH), 6.46–7.57 [H-15 and
H-16, 2q, J$_{15,16}$ (*trans*) 7.7, J$_{15,16}$ (*cis*) 2.6, J$_{16,16}$ 19.2]
                                            (Shotter *et al.*, 1973)

$C_{23}H_{20}O_4$

    (**414**) Methyl 15,16-dihydro-17-oxo-16-(3-oxobutyl)cyclopenta[a]-
phenanthrene-16-carboxylate

    MW 360; mp 170°C   (Nasipuri and Roy, 1961)

$C_{23}H_{22}O_4$

    (**404**) Ethyl 17-(3,11-dimethoxycyclopenta[a]phenanthrylidene)-
acetate

    MW 362; mp 192°C   (Robinson and Slater, 1941)

$C_{23}H_{24}O_2$

    (**395**) 15,16-Dihydro-11-*n*-hexoxycyclopenta[a]phenanthren-17-one

    MW 332; mp 136–137°C

    λ_{max} 246 (4.96), 279 (4.78), 303 (4.30), 349 (4.07)

                            (Bhatt, unpublished data)

$C_{24}H_{15}NO_3$

    11-Benzoxazol-2-yloxy-15,16-dihydrocyclopenta[a]phenanthren-17-
one [30835-62-2]

    MW 365; mp 237–238°C

    λ_{max} 229, 263, 285, 300, 338, 355, 373 nm   (Coombs and Jaitly, 1971)

$C_{24}H_{16}$ (**420**) 17-Benzylidenecyclopenta[a]phenanthrene [5830-62-6]

    MW 292; Orange needles, mp 262-263°C

    λ_{max} 249 (4.52), 328 (4.65), 384 (4.07) nm

    ν_{max} 12.05, 12.47, 13.12, 13.38, 14.44 μm   (Coombs, 1966*b*)

$C_{24}H_{16}O$ (**330**) 17-Methyl-16-phenylcyclopenta[a]phenanthren-15-one

    [27983-36-4]

    MW 320   (Mladenova-Olinova *et al.*, 1970)

$C_{24}H_{18}O_2$

    (**146**) 16,17-Dihydro-15-hydroxy-15*H*-cyclopenta[a]phenanthrene
benzoate

    MW 338; mp 176–177°C   (Badger *et al.*, 1952)

$C_{24}H_{18}O_4S$

    11-Hydroxy-17-oxo-cyclopenta[a]phenanthrene tosylate [54206-57-4]

                           (Kawarura *et al.*, 1974)

$C_{24}H_{20}$ (**423**) 17-Benzyl-16,17-dihydro-15*H*-cyclopenta[a]phenanthrene

    [5830-61-5]

    MW 260; mp 156–157°C

    λ_{max} 216 (4.46), 260 (4.81), 281 (4.20), 289 (4.08), 301 (4.14),
320 (2.77), 336 (2.98), 352 (3.00) nm

    ν_{max} 12.10, 12.36, 12.96, 13.30, 13.48, 14.28 μm   (Coombs, 1966*b*)

$C_{24}H_{20}O_3S$

    (**147**) 16,17-Dihydro-15-hydroxy-15*H*-cyclopenta[a]phenanthrene
tosylate

    MW 388   (Coombs and Hall, 1973)

$C_{24}H_{20}O_3S$

    (**145**) 16,17-Dihydro-17-hydroxy-15*H*-cyclopenta[a]phenanthrene
tosylate [5837-15-0]

    MW 388; Leaflets, mp 178–179°C

    λ_{max} 220 (4.48), 259 (4.83), 279 (4.23), 288 (4.09), 300 (4.15) nm

ν_{max} 11.40, 12.24, 12.80, 12.95, 14.00, 14.30, 14.68 μm

(Coombs, 1966*b*)

$C_{24}H_{22}O_4$

(**415**) Methyl 15,16-dihydro-17-oxo-16-(3-oxopentyl)cyclopenta[a]-phenanthrene-16-carboxylate

MW 374;   mp 157°C   (Nasipuri and Roy, 1961)

$C_{24}H_{22}O_7$

(**461**) 1α,2β,15-Triacetoxy-1,2,15,16-tetrahydro-11-methylcyclopenta[a]phenanthren-17-one

MW 422;   mp 170–171°C

λ_{max} 268 (4.64), 322 (4.05), 333 (4.07), 370 (3.50) nm

ν_{max} 5.75, 5.85, 9.80 μm

δ H-1, 7.11 ($J_{1,2}$ 2); H-2, 5.47 ($J_{1,2}$ 2, $J_{2,3}$ 6); H-3, 6.28 ($J_{2,3}$ 5, $J_{3,4}$ 9); H-4, 6.95 ($J_{3,4}$ 9); H-6, 7.55 ($J_{6,7}$ 9); H-7, 8.11 ($J_{6,7}$ 9); H-12, 7.56; H-15, 6.70 ($J_{15,16}$ 1.5, $J_{15,16}$ 6); H-16, 3.28 ($J_{15,16}$ 6, $J_{16,16}$ 19); H-16, 2.62 ($J_{15,16}$ 1.5, $J_{16,16}$ 19); 11-CH$_3$, 2.93

(Coombs and Crawley, 1974)

$C_{25}H_{18}O_2$

(**208**) 16-Benzylidene-15,16-dihydro-3-methoxycyclopenta[a]-phenanthren-17-one

MW 350;   Yellow needles, mp 223–224°C

(Koebner and Robinson, 1941)

$C_{25}H_{22}O_2$

(**207**) 16-Benzylidene-11,12,13,14,15,16-hexahydro-3-methoxy-cyclopenta[a]phenanthren-17-one

MW 354   (Koebner and Robinson, 1941)

$C_{25}H_{22}O_3S$

(**149**) 16,17-Dihydro-17-hydroxy-11-methyl-15*H*-cyclopenta[a]-phenanthrene tosylate

MW 402

ν_{max} 9.71, 9.90 μm   (Coombs and Hall, 1973)

$C_{26}H_{21}N$ (**421**) 17-*p*-Dimethylaminobenzylidenecyclopenta[a]phenanthrene [5831-06-1]

MW 347;   Yellow crystals, mp 248–250°C

λ_{max} 371 (4.18), 434 (4.58) nm

ν_{max} 12.15, 12.32, 12.58, 13.24, 13.50 μm   (Coombs, 1966*b*)

$C_{26}H_{30}$ (**151**) 17-Methyl-17-[2(6-methyl)-heptyl]-cyclopenta[a]phenanthrene

MW 342;   mp 138–139°C, $[\alpha]_D^{26°}$ $-75°$ (CHCl$_3$)

λ_{max} 221 (4.83), 241.5 (4.56), 265 (4.66), 294.5 (4.05), 306.5 (4.18), 319.5 (4.18), 345 (3.07), 362 (2.98) nm

ν_{max} (KBr) 12.18, 12.63, 13.24 μm

δ 0.59 (d,J 6.5), 0.88 (d,J 6.0), 1.38(s), 6.4–8.8(m)

(Dannenberg *et al.*, 1964)

$C_{26}H_{32}$ (**27**) 15,16-Dihydro-17-methyl-17-[2(6-methyl)-heptyl]-cyclopenta[a]-phenanthrene [80382-29-2]

MW 344

δ 0.74 (3H,d,J 6.5), 0.88 (6H,d,J 6.5), 1.33 (3H,s), 2.29 (2H,m), 3.23 (2H,m), 7.43–8.58 (8H,m)

m/z 344 (M$^+$, 4%), 231 (M$^+$-C$_8$H$_{17}$, 100%),
216 (M$^+$-C$_8$H$_{17}$-CH$_3$, 8%)   (Ludwig *et al.*, 1981)

C$_{27}$H$_{30}$ **(170)** 17-Methyl-17-[2(5,6-dimethyl)hept-3-enyl]-cyclopenta[a]phenanthrene [13914-42-6]
MW 354; mp 131°C
λ_{max} 222 (4.84), 242.5 (4.58), 267.5 (4.67), 295 (4.06), 307 (4.19), 320 (4.18), 346 (3.08) nm
ν_{max} (KBr) 12.17, 12.61, 13.21 μm
     (Dannenberg and Hebenbrock, 1966)

C$_{27}$H$_{32}$ **(152)** 1,17-Dimethyl-17-[2(6-methyl)-heptyl]-cyclopenta[a]phenanthrene
MW 356; oil, $[\alpha]_D^{13°}$ $-75.7°$ (CHCl$_3$)
λ_{max} 224 (4.74), 245 (4.46), 264 (4.69), 297 (4.06), 309 (4.25), 322 (4.25), 347 (2.94), 364 (2.70) nm
ν_{max} 12.14, 13.27 μm
δ 6.4–8.8 (aromatic and olefinic protons), 3.12 (1-methyl), 1.38 (17-methyl)   (Dannenberg *et al.*, 1964)

C$_{27}$H$_{32}$ **(153)** 4,17-Dimethyl-17-[2(6-methyl)-heptyl]-cyclopenta[a]-phenanthrene [26231-18-5]
MW 356; mp 152°C, $[\alpha]_D^{23°}$ $-57.8°$ (CHCl$_3$)
λ_{max} 224 (4.75), 237 (4.43), 244 (4.56), 272.5 (4.59), 280 (4.46), 298 (4.06), 310 (4.24), 323 (4.23), 347 (3.01), 364 (2.79) nm
     (Dannenberg and Neumann, 1961*b*)

C$_{27}$H$_{34}$ **(30)** 15,16-Dihydro-1,17-dimethyl-17-[2-(6-methyl)-heptyl]-cyclopenta[a]phenanthrene [80382-27-0]
MW 358; oil, $[\alpha]_D^{25°}$ $-22.4°$ (CHCl$_3$)
λ_{max} 213 (4.45), 226.5 (4.25), 257 (4.89), 282 (4.13), 293 (4.08), 305.5 (4.18), 337 (2.70), 353 (2.60), 364 (2.64) nm
ν_{max} (CS$_2$) 12.19, 13.23, 13.96 μm (Dannenberg *et al.*, 1964)
δ 0.78 (3H,d,J 6.8), 0.91 (6H,d,J 6.8), 1.38 (3H,s), 2.34 (2H,m), 3.17 (3H,s), 392. (2H,m), 7.50–8.72 (7H,m)
m/z 358 (M$^+$, 4%), 245 (M$^+$-C$_8$H$_{17}$, 100%), 230 (M$^+$-C$_8$H$_{17}$-CH$_3$, 10%), 215 (M$^+$-C$_8$H$_{17}$-2CH$_3$, 10%)   (Ludwig *et al.*, 1981)

C$_{27}$H$_{34}$ **(33)** 15,16-Dihydro-4,17-dimethyl-17-[2(6-methyl)-heptyl]cyclopenta[a]phenanthrene [80382-25-8]
MW 358; mp 140°C, $[\alpha]_D^{23°}$ -11.8 (CHCl$_3$)
λ_{max} 216 (4.58), 255 (4.71), 263 (4.79), 283.5 (4.13), 294 (4.10), 306 (4.22), 322 (2.76), 337.5 (2.81), 354 (2.69) nm (Dannenberg and Neumann, 1961*b*)
δ 0.73 (3H,d,J 6.8), 0.87 (6H,d,J 6.5), 1.34 (3H,s), 2.31 (2H,m), 2.75 (3H,s), 3.29 (2H,m), 7.50–8.57 (7H,m)
m/z 358 (M$^+$, 4%), 245 (M$^+$-C$_8$H$_{17}$, 100%), 230 (M$^+$-C$_8$H$_{17}$-CH$_3$, 8%), 215 (M$^+$-C$_8$H$_{17}$-2CH$_3$, 8%)   (Ludwig *et al.*, 1981)

C$_{27}$H$_{34}$O$_2$
15,16-Dihydro-15,16-dihydroxy-4,17-dimethyl-17-[2(6-methyl)-heptyl]cyclopenta[a]phenanthrene
MW 390; mp 87°C
λ_{max} 216 (4.53), 229 (4.23), 253 (4.72), 261 (4.80), 282 (4.16),

292.5 (4.13), 305 (4.23), 320 (2.76), 336 (2.74), 352 (2.42) nm

ν_{max} (KBr) 2.96, 9.40 μm   (Dannenberg and Neumann, 1961*a*)

$C_{29}H_{38}$ (**32**) 15,16-Dihydro-1,17-dimethyl-17-[2-(5-ethyl-6-methyl)-heptyl]cyclopenta[a]phenanthrene [80382-28-1]

MW 386

δ 0.75 (3H,d,J 6.8), 0.84 (6H,d,J 6.8), 0.86 (3H,t,J 7.6),
1.35 (3H,s), 2.31 (2H,m), 3.13 (3H,s), 3.28 (2H,m),
7.44–8.78 (7H,m)

m/z 386 (M$^+$, 3%), 245 (M$^+$-$C_{10}H_{21}$, 100%), 230 (M$^+$-$C_{10}H_{21}$-CH_3,
7%), 215 (M$^+$-$C_{10}H_{21}$-2CH$_3$, 7%)   (Ludwig *et al.*, 1981)

$C_{29}H_{38}$ (**35**) 15,16-Dihydro-4,17-dimethyl-17-[2-(5-ethyl-6-methyl)heptyl]cyclopenta[a]phenanthrene

MW 386

δ 0.75 (3H,d,J 6.5), 0.86 (3H,t,J 6.5), 0.87 (6H,d,J 6.5),
1.33 (3H,s), 2.72 (3H,s), 3.30 (2H,m), 7.30–8.25 (7H,m)

m/z 386 (M$^+$, 4%), 245 (M$^+$-$C_{10}H_{21}$, 100%), 230 (M$^+$-$C_{10}H_{21}$-CH_3,
7%), 215 (M$^+$-$C_{10}H_{21}$-2CH$_3$, 7%)   (Ludwig *et al.*, 1981)

$C_{31}H_{38}O_4$

15,16-Diacetoxy-15,16-dihydro-4,17-dimethyl-17-[2(6-methyl)-heptyl]cyclopenta[a]phenanthrene

MW 474; $[\alpha]_D^{23°}$ +29° (ethanol)

λ_{max} 216 (4.58), 221 (4.40), 253 (4.73), 261 (4.80), 282.5 (4.20),
293 (4.17), 305.5 (4.25), 320 (2.94), 336 (2.93), 352 (2.83) nm

ν_{max} 5.76, 8.10, 9.5, 12.17, 12.55, 13.10 μm

(Dannenberg and Neumann, 1961*a*)

$C_{36}H_{26}O_3$

(**217**) Bis(15,16-dihydro-17-oxocyclopenta[a]phenanthr-12-ylmethyl)
ether [5837-22-0]

MW 506; mp 229–233°C

λ_{max} 219, 267.5, 286, 298, 338, 353, 371 nm

ν_{max} 5.92, 12.32, 13.36, 13.68, 14.50 μm   (Coombs, 1966*a*)

$C_{36}H_{28}$ (**129**) 16-[17-(16,17-Dihydro-17-methyl-15*H*-cyclopenta[a]-phenanthryl)]-17-methyl-15*H*-cyclopenta[a]phenanthrene

λ_{max} 261.5 (4.76), 273 (4.80), 283.5 (4.92), 300.5 (4.44), 324 (4.13) nm

ν_{max} 11.60, 12.32, 13.40, 13.88 μm   (Coombs, 1966*b*)

$C_{39}H_{30}O_6$

(**428**) 16,16'-Di(17-oxo-3,11-dimethoxycyclopenta[a]phenanthryl)-
methine

MW 594; mp 301–302°C   (Robinson and Rydon, 1939)

5.4   Index relating serial numbers assigned to cyclopenta[a]-phenanthrenes appearing in the text, tables, and figures to their molecular formulae

Serial No.	Molecular formula	Serial No.	Molecular formula	Serial No.	Molecular formula
1	$C_{17}H_{14}$	3	$C_{17}H_{12}$	7	$C_{18}H_{16}$
2	$C_{17}H_{12}$	4	$C_{17}H_{12}O$	11	$C_{18}H_{16}O$

Serial No.	Molecular formula	Serial No.	Molecular formula	Serial No.	Molecular formula
13	$C_{20}H_{26}O$	76	$C_{21}H_{22}$	136	$C_{19}H_{16}$
14	$C_{20}H_{20}O$	80	$C_{19}H_{14}O_3$	137	$C_{20}H_{18}$
16	$C_{19}H_{24}O$	82	$C_{17}H_{16}O$	138	$C_{19}H_{16}O$
17	$C_{19}H_{18}O$	83	$C_{18}H_{16}$	139	$C_{19}H_{18}$
22	$C_{18}H_{22}O_2$	84	$C_{20}H_{18}O_4$	140	$C_{19}H_{18}$
23	$C_{17}H_{12}O_2$	85	$C_{19}H_{18}O_3$	141	$C_{20}H_{20}$
24	$C_{18}H_{14}O_2$	86	$C_{18}H_{18}O$	142	$C_{19}H_{18}O$
26	$C_{18}H_{14}O$	87	$C_{19}H_{18}$	143	$C_{18}H_{14}$
27	$C_{26}H_{32}$	93	$C_{18}H_{22}O$	145	$C_{24}H_{20}O_3S$
30	$C_{27}H_{34}$	94	$C_{18}H_{16}$	146	$C_{24}H_{18}O_2$
32	$C_{29}H_{38}$	96	$C_{17}H_{18}O$	147	$C_{24}H_{20}O_3S$
33	$C_{27}H_{34}$	97	$C_{18}H_{16}$	148	$C_{18}H_{12}O_2$
35	$C_{29}H_{38}$	98	$C_{18}H_{16}$	149	$C_{25}H_{22}O_3S$
36	$C_{20}H_{20}$	99	$C_{19}H_{18}$	150	$C_{18}H_{14}$
37	$C_{21}H_{22}$	100	$C_{18}H_{16}$	151	$C_{26}H_{30}$
38	$C_{17}H_{14}O$	101	$C_{19}H_{18}$	152	$C_{27}H_{32}$
39	$C_{22}H_{24}$	102	$C_{17}H_{12}O$	153	$C_{27}H_{32}$
44	$C_{17}H_{18}$	103	$C_{17}H_{16}O_2$	162	$C_{20}H_{20}O$
45	$C_{18}H_{16}$	104	$C_{17}H_{12}O_2$	164	$C_{20}H_{24}O$
46	$C_{18}H_{16}$	105	$C_{19}H_{18}$	165	$C_{20}H_{18}O$
48	$C_{19}H_{22}$	107	$C_{18}H_{16}$	170	$C_{27}H_{30}$
49	$C_{18}H_{14}O$	109	$C_{21}H_{18}O_4$	172	$C_{19}H_{17}Cl$
50	$C_{19}H_{16}O$	110	$C_{19}H_{18}$	174	$C_{17}H_{14}O$
51	$C_{20}H_{18}O$	111	$C_{19}H_{16}O_3$	176	$C_{17}H_{14}$
52	$C_{19}H_{18}$	112	$C_{19}H_{16}O_3$	179	$C_{17}H_{14}O$
53	$C_{20}H_{20}$	114	$C_{17}H_{16}O_2$	185	$C_{17}H_{10}O_2$
56	$C_{19}H_{22}O$	115	$C_{17}H_{16}O_2$	186	$C_{19}H_{14}O_4$
57	$C_{19}H_{18}O$	116	$C_{17}H_{14}O_2$	190	$C_{20}H_{16}O_4$
58	$C_{19}H_{18}O$	118	$C_{21}H_{20}O_6$	193	$C_{17}H_{14}O_2$
59	$C_{18}H_{16}O$	123	$C_{20}H_{24}O$	194	$C_{18}H_{16}O_3$
61	$C_{18}H_{16}O$	124	$C_{21}H_{26}O_2$	199	$C_{19}H_{20}O_3$
62	$C_{19}H_{18}O$	125	$C_{21}H_{26}$	200	$C_{19}H_{24}O_3$
63	$C_{19}H_{22}O$	126	$C_{20}H_{20}O$	201	$C_{19}H_{18}O_3$
66	$C_{18}H_{16}O_2$	127	$C_{21}H_{22}O$	202	$C_{20}H_{20}O_4$
67	$C_{18}H_{16}$	128	$C_{18}H_{14}$	203	$C_{21}H_{22}O_4$
68	$C_{19}H_{18}$	129	$C_{36}H_{28}$	204	$C_{22}H_{24}O_5$
69	$C_{20}H_{20}$	130	$C_{18}H_{14}O$	205	$C_{17}H_{16}O$
70	$C_{18}H_{16}$	131	$C_{19}H_{16}O$	206	$C_{17}H_{12}O_2$
71	$C_{19}H_{18}$	132	$C_{18}H_{14}O_2$	207	$C_{25}H_{22}O_2$
72	$C_{20}H_{16}O_3$	133	$C_{18}H_{14}$	208	$C_{25}H_{18}O_2$
73	$C_{20}H_{18}O$	134	$C_{19}H_{16}O$	209	$C_{20}H_{20}O_3$
74	$C_{20}H_{20}O$	135	$C_{19}H_{16}$	210	$C_{21}H_{22}O_3$

Serial No.	Molecular formula	Serial No.	Molecular formula	Serial No.	Molecular formula
211	$C_{19}H_{16}O$	332	$C_{19}H_{18}O_3$	384	$C_{17}H_{14}O$
212	$C_{21}H_{20}O$	333	$C_{19}H_{16}O_2$	387	$C_{19}H_{16}O_3$
213	$C_{20}H_{22}O_4$	334	$C_{18}H_{14}O$	388	$C_{20}H_{18}$
214	$C_{22}H_{22}O_4$	335	$C_{17}H_{10}O_3$	389	$C_{16}H_{16}O_2$
215	$C_{18}H_{14}O_2$	336	$C_{18}H_{12}O_3$	390	$C_{19}H_{16}O_2$
216	$C_{20}H_{18}O_4$	337	$C_{17}H_{14}O_3$	391	$C_{20}H_{18}O_2$
217	$C_{36}H_{26}O_3$	338	$C_{18}H_{16}O_3$	392	$C_{20}H_{18}O_2$
227	$C_{20}H_{16}O_3$	339	$C_{17}H_{12}O_2$	393	$C_{21}H_{20}O_2$
228	$C_{21}H_{21}O_5P$	340	$C_{18}H_{14}O_2$	394	$C_{22}H_{22}O_2$
229	$C_{22}H_{23}O_5P$	341	$C_{19}H_{14}O_2$	395	$C_{23}H_{24}O_2$
230	$C_{18}H_{14}O$	342	$C_{20}H_{16}O_2$	396	$C_{17}H_{12}O_2$
233	$C_{17}H_{18}O_2$	343	$C_{19}H_{14}O_3$	397	$C_{19}H_{14}O_3$
235	$C_{19}H_{18}O_3$	344	$C_{20}H_{16}O_3$	400	$C_{20}H_{20}O_2$
237	$C_{17}H_{16}O$	345	$C_{17}H_{12}O_2$	402	$C_{18}H_{14}O$
238	$C_{18}H_{18}O$	346	$C_{18}H_{14}O_2$	403	$C_{22}H_{20}O_3$
249	$C_{18}H_{16}O$	347	$C_{19}H_{16}O$	404	$C_{23}H_{22}O_4$
250	$C_{19}H_{18}O$	348	$C_{19}H_{17}NO$	405	$C_{21}H_{18}O_2$
251	$C_{20}H_{20}O$	349	$C_{17}H_{15}N$	406	$C_{22}H_{20}O_2$
252	$C_{18}H_{16}O$	351	$C_{21}H_{21}NO_2$	407	$C_{19}H_{16}O_2$
253	$C_{19}H_{16}O$	353	$C_{19}H_{20}O$	408	$C_{20}H_{18}O_2$
254	$C_{20}H_{18}$	354	$C_{19}H_{17}NO$	409	$C_{20}H_{18}O_2$
255	$C_{19}H_{18}$	355	$C_{18}H_{13}BrO$	410	$C_{21}H_{20}O_2$
256	$C_{20}H_{20}$	356	$C_{17}H_{10}Br_2O$	414	$C_{23}H_{20}O_4$
257	$C_{18}H_{16}O$	357	$C_{18}H_{12}Br_2O$	415	$C_{24}H_{22}O_4$
302	$C_{18}H_{14}O$	358	$C_{17}H_{11}BrO$	416	$C_{21}H_{14}$
303	$C_{18}H_{14}O$	359	$C_{18}H_{13}BrO$	418	$C_{18}H_{12}O_2$
304	$C_{18}H_{14}O$	362	$C_{17}H_{10}Br_2O$	419	$C_{22}H_{20}O_2$
305	$C_{18}H_{14}O$	363	$C_{17}H_{10}O$	420	$C_{24}H_{16}$
306	$C_{18}H_{14}O$	364	$C_{18}H_{12}O$	421	$C_{26}H_{21}N$
307	$C_{18}H_{14}O_2$	365	$C_{19}H_{14}O_3$	422	$C_{20}H_{16}$
308	$C_{18}H_{14}O_2$	366	$C_{20}H_{16}O_3$	423	$C_{24}H_{20}$
309	$C_{19}H_{16}O$	367	$C_{18}H_{14}O_2$	424	$C_{20}H_{16}$
310	$C_{18}H_{12}O$	368	$C_{19}H_{16}O_2$	425	$C_{20}H_{18}$
311	$C_{19}H_{16}O_2$	369	$C_{17}H_{12}O_2$	426	$C_{19}H_{16}O_3$
313	$C_{18}H_{22}O$	370	$C_{18}H_{14}O_2$	427	$C_{18}H_{20}O_2$
318	$C_{17}H_{11}BrO$	376	$C_{17}H_{14}O_2$	428	$C_{39}H_{30}O_6$
322	$C_{18}H_{13}ClO_2$	377	$C_{18}H_{16}O_2$	429	$C_{20}H_{16}O_4$
324	$C_{17}H_{14}O_2$	378	$C_{17}H_{14}O_2$	430	$C_{20}H_{15}NO_3$
325	$C_{17}H_{16}O$	379	$C_{18}H_{16}O_2$	437	$C_{18}H_{20}O_2$
326	$C_{17}H_{18}$	380	$C_{17}H_{12}O$	438	$C_{17}H_{20}O$
328	$C_{23}H_{16}O$	381	$C_{18}H_{14}O$	439	$C_{18}H_{22}O_2$
330	$C_{24}H_{16}O$	382	$C_{17}H_{14}O_2$	440	$C_{17}H_{18}$

Serial No.	Molecular formula	Serial No.	Molecular formula	Serial No.	Molecular formula
441	$C_{18}H_{20}O$	454	$C_{18}H_{16}O_4$	462	$C_{18}H_{18}O_4$
442	$C_{17}H_{16}$	455	$C_{18}H_{16}O_4$	463	$C_{18}H_{14}O_4$
443	$C_{18}H_{18}$	456	$C_{18}H_{16}O_4$	464	$C_{22}H_{18}O_6$
444	$C_{17}H_{22}O$	457	$C_{18}H_{16}O_3$	465	$C_{18}H_{14}O_3$
445	$C_{22}H_{30}O_3$	458	$C_{18}H_{14}O_2$	466	$C_{22}H_{18}O_5$
446	$C_{22}H_{20}O_4$	459	$C_{18}H_{16}O_3$	467	$C_{20}H_{20}$
447	$C_{19}H_{16}O_2$	460	$C_{18}H_{16}O_5$	468	$C_{19}H_{16}O_2$
448	$C_{18}H_{16}O$	461	$C_{24}H_{22}O_7$	469	$C_{20}H_{16}O_3$

5.5 References

Bachmann, W. E. & Holman, R. E. (1951). Synthesis of compounds related to equilenin. *J. Am. Chem. Soc.*, **73**, 3660–5.

Bachmann, W. E. & Kloetzel, M. C. (1937). Phenanthrene derivatives. VII. The cyclization of β-phenanthrylpropionic acid. *J. Am. Chem. Soc.*, **59**, 2207–13.

Bachmann, W. E., Gregg, R. A. & Pratt, E. F. (1943). Synthesis of compounds related to sex hormones. *J. Am. Chem. Soc.*, **65**, 2314–18.

Badger, G. M., Carruthers, W. & Cook, J. W. (1952). New derivatives of 1:2-cyclopentenophenanthrene. *J. Chem. Soc.*, 4996–5000.

Bardhan, J. C. (1936). Studies in the sterol–oestrone group. Part 1. A synthesis of 3'-keto-3:4-dihydro-1:2-cyclopentenophenanthrene. *J. Chem. Soc.*, 1848–51.

Bergmann, E. & Hillemann, H. (1933). γ-Methyl-1,2-cyclopenteno-phenanthren. *Ber.*, **66**, 1302–6.

Bharucha, M. S., Weiss, E. & Reichstein, T. (1962). Producte de Dehydrierung von Stropanthidin und 5-pregnen-3,20-diol mit Selen. *Helv. Chim. Acta*, **62**, 103–29.

Bhatt, T. S., Hadfield, S. T. & Coombs, M. M. (1982). Carcinogenicity and mutagenicity of some alkoxy cyclopenta[a]phenanthren-17-ones: effect of obstructing the bay-region. *Carcinogenesis*, **3**, 677–80.

Birch, A. J. & Robinson, R. (1944). Experiments on the synthesis of substances related to steroids. Part XLIII. *J. Chem. Soc.*, 503–6.

Bowie, J. H. (1966). Electron impact studies 1. High resolution mass spectra of some unsaturated cyclic ketones. *Aust. J. Chem.*, **19**, 1619–26.

Brown, K. S. & Kupchan, S. M. (1962). The structure of cyclobuxine. *J. Am. Chem. Soc.*, **83**, 4590–1.

Brown, W. & Turner, A. B. (1971). Applications of high potential quinones. Part VII. The synthesis of steroidal phenanthrenes by double methyl migration. *J. Chem. Soc. (C)*, 2566–72.

Buchta, E. & Kraetzer, H. (1962). Polycyclic compounds X. 5-methyl-naphtho[2',1':1,2]fluorene. *Ber.*, **95**, 1820–5.

Buchta, E. & Ziemer, H. (1956). Versuche zur Synthese von Steroiden. XII. Partiell Hydrierte Tri- und Tetracyclische Verbindungen. *Annalen*, **601**, 155–69.

Butenandt, A. & Suranyi, L. A. (1942). Uberfuhrung von steroidhormonen in methylhomologe des cyclopentenophenanthrenes. *Ber.*, **75B**, 597–606.

Butenandt, A., Dannenberg, H. & von Dresler, D. (1946a). Methylhomologe des 1,2-Cyclopentenophenanthrens. II. Mitteilung:

Synthese des 3-Methyl-,4-Methyl-, und 3,4-dimethyl-1,2-cyclopentenophenanthrens. *Z. Naturforsch.*, **1**, 151–6.

Butenandt, A., Dannenberg, H. & von Dresler, D. (1946*b*). Methylhomologen des 1,2-cyclopentenophenanthrens. III. Mitteilung: Synthese des 9,10-dimethyl-1,2-cyclopentenophenanthrens. *Z. Naturforsch.*, **1**, 222–6.

Butenandt, A., Dannenberg, H. & von Dresler, D. (1946*c*). Methylhomologe des 1,2-cyclopentenophenanthrens. IV. Mitteilung: Synthese des 6-methyl und 3,6-dimethyl-1,2-cyclopentenophenanthrens. *Z. Naturforsch.*, **1**, 227–9.

Butenandt, A., Dannenberg, H. & von Dresler, D. (1949*a*). Methylhomologe des 1,2-cyclopentenophenanthrens. V. Mitteilung: Synthese des 10-methyl-1,2-cyclopentenophenanthrens. *Z. Naturforsch.*, **4b**, 69–76.

Butenandt, A., Dannenberg, H. & von Dresler, D. (1949*b*). Methylhomologe des 1,2-cyclopentenophenanthrenes. VI. Mitteilung: Synthese des 8-methyl und 3,8-dimethyl-1,2-cyclopentenophenanthrens. *Z. Naturforsch.*, **4b**, 77–9.

Butenandt, A., Dannenberg, H., Bieneck, E. & Steidle, W. (1950). Methylhomologe des 1,2-cyclopentenophenanthrenes. VII. Mitteilung: Synthese des 5-methyl-1,2-cyclopentenophenanthrens. *Z. Naturforsch.*, **5b**, 405–9.

Butz, L. W., Gaddis, A. M., Butz, E. W. T. & Davis, R. E. (1940). The total synthesis of a non-benzenoid steroid. *J. Am. Chem. Soc.*, **62**, 995–6.

Cagara, C. & Siewinski, A. (1975). Microbiological transformations. VII. Microbiological reduction of (+ −)-14β-1,3,5(10),6,8-gonapentaene-11-on-17α-ol and (+ −)-14β-1,3,5(10),6,8-gonapentaene-11-on-17β-ol with *Rhodotorula mucilaginosa* strain. *Bull. Acad. Pol. Sci., Sér. Sci. Chim.*, **23**, 815–20.

Chaffee, A. L. & Jones, R. B. (1983). Polycyclic aromatic hydrocarbons in Australian coals. 1. Angularly fused pentacyclic tri- and tetra-aromatic components of Victorian brown coal. *Geochim. Cosmochim. Acta*, **47**, 2142–55.

Chinn, L. J. & Mihina, J. S. (1965). Formation of 17α-ethyl-17-methyl-8,9,13,14-gona-1,3,5(10)-trien-3-ol from 17α-ethyl-19-nortestosterone. An unusual transformation. *J. Org. Chem.*, **50**, 257–9.

Chuang, C. K., Ma, C. M., Tien, Y. L. & Huang, Y. T. (1939). Synthetic studies in the sterol and sex hormone group. III. Synthesis of 7-hydroxy-3'-keto-3,4-dihydrocyclopenteno-1',2', 1,2-phenanthrene and its methyl ether. *Ber.*, **72B**, 949–53.

Clar, E. (1952). *Aromatische Kohlenwasserstoffe*, 2nd edn. Springer-Verlag: Berlin.

Cohen, A., Cook, J. W. & Hewett, C. L. (1935). The synthesis of compounds related to the sterols, bile acids, and oestrus-producing hormones. Part VI. Experimental evidence of the complete structure of oestrin, equilin, equilenin. *J. Chem. Soc.*, 445–55.

Cook, J. W. & Girard, A. (1934). Dehydrogenation of oestrin. *Nature*, **133**, 377–8.

Cooke, J. W. & Hewett, C. L. (1933). The synthesis of compounds related to sterols, bile acids and oestrus-producing hormones. Part 1. 1:2-Cyclopentenophenanthrene. *J. Chem. Soc.*, 1098–111.

Coombs, M. M. (1965). A new synthesis of 3'-oxo-1,2-cyclopentenophenanthrene. *Chem. Ind. (London)*, 270–1.

Coombs, M. M. (1966*a*). Potentially carcinogenic cyclopenta[a]-
phenanthrenes. Part I. A new synthesis of 15,16-dihydro-17-
oxocyclopenta[a]phenanthrene and the phenanthrene analogue of 18-
noroestrone methyl ether. *J. Chem. Soc. (C)*, 955–62.

Coombs, M. M. (1966*b*). Potentially carcinogenic cyclopenta[a]-
phenanthrenes. Part II. Derivatives containing further unsaturation in ring
D. *J. Chem. Soc. (C)*, 963–8.

Coombs, M. M. (1969). Potentially carcinogenic cyclopenta[a]phenanthrenes.
Part III. Oxidation studies. *J. Chem. Soc. (C)*, 2484–8.

Coombs, M. M. & Bhatt, T. S. (1973). Potentially carcinogenic
cyclopentaphenanthrenes. Part VI. 1,2,3,4-Tetrahydro-17-ketones. *J.
Chem. Soc. Perkin Trans. I*, 1255–8.

Coombs, M. M. & Crawley, F. E. H. (1974). Potentially carcinogenic
cyclopenta[a]phenanthrenes. Part IX. Characterisation of a 5,10-
epoxybenzocyclodecene as a major urinary metabolite of the carcinogen
15,16-dihydro-11-methylcyclopenta[a]phenanthren-17-one. *J. Chem. Soc.
Perkin Trans. I*, 2330–5.

Coombs, M. M. & Hall, M. (1973). Potentially carcinogenic
cyclopenta[a]phenanthrenes. Part VII. Ring-D diols and related
compounds. *J. Chem. Soc. Perkin Trans. I*, 1255–8.

Coombs, M. M. & Jaitly, S. B. (1971). Potentially carcinogenic
cyclopenta[a]phenanthrenes. Part V. Synthesis of 15,16-dihydro-7-
methylcyclopenta[a]phenanthren-17-one. *J. Chem. Soc. (C)*, 230–4.

Coombs, M. M. & Vose, C. (1974). A novel and convenient conversion of
17-keto-steroids into their 18-nor derivatives. *J. Chem. Soc., Chem.
Commun.*, 602–3.

Coombs, M. M., Bhatt, T. S. & Croft, C. J. (1973*b*). Correlation between
carcinogenicity and chemical structure in cyclopenta[a]phenanthrenes.
Cancer Res., **33**, 832–7.

Coombs, M. M., Bhatt, T. S., Kissonerghis, A.-M. & Vose, C. W. (1980).
Mutagenic and carcinogenic metabolites of the carcinogen 15,16-dihydro-
11-methylcyclopenta[a]phenanthren-17-one. *Cancer Res.*, **40**, 882–6.

Coombs, M. M., Hall, M. & Vose, C. W. (1973*a*). Potentially carcinogenic
cyclopenta[a]phenanthrenes. Part VIII. Bromination of 17-ketones. *J.
Chem. Soc. Perkin Trans. I*, 2336–40.

Coombs, M. M., Hall, M., Siddle, V. A. & Vose, C. W. (1975). Potentially
carcinogenic cyclopenta[a]phenanthrenes. Part X. Oxygenated derivatives
of the carcinogen 15,16-dihydro-11-methylcyclopenta[a]phenanthren-17-one
of metabolic interest. *J. Chem. Soc. Perkin Trans. I*, 265–70.

Coombs, M. M., Jaitly, S. B. & Crawley, F. E. H. (1970). Potentially
carcinogenic cyclopenta[a]phenanthrenes. Part IV. Synthesis of 17-ketones
by the Stobbe condensation. *J. Chem. Soc. (C)*, 1266–71.

Coombs, M. M., Kissonerghis, A.-M., Allen, J. A. & Vose, C. W. (1979).
Identification of the proximate and ultimate forms of the carcinogen 15,16-
dihydro-11-methylcyclopenta[a]phenanthren-17-one. *Cancer Res.*, **39**,
4160–5.

Coombs, M. M., Russell, J. C., Jones, J. R. & Ribeiro, O. (1985). A
comparative examination of the *in vitro* metabolism of five
cyclopenta[a]phenanthrenes of varying carcinogenic potential.
Carcinogenesis, **6**, 1217–22.

Corey, E. J. & Estreicher, H. (1981). 3-Nitroalkenones, synthesis and use as
reverse affinity cycloalkynone equivalents. *Tetrahedron Lett.*, **22**, 603–6.

128   *Physical and spectral properties*

Dao, L. H., Hopkinson, A. C. & Lee-Ruff, E. (1978). Acid-catalysed rearrangements of cyclobutanones. IV. A novel synthesis of a steroid. *Tetrahedron Lett.*, 1413–14.

Dannenberg, H. (1950). Attempts to synthesise 'steranthrene'. I. 5-Propyl-3-methylcholanthrene. *Annalen*, **568**, 100–16.

Dannenberg, H. & Dannenberg-von Dresler, D. (1964). Relation between steroids and carcinogenic compounds. IV. Cholanthrene-5-acetic and propionic acids, their synthesis and carcinogenic action. *Z. Naturforsch.*, **198**, 801–6.

Dannenberg, H. & Hebenbrock, K. F. (1966). Dehydrogenation of steroids. XIII. Formation of dehydrogenated steroid-chloranildiene addition compounds. *Annalen*, **700**, 106–13.

Dannenberg, H. & Neumann, H. G. (1961a). Dehydrierung von 4-methyl-$\Delta^{1,3,5(10)}$-19-norcholestratrien mit chloranil. *Chem. Ber.*, **94**, 3085–94.

Dannenberg, H. & Neumann, H. G. (1961b). Verhalten der angularen Methylgruppen von Steroiden bei der Dehydrierung mit Chloranil. *Chem. Ber.*, **94**, 3094–109.

Dannenberg, H. & Neumann, H. G. (1964). Dehydrogenation of steroids. IX. Dependence of dehydrogenation with quinones on the quinone, reaction medium and steroid. *Annalen*, **675**, 109–25.

Dannenberg, H. & Steidle, W. (1954). Zur Systematik der UV-absorption. II. Mitt. Die Methylhomologen des 1,2-cyclopenophenanthrens. *Z. Naturforsch.*, **9b**, 294–7.

Dannenberg, H., Dannenberg-von Dresler, D. & Neumann, H.-G. (1960). Dehydrierung von steroiden, 111. 1:2-Cyclopentadienophenanthrene. *Annalen*, **636**, 74–87.

Dannenberg, H., Neumann, H. G. & Dannenberg-von Dresler, D. (1961). Dehydrierung von cholesterin mit choranil. *Annalen*, **674**, 152–67.

Dannenberg, H., Neumann, H. G. & Dannenberg-von Dresler, D. (1964). Dehydrierung von cholesterin mit chloranil. *Annalen*, **674**, 152–67.

Dannenberg, H., Schiedt, U. & Steidle, W. (1953). Zusammenhange zwischen Infrarot-Spektrum und Konstitution von kondensierten Aromaten. *Z. Naturforsch.*, **8b**, 269–76.

Dannenberg, H., Sonnenbichler, J. & Gross, H. J. (1965). 3-Amino and 9-acetamido-1,2-cyclopentenophenanthrene. *Annalen*, **684**, 200–9.

Diels, O. & Gadke, W. (1927). Uber die bildung von chrysen bei der dehydrierung des cholesterins. *Ber.*, **60**, 140–7.

Diels, O. & Rickert, H. F. (1935). Uber den identitats-nachweis des dehydrierungs-kohlenwasserstoffes $C_{18}H_{16}$ aus sterinien und geninan mit γ-methylcyclopentenophenanthrene. *Ber.*, **68**, 267–72.

Fieser, L. F. & Hershberg, E. B. (1936). The synthesis of phenanthrene and hydrophenanthrene derivatives. VII. 5,9-Dimethoxy-1′,3′-diketo-1,2-cyclopentenophenanthrene. *J. Am. Chem. Soc.*, **58**, 2382–5.

Fieser, L. F., Fieser, M. & Hershberg, E. B. (1936). The synthesis of phenanthrene and chrysophenanthrene derivatives. VI. 1′,3′-diketocyclopentenophenanthrene. *J. Am. Chem. Soc.*, **58**, 2322–5.

Gamble, D. J. C. & Kon, G. A. R. (1935). Synthesis of polycyclic compounds related to steroids. Part III. 9-Methyl and 3′,9-dimethyl-cyclopentenophenanthrene. *J. Chem. Soc.*, 443–5.

Harper, S. H., Kon, G. A. R. & Ruzica, F. C. J. (1934). Synthesis of polycyclic compounds related to the steroids. Part II. Diels' hydrocarbon $C_{18}H_{16}$. *J. Chem. Soc.*, 124–8.

Hawthorne, J. R. & Robinson, R. (1936). Experiments on the synthesis of substances related to the sterols. Part XIII. Hydrocyclopentenophenanthrene derivatives. *J. Chem. Soc.*, 763–5.

Hoffelmer, K., Lisbet, H. & Schmidt, L. (1964). Aromatic cracking products of steroids. *Zeit. Ernaehungswiss*, **5**, 16–21.

Hoffsomner, R. D., Taub, D. & Wendler, N. L. (1966). Rearrangement in the oestrone series. *Chimia*, **20**, 251.

Inhoffen, H. H., Stoeck, G. & Kolling, G. (1949). The migration of the angular methyl group at carbon atom 10 in the steroids. Preparation of 1,17-dimethyl-15,16-dihydrocyclopenta[a]phenanthrene. *Chem. Ber.*, **82**, 263–6.

Jacob, G., Cagniant, D. & Cagniant, R. (1971). Recherches dans le domaine du dihydro-16,17-15*H*-cyclopenta[a]phenanthrene. *C. R. Hebd. Séances Acad. Sci., Sér. C*, **272**, 650–2.

Johns, W. F. (1958). Synthesis of 18,19-dinor steroids. *J. Am. Chem. Soc.*, **80**, 6456–7.

Johnson, W. S. & Peterson, J. W. (1945). The Stobbe condensation with 1-keto-1,2,3,4-tetrahydrophenanthrene. A synthesis of 3′-keto-3,4-dihydro-1,2-cyclopentenophenanthrene. *J. Am. Chem. Soc.*, **67**, 1366–8.

Jung, M. E. & Hudspeth, J. P. (1978). Anionic oxy-Cope rearrangements with aromatic substrates in bicyclo [2.2.1]heptene systems. Facile synthesis of *cis*-hydrindone derivatives, including steroid analogues. *J. Am. Chem. Soc.*, **100**, 4309–11.

Kawarura, M., Abe, K. & Hirami, Y. (1974). Synthesis of hydrocarbons by desulphurisation of 4-hydroxy-3′-keto-1,2-cyclopentenophenanthrene toxylate. *Kochi Joshi Daigaku Kujo, Shizen Kagaku Hen*, **22**, 19–23 (*Chem. Abst.*, **81**, 120303v).

Koebner, A. & Robinson, R. (1938). Experiments on the synthesis of substances related to sterols. Part XXII. Synthesis of x-norequilenin methyl ether. *J. Chem. Soc.*, 1994–7.

Koebner, A. & Robinson, R. (1941). Experiments on the synthesis of substances related to the sterols. Part XXXVI (Continuation of Part XXII). *J. Chem. Soc.*, 566–9.

Kon, G. A. R. (1933). Synthesis of polycyclic compounds related to steroids, Part I. *J. Chem. Soc.*, 1081–7.

Kon, G. A. R. & Ruzicka, F. C. J. (1935). Synthesis of polycyclic compounds related to the sterols. Part V. Methoxy and hydroxy derivatives of phenanthrene. *J. Chem. Soc.*, 187–92.

Kon, G. A. R. & Woolman, A. M. (1939). Sapogenins. Part III. The dehydrogenation products of methylsarsasopogenin and methylcholesterol. *J. Chem. Soc.*, 794–800.

Laflamme, R. E. & Hites, R. A. (1979). Tetra- and pentacyclic, naturally occurring, aromatic hydrocarbons in recent sediments. *Geochim. Cosmochim. Acta*, **43**, 1687–91.

Lee-Ruff, E., Hopkinson, A. C. & Dao, Le H. (1981). Acid-catalysed rearrangements of cyclobutanones. VI Synthesis of chrysenes and steroid-like substances. *Can. J. Chem.*, **59**, 1675–84.

Lee-Ruff, E., Hopkinson, A. C., Kazarians-Moghaddam, H., Gupta, B. & Kutz, M. (1982). Acid catalysed rearrangements of cyclobutanols. Synthesis of chrysenes, cyclopenta[a]phenanthrenes and diarylmethanes. *Can. J. Chem.*, **60**, 154–9.

Loke, K. H., Marrian, G. F., Johnson, W. S., Meyer, W. L. & Cameron, D. D. (1958). Isolation and identification of 18-hydroxy-oestrone from the urine of pregnant women. *Biochim. Biophys. Acta*, **28**, 214.

Ludwig, B., Hussler, G., Wehrung, P. & Albrecht, P. (1981). C_{26}- C_{29} triaromatic steroid derivatives in sediments and petroleums. *Tetrahedron Lett.*, **22**, 3313-16.

Mejer, S. & Kalinowska, K. (1969). Reduction of (+ −)-14β-gona-1,3,5(10),6,8-pentaene-11,17-dione with lithium aluminium hydride. *Bull. Acad. Pol. Sci., Sér. Sci. Chim.*, **17**, 145-9.

Mladenova-Orlinova, L., Ivanov, C. & Aleksiev, B. V. (1970). Preparation and dehydration of phenanthyl-substituted hydroxypropanoic and hydroxy-butanoic acids. *Dokl. Bolg. Akad. Nauk*, **23**, 73-6.

Nasipuri, D. & Roy, D. N. (1961). Polycyclic systems. Part IX. A new synthesis of indeno (2′,3′:1,2)phenanthrene. *J. Chem. Soc.*, 3361-6.

Nazarov, I. N. & Kotlyarevskii, I. L. (1953). Synthesis of compounds related to estrone by the method of diene condensation. *Izv. Akad. Nauk S.S.S.R., Otdel, Khim. Nauk*, 1100-10.

Rahman, A. & Rodriguez, N. M. (1969). Total synthesis of 1,2-cyclopentenophenanthrene. *Chem. Ind.* (London), **52**, 1870-1.

Ribeiro, O., Hadfield, S. T., Clayton, A. F. Vose, C. W. & Coombs, M. M. (1983). Potentially carcinogenic cyclopenta[a]phenanthrenes. Part 11. Synthesis of the 1-methyl, 1,11-methano, and 7,11-dimethyl derivatives of 15,16-dihydrocyclopenta[a]phenanthren-17-one. *J. Chem. Soc. Perkin Trans. I*, 87-91.

Riegel, B., Gold, M. H. & Kubio, M. A. (1943). Synthesis of 3′-alkyl-1,2-cyclopentenophenanthrenes. *J. Am. Chem. Soc.*, **65**, 1772-6.

Riegel, B., Sigel, S. & Kritchevsky, D. (1948). The synthesis of 3-alkyl-1,2-cyclopentenophenanthrenes. *J. Am. Chem. Soc.*, **70**, 2950-2.

Robinson, R. (1938). Experiments on the synthesis of substances related to sterols. Part XXI. A new synthesis of keto*cyclo*pentenophenanthrenes. *J. Chem. Soc.*, 1390-7.

Robinson, R. & Rydon, H. N. (1939). Experiments on substances related to the sterols. Part XXVII. The synthesis of α-noroestrone. *J. Chem. Soc.*, 1394-405.

Robinson, R. & Slater, S. N. (1941). Experiments on the synthesis of substances related to the sterols. Part XXIX. *J. Chem. Soc.*, 376-85.

Ruzicka, L. & Goldberg, M. W. (1937). Polyterpene und polyterpenoide. CXVII. Zur Kenntnis der bedingungen und des mechanisms des dehydrierung der homologen sterine und des cholsaur. *Helv. Chim. Acta*, **20**, 1245-53.

Ruzicka, L., Ehmann, L., Goldberg, M. W. & Hosli, H. (1933). Synthesis of 1,2-cyclopentenophenanthrene and its α- and β-methyl derivatives and of chrysene. *Helv. Chim. Acta*, **16**, 812-32.

Schontube, E. & Janak, J. (1968). Analytical significance of dehydrogenation of steroids with selenium: contribution to the problem of Diels' hydrocarbon content in products of steroid dehydrogenation. *Collect. Czech. Chem. Commun.*, **33**, 193-209.

Sen Gupta, S. C. & Bhattacharyya, A. (1954). Synthesis of polynuclear hydrocarbons with fused cyclopentane ring III. Application of the Diels-Alder reaction. *J. Indian Chem. Soc.*, **31**, 897-903.

Shi, J. Y., Mackenzie, A. S., Alexander, R., Eglinton, G., Gowar, A. P., Wolff, G. A. & Maxwell, J. R. (1982). A biological marker investigation of petroleums and shales from the Shengli oilfield, The People's Republic of China. *Chem. Geol.*, **35**, 1-31.

Shotter, R. G., Johnson, K. M. & Williams, H. J. (1973). Polyphosphoric catalysed cyclization of aryl stryryl ketones. *Tetrahedron*, **29**, 2163-6.

Siewinski, A., Dmochowska, J. & Mejer, S. (1969). Microbiol
transformations. III. Microbiol reduction of $(+ -)$-14β-gona-
1,3,5(10),6,8,pentaene-11,17-dione by *Rhodotorula mucilaginosa*. *Bull.
Acad. Pol. Sci., Sér. Sci. Chim.*, **17**, 151–4.

Süss, O. (1953). Uber die Lichtreaktion der o-chinondiazide photosynthese
von cyclopentadienabkommlingen 4. Mitteilung. Uber die natur der
Lichtzersetzungs produkte von diazoverbindungen. *Annalen*, **579**, 133–58.

Tamayo, M. L. & Martin, J. (1952). Derivatives of cyclopentenophenanthrene. I. The condensation of 1-vinylhydrinene with *p*-benzoquinone.
Anales real Soc. espan. fís. y chim., **48b**, 693–8.

Tatta, K. R. & Bardham, J. C. (1968). Synthesis of polycyclic compounds.
Part VIII. Friedel–Crafts acylation with anhydrides of tricarboxylic acids.
Synthesis of 16,17-dihydro-17-methyl-15*H*-cyclopenta[a]phenanthrene. *J.
Chem. Soc. (C)*, 893–900.

Turner, D. L. (1949). Some aryl-substituted cyclopentenones; a new synthesis
of the cyclopentenophenanthrene structure. *J. Am. Chem. Soc.*, **71**,
612–15.

Vose, C. W. & Coombs, M. M. (1977). Mass spectrometry of
cyclopenta[a]phenanthrenes. Metabolites formed *in vitro* and *in vivo* from
the carcinogen 15,16-dihydro-11-methylcyclopenta[a]phenanthrene-17-one.
Biomed. Mass Spectrom., **4**, 48–51.

Wiebers, J. L., Abbott, P. J., Coombs, M. M. & Livingston, D. C. (1981).
Mass spectral characterisation of the major DNA-carcinogen adduct
formed from the metabolically activated carcinogen 15,16-dihydro-11-
methylcyclopenta[a]phenanthren-17-one. *Carcinogenesis*, **2**, 637–43.

Wilds, A. C. (1942). The synthesis of 2'-ketodihydro-1,2-
cyclopentenophenanthrene and derivatives of phenanthro[1,2-b]furan. *J.
Am. Chem. Soc.*, **64**, 1421–9.

Wilk, M. & Taupp, W. (1969). Dehydrogenation of cholesterol in the
activated, adsorbed state under normal conditions and application to the
study of endogenesis of carcinogenic, polycyclic hydrocarbons. *Z.
Naturforsch.*, **B.24**, 16–23.

Woodward, R. B., Inhoffen, H. H., Larsen, H. O. & Menzel, K. H. (1953).
Synthesis of 3',8-dimethyl-1,2-cyclopentenophenanthrene. *Chem. Ber.*, **86**,
594–600.

6

Carcinogenicity and mutagenicity of cyclopenta[a]phenanthrenes

6.1 Structure/carcinogenic activity relationships

As has been discussed in Chapter 1, simple cyclopenta[a]-phenanthrene hydrocarbons became of interest during the establishment of the correct structure of the sterols in the 1930s. This coincided with the isolation of benzo[a]pyrene from coal tar in 1933, and the intense interest in carcinogenic polycyclic hydrocarbons which followed soon showed that their structures were based mainly upon the phenanthrene ring system extended with one or more fused aromatic ring(s). Diels' hydrocarbon (16,17-dihydro-17-methyl-15H-cyclopenta[a]phenanthrene,**7**) was shown to be inactive as a carcinogen (Craciun *et al.*, 1939; Butenandt and Suranyi, 1942), and this reinforced the idea that additional fused benzo rings, as for example in the benz[a]anthracenes, were essential for carcinogenic activity. However, it also became apparent that correct methyl substitution can have dramatic effects on activity; thus whilst benz[a]anthracene is essentially inactive, its 7,12-dimethyl derivative is one of the most potent carcinogens known. This prompted Butenandt to synthesize the aryl methyl isomers of Diels' hydrocarbon and to test them, together with six dimethyl and trimethyl homologues, for carcinogenicity in the mouse (Butenandt and Dannenberg, 1953) both by skin painting and injection experiments. For the former, mice of the Bl.Hl. strain of known cancer incidence (Kaufmann *et al.*, 1942) as well as mice of mixed strain from a commercial source were employed. The animals received two drops of a 0.4% solution of the test compound in benzene twice weekly on their dorsal skin, and the experiments lasted from 275 to 714 days with the results shown in Table 8. Only compounds bearing methyl groups at C-7 or C-11 were carcinogens; the 7-methyl (**94**) and 11-methyl (**83**) isomers were of similar activity with tumour incidences of 14.3 and 15.4%, respectively, whereas the 11,12-dimethyl hydrocarbon

Table 8. *Skin tumour induction in mice with methyl homologues of 16,17-dihydro-15H-cyclopenta[a]phenanthrene*

Compound	No. and (strain of mice used)	Tumours at site of application		No. of mice with tumour/ Total no. of mice
		papillomas	carcinomas	
unsubstituted (**1**)	22 (Bl.Hl.)	0	0	—
1-methyl (**107**)	21 (mixed)	0	0	—
2-methyl (**98**)	18 (Bl.Hl.)	0	0	—
2-methyl (**98**)	10 (mixed)	0	0	—
4-methyl (**100**)	15 (mixed)	0	0	—
6-methyl (**67**)	10 (Bl.Hl.)	0	0	—
7-methyl (**94**)	35 (mixed)	1	4	5/35
11-methyl (**83**)	20 (Bl.Hl.)	1	1	2/13
12-methyl (**97**)	13 (Bl.Hl.)	0	0	—
17-methyl (**7**) (Diels' hydrocarbon)	25 (Bl.Hl.)	0	0	—
4,17-dimethyl (**110**)	10 (mixed)	0	0	—
2,12-dimethyl (**99**)	16 (Bl.Hl.)	0	0	—
2,12-dimethyl (**99**)	25 (mixed)	0	0	—
4,12-dimethyl (**101**)	14 (mixed)	0	0	—
6,7-dimethyl (**105**)	11 (Bl.Hl.)	0	0	—
6,7-dimethyl (**105**)	10 (mixed)	0	0	—
11,12-dimethyl (**87**)	10 (Bl.Hl.)	0	1	1/10
6,17,17-trimethyl (**69**)	11 (Bl.Hl.)	0	0	—

Table 9. *Skin-painting and injection experiments with unsaturated D-ring cyclopenta[a]phenanthrenes*

Compound	No. and (strain of mice used)	Route of application	Tumours at the site of application		No. of mice with tumour
			papillomas	carcinomas	
17-methyl-15*H*- (133)	15 (Swiss)	topical	0	1	1/15
	10 (mixed)	topical	1	6	7/10[a]
15-methyl-17*H*- (128)	15 (Swiss)	topical	1	8	9/15[b]
17-isopropyl-15*H*- (388)	15 (Swiss)	topical	0	3	3/15
17-methyl-15*H*- (133)	10 (Swiss)	injection		3 spindle cell sarcomas	
	10 (mixed)	injection		0	
15-methyl-17*H*- (128)	10 (Swiss)	injection		1 carcinoma	
17-isopropyl-15*H*- (388)	10 (Swiss)	injection		0	

a, mean latent period, 73 weeks; *b*, mean latent period, 83 weeks.

(**87**) was less active (tumour incidence 10%). No latent periods were given and the use of two different strains of mice complicates interpretation, but it is evident that these hydrocarbons are only weakly carcinogenic. This was supported by the observation that no local tumours were induced by injection of these compounds into Bl.Hl. mice (5 mg in oil).

Three cyclopenta[a]phenanthrenes containing a conjugated double bond in ring-D, namely 17-methyl-15*H*- (**133**), 17-isopropyl-15*H*- (**388**), and 15-methyl-17*H*-cyclopenta[a]phenanthrene (**128**) (Table 9), were also tested for carcinogenicity in mice of mixed strain and Swiss mice with low spontaneous tumour incidence (Dannenberg, 1960) by the methods already described. Introduction of a conjugated D-ring double bond was accompanied by the appearance of weak carcinogenicity; all three compounds were active by topical application, although their activity was low as judged by their long mean latent periods. The least active was the isopropyl hydrocarbon, and this failed to induce tumours on injection. Quinone dehydrogenation of sterols (Dannenberg *et al.*, 1956) leads to this type of hydrocarbon, and Dannenberg felt that their carcinogenicity might be connected with the possibility of the reactive D-ring double bond behaving as a 'K-region'. Thus two independent structural factors give rise to carcinogenicity in the cyclopenta[a]phenanthrene series, namely methyl substitution at C-7 or C-11 and extension of the conjugation of the phenanthrene ring system into the D-ring. However, it was not established whether these two influences were additive.

A chance came to test this using a series of 17-ketones which were originally synthesized for another purpose (see below). As shown in Fig. 21 these were converted by means of the Grignard reaction into the corresponding 17-methyl-15*H*-cyclopenta[a]phenanthrenes which were further reduced catalytically to their 16,17-dihydro derivatives. The 12 compounds thus obtained, together with three related hydrocarbons (Fig. 53), were tested for carcinogenicity (Coombs and Croft, 1966, 1969). A standardized method was set up employing Swiss mice of the T.O. (Theiler's Original) strain outbred within a closed colony in the laboratories of the Imperial Cancer Research Fund for many years. They were housed 10 to a cage on sawdust bedding and had free access to a standard solid laboratory diet and water at all times. At the beginning of the experiment they were three months old, and they were used in formally randomized groups of 20 (10 male and 10 female) for each compound. One drop of a toluene solution (0.5% w/v) of the compound was applied to the shaved dorsal skin (1 drop = 6 μL = 30 μg = 120 nmol) twice weekly for one year. The mice were observed for a second year and experiments were terminated at two years ($\sim$730 days). Survival was excellent; more than 40% of the animals were still alive at this time in the untreated and solvent control groups, and 90% survived to 18 months. No skin tumours were seen on any mice painted with toluene alone and their survival was the same as those of the untreated group. The date of appearance, position, and size of all skin tumours were recorded both when the animals were painted during the first year, and once a week during the second year. The times of appearance of the first skin tumours were used to calculate mean latent periods; at this time the tumour was less than 1 mm in diameter, but it was scored only if it persisted and grew in size. When the tumour exceeded 1 cm in diameter the animal was killed and autopsied, as were all the mice remaining at the end of the experiment. Occasionally seriously sick animals were killed and autopsied to avoid loss of the tumour material. All skin tumours and surrounding tissue were examined by routine histology and classified as papillomas unless there was evidence of penetration of the *panniculus carnosus* muscle, when they were classed as carcinomas.

Table 10 summarizes the results of this experiment. The last column lists Iball indices calculated for these compounds from the observed mean latent periods and tumour incidences as follows:

$$\text{Iball index} = \frac{\text{percentage of animals with tumour}^*}{\text{mean latent period in days}} \times 100$$

*based on the number of animals alive at the time of the appearance of the first skin tumour in that group

Fig. 53. Cyclopenta[a]phenanthrenes tested for carcinogenicity by skin painting (Coombs and Croft, 1969).

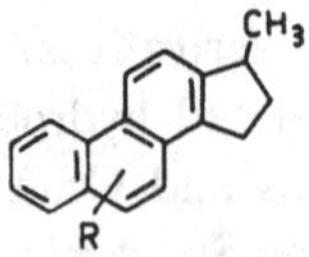

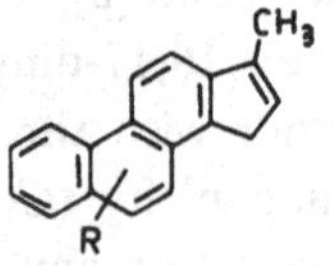

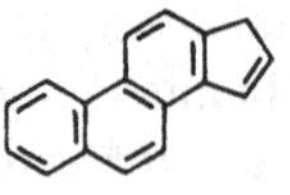

	R	
7	H	133
17	3-OCH$_3$	134
139	11-CH$_3$	135
140	12-CH$_3$	136
141	11,12-(CH$_3$)$_2$	137
142	11-OCH$_3$	138

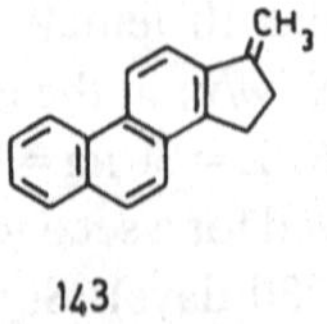

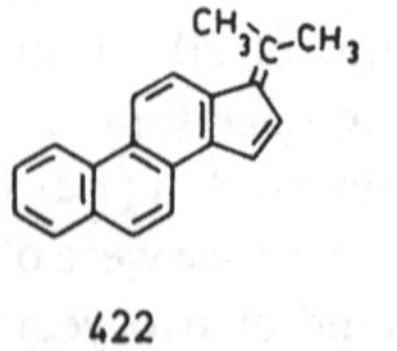

143   422

Table 10. *Skin tumour induction with some cyclopenta[a]phenanthrene hydrocarbons and methoxy analogues*

Compound	No. of mice with skin tumours at site of application		Percentage tumour incidence	Iball index
	papillomas	carcinomas		
16,17-dihydro-15H-cyclopenta[a]phenanthrenes				
17-methyl (Diels' hydrocarbon **7**)	0	0	0	—
11,17-dimethyl (**139**)	0	2	10	3
12,17-dimethyl (**140**)	0	0	0	—
11,12,17-trimethyl (**141**)	0	6	30	12
3-methoxy-17-methyl (**17**)	0	0	0	—
11-methoxy-17-methyl (**142**)	0	1	5	1
15H-cyclopenta[a]phenanthrenes				
17-methyl (**133**)	3	3	30	8
11,17-dimethyl (**135**)	1	16	85	27
12,17-dimethyl (**136**)	1	2	15	7
11,12,17-trimethyl (**137**)	1	14	75	23
3-methoxy (**134**)	0	1	5	2
11-methoxy (**138**)	1	4	25	11
17H-cyclopenta[a]phenanthrene (**2**)	0	0	0	—
17-methylene-15,16-dihydro (**143**)	1	4	25	5
17-isopropylidenecyclopenta[a]phenanthrene (**422**)	0	0	0	—

For this index 'tumours' include both papillomas and carcinomas at the site of application, and the latent period is the time elapsed between the beginning of the treatment and the first appearance of the first skin tumour on each mouse. The mean latent period is the average latent period for all the animals in that group. This index is a better measure of carcinogenicity than tumour incidence alone because it also takes latent periods into account, although, of course, it does not include other important parameters such as the total number of tumours per animal, the carcinoma/papilloma ratio, or the rate of tumour growth. However, it has the merit of allowing comparisons to be made readily, and is probably a valid procedure for a series of closely related compounds such as the one at present under discussion because these compounds all have very similar physical properties, especially solubility.

Substitution of a methyl group at C-17 in 16,17-dihydro-15*H*-cyclopenta[a]phenanthrene does not lead to activity because Diels' hydrocarbon (7) fails to induce skin tumours, as others have found. In agreement with Butenandt and Dannenberg, introduction of a methyl group at C-11 into Diels' hydrocarbon leads to weak carcinogenicity (compounds **139** and **141**) whereas introduction of this group at C-12 does not (compound **140**). A methoxy group at the biologically important C-3 position is ineffective, but again it is weakly activating at C-11. Also in agreement with the latter author (Dannenberg, 1960), introduction of a 16(17)-double bond into Diels' hydrocarbon to yield 17-methyl-15*H*-cyclopenta[a]phenanthrene (**133**) is accompanied by the appearance of weak activity; the tumour incidence of this compound reached 30%, but its mean latent period was very long resulting in a low Iball index. The isomeric 17-methylene hydrocarbon (**143**) was of similar activity, but as it is known to isomerize readily to the 16(17)-isomer (**133**) the meaning of this is unclear. 17*H*-Cyclopenta[a]phenanthrene (**2**) lacking a D-ring methyl group was inactive as was the isopropylidene hydrocarbon (**422**). However, introduction of a methyl group at C-11 in these unsaturated ring-D compounds dramatically enhanced activity; thus 11,17-dimethyl-15*H*-cyclopenta[a]phenanthrene (**135**) and its 11,12,17-trimethyl homologue (**137**) were moderately strong carcinogens. It is interesting that in this series a methoxy group at C-11 has only a marginally activating effect, while at C-3 it appears to cause deactivation. Thus it is clear that ring-D unsaturation and 11-methyl group substitution are additive *vis-à-vis* induction of carcinogenicity in this series.

The 17-ketones corresponding to these hydrocarbons were also tested in this experiment to determine whether conjugation by a carbonyl group at C-17 would have an enhancing effect similar to that shown by a 16(17)-

double bond. A carbonyl group at this position is, of course, a feature of many naturally occurring steroids. The results of this test are shown in Table 11. It is immediately obvious that conjugation of a carbonyl group has a considerable enhancing effect on carcinogenicity. In fact 15,16-dihydro-11-methylcyclopenta[a]phenanthren-17-one (**26**) was the most potent carcinogen to be tested, and was more active than the analogous ring-D unsaturated hydrocarbon (**135**). The 11,12-dimethyl and 11-methoxy ketone (**131** and **132**) were also strong carcinogens whilst the unsubstituted ketone (**4**) and its 12-methyl (**130**) and 3-methoxy (**24**) derivatives were devoid of activity. The 11-acetoxy-17-ketone (**80**) appeared to be marginally active, but the 11-phenol (**206**) was too insoluble to be tested in this way. The high activity of the 11-methyl-17-ketones was unexpected because introduction of oxygen substituents into polycyclic aromatic hydrocarbons often has the reverse effect. This series also differs from the 16(17)-ene series in that the parent 17-ketone (**4**) is inactive, as are its 12-methyl and 3-methoxy derivatives, whilst the 11-methoxy derivative is considerably more carcinogenic than the corresponding hydrocarbon derivative (**138**).

The high activity of the 11-methyl-17-ketone (**26**) prompted a much more thorough study of the structure/carcinogenicity relationships in this series of 17-ketones. All the aryl methyl isomers were synthesized and tested, as were a range of related compounds listed in Table 12 which shows the results of testing these compounds by the standard method (Coombs *et al.*, 1973, 1979; Hadfield *et al.*, 1984; Kashino *et al.*, 1986). The 11-methyl-17-ketone (**26**), used as a positive control, was again shown to be a potent carcinogen, whereas the 2-, 3-, 4-, and 6-methyl

Table 11. *Skin tumour induction with some 15,16-dihydrocyclo-penta[a]phenanthren-17-ones*

Compound	No. of mice with skin tumours at site of application		Percentage tumour incidence	Iball index
	papillomas	carcinomas		
unsubstituted (**4**)	0	0	0	—
11-methyl (**26**)	1	13	70	36
12-methyl (**130**)	0	0	0	—
11,12-dimethyl (**131**)	2	11	65	30
3-methoxy (**24**)	0	0	0	—
11-methoxy (**132**)	2	9	55	25
11-acetoxy (**80**)	1	1	10	3

Table 12. *Skin tumour induction with some further derivatives and analogues of 15,16-dihydrocyclopenta[a]phenanthren-17-one by repeated application*

Compound	No. of mice with skin tumour(s) at the site of application		Percentage tumour incidence	Iball index
	papillomas	carcinomas		
1-methyl-17-ketone (**302**)	1	0	5	(1)[a]
2-methyl-17-ketone (**303**)	0	0	0	—
3-methyl-17-ketone (**304**)	0	0	0	—
4-methyl-17-ketone (**305**)	0	0	0	—
6-methyl-17-ketone (**306**)	0	0	0	—
7-methyl-17-ketone (**230**)	0	6	30	10
11-methyl-17-ketone (**26**)	0	18	90	46
11-ethyl-17-ketone (**211**)	3	3	30	8
11-*n*-butyl-17-ketone (**212**)	0	0	0	—
1,11-methano-17-ketone (**310**)	6	2	40	(16)[a]
7,11-dimethyl-17-ketone (**309**)	2	11	65	(49)[b]
6-methoxy-11-methyl-17-ketone (**468**)	2	9	55	14
11-methoxy-7-methyl-17-ketone (**447**)	0	10	50	17
11,12-dihydro-11-methyl-17-ketone (**252**)	0	0	0	—
1,2,3,4-tetrahydro-11-methyl-17-ketone (**238**)	0	0	0	—
unsubstituted -15-ketone (**102**)	0	0	0	—
11-methyl-15-ketone (**334**)	3	1	20	5
1,2,3,4-tetrahydrochrysen-1-one (**449**)	0	0	0	—
1,2,3,4-tetrahydro-11-methylchrysen-1-one (**450**)	1	16	85	45
11-methyl-17-ol (**448**)	2	10	60	23

All compounds were applied as before at a dose of 120 nmol twice weekly for one year with observation for a second year except: *a*, the dose was 200 nmol twice weekly for one year; and *b*, the dose was 200 nmol twice weekly for 10 weeks only. Observation was continued for up to two years in both cases as usual.

isomers were inactive. The 1-methyl-17-ketone (**302**) appeared to possess marginal carcinogenic activity because one mouse developed a papilloma at the site of application; this has never been observed with mice in control groups treated repeatedly with the vehicle (toluene) alone. The 7-methyl-17-ketone (**230**) was moderately active, so that these structure/activity relationships resemble those found by Butenandt and Dannenberg for the corresponding hydrocarbons, with the exception that in the ketone series the 11-methyl compound is much more active than its 7-methyl isomer. The 11-ethyl-17-ketone (**211**) was much less carcinogenic than its methyl homologue, and the 11-*n*-butyl-17-ketone (**212**) was inactive. This order of decreasing carcinogenicity with increasing carbon chain length in a bay-region substituent has been observed in several other series of polycyclic aromatic hydrocarbons. As anticipated, the 7,11-dimethyl-17-ketone (**309**) proved to be a powerful carcinogen, probably more active than its 11-methyl homologue. Unfortunately, owing to shortage of material repeated applications of this dimethyl ketone were continued for only 10 weeks instead of the 50 weeks in the standard regime, but this, nevertheless, resulted in 30 skin tumours, a third of which were malignant, in 13/20 mice with a short mean latent period of 19 weeks. There is little doubt that both the number of tumours and the tumour incidence would have been higher if topical applications had been continued as usual for one year. Introduction of a 6-methoxy group into the 11-methyl ketone to give compound (**468**) considerably diminished its activity, whereas introduction of an 11-methoxy group into the 7-methyl-17-ketone to give compound (**447**) led to an increase in activity, although not to the extent that might have been predicted.

Interruption of conjugation in the phenanthrene ring system abolished carcinogenicity; thus neither the 11,12-dihydro-11-methyl-17-ketone (**252**) nor the 1,2,3,4-tetrahydro derivative (**238**) were active. It is, therefore, probable that an intact phenanthrene system is the smallest polycyclic aromatic ring system that can give rise to carcinogenicity upon correct substitution. Transposition of the 17-carbonyl group to C-15 (compound **334**) markedly reduced activity; in fact this ketone was a weak carcinogen, like the corresponding saturated D-ring hydrocarbon (**139**). This is surprising because Dannenberg (1960) demonstrated that in the unsaturated D-ring hydrocarbon series both 15-methyl-17*H*- and 17-methyl-15*H*-cyclopenta[a]phenanthrenes were carcinogenic and of comparable activity. As expected the unsubstituted -15-ketone (**102**) was inactive. Linkage of the C-1 and C-11 positions by a methylene bridge did not destroy activity, for 15,16-dihydro-1,11-methanocyclopenta[a]phenanthren-17-one (**310**) is moderately carcinogenic, although it does not possess a bay-region. Expansion of the five-membered ring by one carbon atom to yield 11-methyl-1,2,3,4-tetrahydrochrysen-1-one (**450**) retained activity unchanged; thus the Iball indices of this ketone and of 15,16-dihydro-11-methylcyclopenta[a]phenanthren-17-one (**26**) were essentially the same. The unsubstituted 1,2,3,4-tetrahydrochrysen-1-one (**449**) was inactive.

The unexpectedly high activity of this chrysenone (**450**) was further investigated by converting it into a series of hydrocarbons including 1,11-dimethylchrysene (**453**) by means of the Grignard reaction followed by dehydration, dehydrogenation, or reduction as outlined in Fig. 54. These compounds were then tested for carcinogenicity by the standard procedure (Coombs *et al.*, 1974) with the results shown in Table 13. The ketone (**450**) was by far the most active, and the least active was the tetrahydrohydrocarbon (**452**); the Iball indices of both were similar to those of the analogous cyclopenta[a]phenanthrenes. However, the 3,4-dihydro hydrocarbon (**451**) was distinctly less carcinogenic than the corresponding 11,17-dimethyl-15*H*-cyclopenta[a]phenanthrene (**135**), and in fact it was the fully aromatic 1,11-dimethylchrysene (**453**) that possessed activity similar to that of (**135**) (see Table 10). This tetrahydro ketone (**450**) is therefore markedly more active than the corresponding aromatic hydrocarbon containing four condensed benzene rings.

The tests so far described all involved repeated application of the test compound and therefore each test with 20 mice required about 100 mg of sample. While this was usually readily possible with synthetic compounds, testing of metabolites, obtained by *in vitro* metabolism and separation by high-pressure liquid chromatography, posed a problem in this respect. Tests by repeated application measure 'complete carcinogenicity', i.e., the sum total of the initiation and promotion caused by the test compound, but it is possible to test for initiation alone using a two-stage initiation–promotion regime. With an initiating dose of 1.6 μmol

Fig. 54

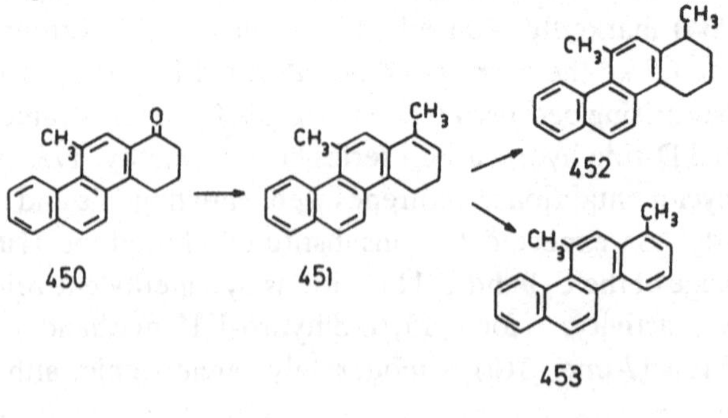

Table 13. *Skin tumours induced in mice by repeated application of some 11-methylchrysene derivatives*

Compound	No. of mice with skin tumour(s) at site of application	Iball index
11-methyl-1,2,3,4-tetrahydrochrysen-1-one (**450**)	17/20	45
1,11-dimethylchrysene (**453**)	15/19	22
1,11-dimethyl-3,4-dihydrochrysene (**451**)	8/20	10
1,11-dimethyl-1,2,3,4-tetrahydrochrysene (**452**)	3/18	4.5

(400 μg) applied once, followed by twice-weekly promotion of the treated area of skin by the application of 10 μL of a 1% v/v solution of croton oil in toluene, it was established that the carcinogen 15,16-dihydro-11-methylcyclopenta[a]phenanthren-17-one (26) produced a tumour incidence and mean latent period similar to those produced by the standard repeated-application method. However, the two-stage method used less than one-tenth of the amount of sample required by the latter, and proved to be useful for studies with metabolites. It was also employed to determine the initiating activity of a range of synthetic compounds (Coombs and Bhatt, 1978; Coombs *et al.*, 1979; Bhatt *et al.*, 1982; Hadfield *et al.*, 1984; Kashino *et al.*, 1986) shown in Table 14.

As was to be expected, the 11-methyl-17-ketone (26) and its 7,11-dimethyl homologue (309) proved to be potent tumour initiators whilst the parent unsubstituted ketone (4) and its 3-methyl derivative (304) were inactive. In line with the results from repeated application of these compounds, the dimethyl compound appeared to be the more active as shown by its shorter mean latent period, and consequently its higher Iball index. Of course, these indices cannot be compared directly with those derived from repeated-application experiments, but they serve the same purpose of providing a convenient guide to the relative initiating potential of a series of closely related compounds. Predictably the 11-methyl-chrysenone (450) was also a very active tumour initiator whereas the unsubstituted chrysenone (449) was inactive. The 1,11-methano-17-ketone (310) was a moderately active initiator, and again the 1-methyl-17-ketone (302) appeared to be marginally active. However, occasionally a papilloma is induced in uninitiated control mice painted with croton oil, so that the meaning of a low Iball index in this system is questionable. Among the 11-alkoxy-17-ketones the methoxy compound (132) was the most active, followed by the 11-ethoxy-17-ketone (390) which was somewhat less so, whilst the *n*-pentoxy, and *n*-hexoxy derivatives were not tumour initiators. Unexpectedly, both the 11-isopropoxy and 11-*n*-butoxy-17-ketones appeared to be very weak tumour initiators, but again these low indices are questionable. The 15-methoxy-17-ketone (367) was not an initiator, but its 11-methyl derivative (368) was active. In this Table the three hydroxy derivatives and the parent 11-methyl-17-ketone used as a positive control are placed together separately. The reason for this is that they were tested together in a separate experiment (Coombs and Bhatt, 1982) in which for solubility reasons acetone–toluene (1:1 v/v) was employed in place of toluene to administer the initiating dose of these compounds. This led to the unexpected result of effectively increasing the initiating activity of this carcinogen, as can be seen from the increased

Table 14. *Initiating activity of some 15,16-dihydrocyclopenta[a]phenanthren-17-ones in the two-stage regime using croton oil as a tumour promoter*

Compound	No. of mice with skin tumours at site of application		Percentage tumour incidence	Iball index[a]
	papillomas	carcinomas		
unsubstituted -17-ketone (**4**)	0	0	0	—
1-methyl-17-ketone (**302**)	2	0	10	3
3-methyl-17-ketone (**304**)	0	0	0	—
11-methyl-17-ketone (**26**)	14	2	80	57
1,11-methano-17-ketone (**310**)	7	5	60	33
7,11-dimethyl-17-ketone (**309**)	10	6	80	66
11-methoxy-17-ketone (**132**)	9	2	55	32
11-ethoxy-17-ketone (**390**)	6	2	40	23
11-*n*-propoxy-17-ketone (**391**)	0	0	0	—
11-isopropoxy-17-ketone (**392**)	2	0	10	4
11-*n*-butoxy-17-ketone (**393**)	4	0	20	5
11-*n*-pentoxy-17-ketone (**394**)	0	0	0	—
11-*n*-hexoxy-17-ketone (**395**)	0	0	0	—
15-methoxy-17-ketone (**367**)	1	0	5	1
15-methoxy-11-methyl-17-ketone (**368**)	3	2	25	15
1,2,3,4-tetrahydrochrysen-1-one (**449**)	0	0	0	—
1,2,3,4-tetrahydro-11-methylchrysen-1-one (**450**)	11	7	90	60
15-hydroxy-11-methyl-17-ketone (**370**)	6	2	40	(13)[b]
16-hydroxy-11-methyl-17-ketone (**346**)	14	6	100	(53)[b]
11-hydroxymethyl-17-ketone (**215**)	7	2	45	(16)[b]
11-methyl-17-ketone (**26**) (positive control)	13	6	95	(63)[b]

a These figures cannot, of course, be compared directly with Iball indices derived from repeated-application experiments.
b Acetone–toluene (1:1 v/v) used to deliver the initiating dose.

Iball index. However, within this small group it is clear that the 16-hydroxy derivative is almost as active as the original carcinogen whereas the 15-hydroxy and 11-hydroxymethyl derivatives are much less active. These hydroxy derivatives are of interest because they also occur as metabolites of this 11-methyl-17-ketone.

In summary it is clear that in the 17-ketone series carcinogenicity is favoured by small electron-releasing groups at C-11 and to a lesser degree at C-7, but not elsewhere in the molecule. On these grounds the 11-phenol   (15,16-dihydro-11-hydroxycyclopenta[a]phenanthren-17-one, **206**) was expected to be carcinogenic, but it was not possible to test it by topical application as usual because it was very sparingly soluble in most organic solvents. It was therefore finely ground and suspended in olive oil for subcutaneous injection into T.O. mice at 10 mg/animal. Subsequent promotion of the dorsal skin remote from the site of injection (shoulder) with 1% v/v croton oil in toluene then led, in two separate but identical experiments, to tumour incidences of 60 and 65% with mean latent periods of 25 and 30 weeks, respectively. Under these conditions of systemic initiation the 11-methyl-17-ketone used as a positive control was very active, giving a 95% dorsal skin tumour incidence with a short mean latent period of 21 weeks.

6.2   The carcinogenicity of 15,16-dihydro-11-methylcyclopenta[a]-phenanthren-17-one

From the foregoing it is apparent that this 11-methyl-17-ketone (**26**) is a potent carcinogen in T.O. mice. This was further studied in two dose/response studies and direct comparisons with the classical polycyclic aromatic hydrocarbon carcinogen benzo[a]pyrene. In the first (Coombs *et al.*, 1979) this ketone was painted on to the dorsal skin twice weekly, using groups of 20 T.O. mice as usual, at doses of 50, 25, 10, and 5 μg per mouse. A further group was treated in the same way with benzo[a]pyrene (5 μg/mouse), and the last group received the 11-methyl-17-ketone at this dosage together with 15 μg of the aryl hydrocarbon hydroxylase inhibitor 7,8-benzoflavone (Kinoshita and Gelboin, 1972). The results of this comparison are displayed in Table 15 and Fig. 55. Comparison of the 11-methyl-17-ketone and benzo[a]pyrene at the same twice-weekly dose (5 μg = 20 nmol) showed that these two compounds are of comparable potency as complete carcinogens on T.O. mouse skin. The figure also shows the curves formed by plotting the time of first appearance of the tumours, and the best line for points given by plotting mean latent periods (*Lp*) against the logarithms of the doses (*d*) using the well-known relationship

Table 15. *Dose/response study with the carcinogen 15,16-dihydro-11-methylcyclopenta[a]phenanthren-17-one by repeated application, and the effect of co-administration of the aryl hydrocarbon hydrolysis inhibitor 7,8-benzoflavone*

Compound	Dose (μg twice weekly)	Percentage tumour incidence	Mean latent period ± s.d.
11-methyl-17-ketone	50	85	23.3 ± 8.1
11-methyl-17-ketone	25	90	28.4 ± 7.7
11-methyl-17-ketone	10	80	31.2 ± 6.8
11-methyl-17-ketone	5	45	34 ± 8.2
11-methyl-17-ketone plus 7,8-benzoflavone (15 μg)	5	15	36.2 ± 8.6
benzo[a]pyrene	5	50	37.5 ± 11.2

$$Lp = a - b\,(\log_{10} d + c)$$

(Bryan and Shimkin, 1941) where a, b, and c are constants. In this case the data fit the equation

$$Lp = 29.40 - 10.803\,(\log_{10} d - 1.199)$$

where Lp is in weeks and d in μg; the correlation coefficient is 0.96. Also shown are the tumours induced by this carcinogen administered together with 7,8-benzoflavone. As found previously (Coombs *et al.*, 1975) this flavone markedly decreased the tumour incidence and increased the mean latent period. When the latter (36.1 weeks) was fitted to this line, it was found that this inhibitor effectively reduced the dose to about half of that administered.

In the second dose/response experiments (Coombs and Bhatt, 1982) single applications of the carcinogen (**26**) were made at doses of 1600, 400, and 200 nmol/mouse to groups of 20 animals which were then promoted with croton oil–toluene twice weekly as usual, with the results shown in Fig. 56. Even at the lowest dose (200 nmol = 50 μg) tumour incidence was 50%; at the highest dose (1600 nmol = 400 μg) both the tumour incidence and mean latent period were similar to those observed on repeated application of 100–200 nmol of this compound twice weekly.

Fig. 55. Induction of skin tumours in T.O. mice by twice-weekly application of benzo[a]pyrene (BaP) (+ — +), the 11-methyl-17-ketone (**26**) (○ — ○), and the relationship between mean latent period and dose for the latter. The solid circles (● — ●) represent tumours produced by this carcinogen when administered together with the aryl hydrocarbon hydroxylase inhibitor 7,8-benzoflavone (BF).

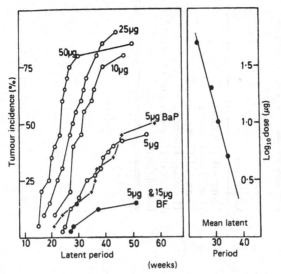

A very similar result was obtained in a previous experiment (Coombs *et al.*, 1979) in which the 11-methyl-17-ketone (**26**) was again compared with benzo[a]pyrene in the two-stage system, with both compounds at a dose of 1600 nmol and subsequent twice-weekly promotion. The effects of the aryl hydrocarbon hydroxylase inhibitor 7,8-benzoflavone and the epoxide hydratase inhibitor 1,1,1-trichloropropene oxide (TCPO) on tumour induction by (**26**) under these conditions were also studied (Table 16). It is apparent that benzo[a]pyrene is somewhat less active as a tumour initiator than the cyclopenta[a]phenanthrene (**26**) in this system. Unexpectedly, co-administration of 7,8-benzoflavone together with the initiating dose of (**26**) had little effect on either tumour incidence or latent period, in marked contrast to its effect upon repeated twice-weekly applications already discussed. It seems probable that the reason for this may reside in the comparatively high initiating dose (1600 nmol) used, in comparison with the twice-weekly dose (20 nmol) employed before (see Fig. 55). In a preliminary experiment (Coombs *et al.*, 1975) it was found that this inhibitor had less effect at a higher dose of (**26**) even though the same ratio of carcinogen:inhibitor was maintained. Appreciable shortening of the mean latent period was obtained when the epoxide hydratase inhibitor TCPO was given with the initiating dose of the

Fig. 56. Appearance of first skin tumours in T.O. mice (groups of 20) treated with a single dose of the carcinogen (as shown) followed by promotion with croton oil applied twice weekly.

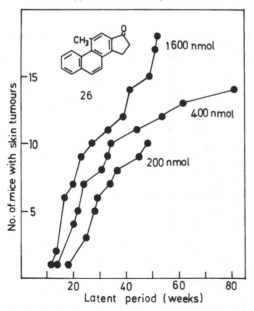

Table 16. *Comparison of tumour induction by 15,16-dihydro-11-methylcyclopenta[a]phenanthrene and benzo[a]pyrene in the two-stage system, and the effects of 7,8-benzoflavone (BF) and 1,1,1-trichloropropene oxide (TCPO) on the former*

Compound	No. of mice with tumours at site of application		Percentage tumour incidence	Mean latent period
	papillomas	carcinomas		
11-methyl-17-ketone (26)	14	4	90	29.9 ± 13.9
11-methyl-17-ketone (26) plus BF	12	4	80	30.6 ± 9.5
11-methyl-17-ketone (26) plus TCPO	17	2	95	23.6 ± 9.7
benzo[a]pyrene	10	3	65	33.5 ± 17.3

carcinogen (**26**). Similar effects have been observed with 3-methyl-cholanthrene (Berry *et al.*, 1977; Burki *et al.*, 1974) and benzo[a]pyrene (Berry *et al.*, 1977). With the latter the inhibitor prevents hydration of the initial 7,8-oxide to the 7,8-diol (Selkirk *et al.*, 1974), but the ultimate carcinogen, the 7,8-dihydroxy-9,10-epoxide is not a substrate for this enzyme (Wood *et al.*, 1976). This suggests that the 11-methyl-17-ketone (**26**) may be activated in a similar manner, via its 3,4-hydroxy-1,2-epoxide.

This ketone (**26**) also behaved like benzo[a]pyrene when croton oil was used as a co-carcinogen. The latter is defined as 'all forms of augmentation of tumour induction, usually brought about by *concurrent* administrations of the carcinogen and the added factor' (Berenblum, 1969). As shown in Table 17, T.O. mice in the usual groups of 20 were treated topically twice weekly with 20 or 200 nmol of the 11-methyl-17-ketone (**26**) or 20 nmol of benzo[a]pyrene dissolved in either toluene or toluene–croton oil (99:1 v/v). At both dose levels of (**26**) 1% croton oil in the solvent markedly reduced the mean latent periods, the difference again being the larger with the lower dose of the carcinogen (**26**). Benzo[a]pyrene behaved in a similar manner, but again appeared to be rather less active than the cyclopenta[a]phenanthrene (**26**) on the basis of tumour incidence, although not on mean latent period (Vose *et al.*, 1981).

In the work described so far skin tumours induced with the 11-methyl-17-ketone (**26**) at the site of application were studied after topical application to the dorsal skin. The first experiment (Table 11) was supported by a small injection experiment shown in Table 18, employing T.O. mice (Coombs and Croft, 1969). Of the three compounds tested, the unsubstituted 17-ketone (**4**) gave no tumours in line with its lack of activity after topical application. The 11-methyl-17-ketone (**26**) was the only compound to yield local sarcomas at the site of injection, although the dose required was high. Both this compound and its 11,12-dimethyl homologue (**131**) gave rise to both papillomas and carcinomas on the skin remote from the site of injection, mainly on the ventral surfaces, without apparent promotion. Ventral skin is thicker and contains considerably more fat than dorsal skin, and it seems probable that this may retard the loss of this lipophilic ketone, thereby allowing it to act over a prolonged period at this site. It is interesting that the more lipophilic benzo[a]pyrene [which dissolves in hexane – the cyclopenta[a]phenanthrenone (**26**) does not], like other polycyclic aromatic hydrocarbons, readily gives rise to local sarcomas after subcutaneous injection. It has already been mentioned, in connection with testing the 11-phenol (**206**), that the 11-methyl-17-ketone acts as a potent systemic initiator after subcutaneous

Table 17. *Co-carcinogenicity experiments with benzo[a]pyrene or the 11-methyl-17-ketone and croton oil*

Compound	Dose (nmol)	Solvent	Percentage of mice with skin tumours at the site of application	Mean latent period (weeks)	Difference in mean latent period (weeks)
11-methyl-17-ketone (**26**)	20	toluene	70	42.7	11.3
11-methyl-17-ketone (**26**)	20	toluene/croton oil	95	31.4	
11-methyl-17-ketone (**26**)	200	toluene	90	26.3	4.9
11-methyl-17-ketone (**26**)	200	toluene/croton oil	100	21.4	
benzo[a]pyrene	20	toluene	30	34.8	8.8
benzo[a]pyrene	20	toluene/croton oil	70	26.0	

Table 18. *Subcutaneous injection experiment with 15,16-dihydrocyclopenta[a]phenanthren-17-one (4) and its 11-methyl (26) and 11,12-dimethyl (131) derivatives*

Compound	Dose injected (mg)	No. of mice injected	No. of mice with local sarcomas	No. of mice with remote skin tumours	
				squamous carcinomas	squamous papillomas
unsubstituted -17-ketone (4)	50	18	0	0	0
11-methyl-17-ketone (26)	50	18	3	5	5
11-methyl-17-ketone (26)	8	21	3	4	4
11,12-dimethyl-17-ketone (131)	8	21	0	3	6

injection of 10 mg of this compound in olive oil, giving a high yield of dorsal skin tumours after promotion of this site remote from the site of injection with croton oil. In order to carry out the long-term experiment to be described (Coombs *et al.*, 1979) it was necessary to avoid the induction of local sarcomas. This was easily achieved by reducing the injected dose to 3 mg; subsequent twice-weekly dorsal promotion with croton oil then led to dorsal skin tumours at the site of promotion in 65% of the animals (see Table 19), but no local sarcomas. The mean latent period for these skin tumours was 33 weeks; no dorsal skin tumours were observed in the absence of croton oil promotion of this area. When mice were injected but otherwise left untreated for six months before the usual promotion was begun, a tumour incidence of 45% was still obtained with the shorter mean latent period of 24 weeks. Iball indices calculated from these tumour incidences and mean latent periods (from the start of promotion) were almost identical (28 for immediate promotion and 27 for delayed promotion), indicating that initiation with this carcinogen is a permanent and irreversible state. These injected animals also developed a number of other tumours, whether they were promoted or not. The eyelids were particularly affected, and head and ventral surface tumours were also noted. This useful property of the carcinogen (**26**) of initiating skin effectively after subcutaneous injection without the induction of local sarcomas has been put to use in two other experiments. In the first (Bhatt *et al.*, 1984), concerned with demonstrating that silica fibre isolated from the seeds of the grass *Phalaris canariensis* can act as a tumour promoter in T.O. mice, among a total of 70 mice injected there were 10 with eyelid and 22 with ventral trunk tumours. It has also made possible skin-transplantation experiments in Balb C mice, which are highly susceptible to the carcinogenicity of this ketone (J. Cox, private communication). Also Abbott (1983) demonstrated that this compound induced skin tumours in C57Bl mice, but not DBA/2 mice, in both the repeated-application (200 nmol twice weekly) and two-stage (1600 nmol once, followed by twice-weekly promotion) regimes. The resistance of DBA/2 mice is difficult to understand because for all three strains (T.O., C57Bl, and DBA/2) total DNA adducts in the treated skin, as well as the pattern of adducts as disclosed by high-pressure liquid chromatography of the derived nucleosides, were very similar. Moreover, the persistences of these DNA adducts *in vivo* were also similar for all three strains. It would be interesting to investigate whether DBA/2 mice lack an onco-gene which is possessed in common by T.O., C57Bl, and Balb C mice, making them susceptible to cancer.

Little work has been carried out with cyclopenta[a]phenanthrenes in

Table 19. Tumours induced in T.O. mice by subcutaneous injection of 15,16-dihydro-11-methylcyclopenta[a]phenanthren-17-one (3 mg/mouse)

Skin tumours appearing on promoted dorsal skin

Group[a]	Promotion	No. of mice with dorsal skin tumours			Mean latent period ± s.d. (weeks)
		total	papillomas	carcinomas	
1	none	0	0	0	—
2	begun 8 days after injection	13	9	4	33 ± 11.7
3	begun 6 months after injection	9	8	1	49 ± 7.0[b]

Tumours other than those appearing on promoted skin

Group	Eyelid	Ear	Head	Ventral surface	Mice with lung adenomas[c]
1	4 (2 pap.)	—	2 pap.	2 (1 mammary carc.)	4
2	4 pap. 2 anaplastic carc. 1 sebaceous adenoma	1 carc.	—	2 pap.	7
3	1 carc. 1 pap.	1 carc.	—	1 pap.	8

a 20 mice per group.
b i.e., 24 weeks from beginning of promotion.
c No lung adenomas among control mice injected with olive oil alone.
pap. = papilloma; carc. = carcinoma.

Table 20. *Mammary tumours induced in rats after intragastric instillation of the 11-methyl-17-ketone (26)*

	No. of rats at time of treatment	at 20 weeks with tumour	alive	at 30 weeks with tumour	alive	at 50 weeks with tumour	alive	at 75 weeks with tumour	alive
Adenocarcinomas									
in rats after (26)	27	2	26	4	26	6	20	—	—
in control rats	96	0	94	0	92	1	85	—	—
		($P = 0.455$)		($P = 0.0019$)		($P = 0.001$)			
Fibroadenomas									
in rats after (26)	27	0	26	0	26	0	20	2	13
in control rats	96	0	94	0	92	3	85	7	70
						($P = 0.5270$)		($P = 0.2845$)	

animals other than mice. However, intragastric instillation of 15,16-dihydro-11-methylcyclopenta[a]phenanthren-17-one (**26**) into 27 virgin female Sprague-Dawley rats (30 mg/rat) induced mammary adeno-carcinomas in six of them, as shown in Table 20 (Coombs *et al.*, 1979). Mammary tumours were detected during the 18th week after treatment, but a single spontaneous adenocarcinoma did not appear among control rats until the 42nd week. Differences in tumour incidence between the two groups were significant at 30 weeks and highly significant at 50 weeks as indicated by the P values calculated by the exact method of Yates (Fisher, 1954). By contrast, benign fibroadenomas occurred later and to a similar extent in both the carcinogen-treated and the untreated control groups. In its ability to induce mammary carcinomas after a single intragastric instillation this compound resembles other potent known carcinogens such as 3-methylcholanthrene (Shay *et al.*, 1949) and 7,12-dimethylbenz[a]anthracene (Huggins, 1961). However, it is less potent than either of the latter in this regard and also in its ability to induce skin tumours in mice after topical application (Coombs and Croft, 1969). The suggestion that the carcinogenicity of aromatic hydrocarbons increases as their structure approaches that of steroids (Yang *et al.*, 1961) is therefore not substantiated. Interperitoneal injection of the cyclopenta[a]-phenanthrenone into 57 male Sprague-Dawley rats (10 mg/rat, in oil) did not induce local sarcomas in any of these animals. In this behaviour it differs markedly from polycyclic aromatic hydrocarbons such as benzo[a]pyrene (Flesher, 1976). However, a third of these animals later developed leukaemia; this disease is caused in rats by hydrocarbons such as 7,12-dimethylbenz[a]anthracene only after injection directly into the bloodstream *via* the caudal vein (Huggins *et al.*, 1978). In addition 25% also suffered liver degeneration, while 50% developed cirrhosis of the kidney including one animal with a reticulosarcoma of this organ (Bhatt, 1986).

6.3   The mutagenicity of cyclopenta[a]phenanthrenes

Over the last decade there has been a great deal of interest shown in the relationship between carcinogenicity and mutagenicity, chiefly in search of short-term tests for carcinogenicity that could supplant the tedious and expensive animal experiments of the type already described. During the intervening period it has become apparent that there is in fact a good correspondence between these two types of biological activity (Ames *et al.*, 1973; Purchase *et al.*, 1976). However, previously this was not obvious, and it then seemed of interest to re-test the 36 cyclopenta[a]phenanthrenes and two chrysenes listed in Table 21 for mutagenicity

Table 21. *Mutagenicity and carcinogenicity of some cyclopenta[a]phenanthrenes and related chrysenes*

Compound	Mutagenicity (no. of revertant TA100 colonies/nmol)	Carcinogenicity (Iball index)	
		Repeated application	Initiation–promotion
Cyclopenta[a]phenanthrenes			
17-methyl-16,17-dihydro-15*H*- (Diels' hydrocarbon, **7**)	0.7*	<1	—
11,17-dimethyl-16,17-dihydro-15*H*- (**139**)	1.5	3	—
3-methoxy-17-methyl-16,17-dihydro-15*H*- (**17**)	<0.2	<1	—
17*H*- (**2**)	4.0*	<1	—
17-methyl-15*H*- (**133**)	1.6	6	—
11,17-dimethyl-15*H*- (**135**)	1.0	27	—
12,17-dimethyl-15*H*- (**136**)	1.0	7	—
11,12,17-trimethyl-15*H*- (**137**)	1.2	23	—
3-methoxy-17-methyl-15*H*- (**134**)	0.7	2	—
11-methoxy-17-methyl-15*H*- (**138**)	0.9	11	—
15,16-dihydro-17-one (**4**)	9.5*	<1	<1
1-methyl-15,16-dihydro-17-one (**302**)	<0.2	1	3
2-methyl-15,16-dihydro-17-one (**303**)	<0.2	<1	—
3-methyl-15,16-dihydro-17-one (**304**)	<0.2	<1	<1
4-methyl-15,16-dihydro-17-one (**305**)	<0.2	<1	<1
6-methyl-15,16-dihydro-17-one (**306**)	<0.2	<1	—
7-methyl-15,16-dihydro-17-one (**230**)	12.3	10	—

Compound			
11-methyl-15,16-dihydro-17-one (**26**)	21.7	46	57
12-methyl-15,16-dihydro-17-one (**130**)	<0.2	<1	—
11,12-dimethyl-15,16-dihydro-17-one (**131**)	1.1	30	33
1,11-methano-15,16-dihydro-17-one (**310**)	1.9	(16)	—
11-ethyl-15,16-dihydro-17-one (**211**)	1.8	8	—
11-*n*-butyl-15,16-dihydro-17-one (**212**)	<0.2	<1	—
3-methoxy-15,16-dihydro-17-one (**24**)	0.2	<1	38
11-methoxy-15,16-dihydro-17-one (**132**)	3.1	25	28
11-ethoxy-15,16-dihydro-17-one (**390**)	1.8	—	<1
11-*n*-propoxy-15,16-dihydro-17-one (**391**)	0.3*	—	4
11-isopropoxy-15,16-dihydro-17-one (**392**)	1.1	—	5
11-*n*-butoxy-15,16-dihydro-17-one (**393**)	<0.2	—	<1
11-*n*-pentoxy-15,16-dihydro-17-one (**394**)	<0.2	—	—
11-methoxy-7-methyl-15,16-dihydro-17-one (**447**)	34.5	17	—
6-methoxy-11-methyl-15,16-dihydro-17-one (**468**)	1.7	14	—
16-hydroxy-11-methyl-15,16-dihydro-17-one (**346**)	18.3	11	—
11-methyl-11,12,15,16-tetrahydro-17-one (**252**)	<0.2	<1	—
16,17-dihydro-15-one (**102**)	6.7*	<1	—
11-methyl-16,17-dihydro-15-one (**334**)	3.7	5	—
Chrysenes			
1,2,3,4-tetrahydro-1-one (**449**)	7.2*	<1	—
11-methyl-1,2,3,4-tetrahydro-1-one (**450**)	7.1	45	

* indicates mutagenic, but not carcinogenic.

since there existed approximately quantitative data on the relative potency of these compounds as carcinogens in mice of a single strain. Initially, it was found that the compounds were not mutagenic in Ames' original *Salmonella typhimurium* strains TA1535 and TA1538, but when these bacteria became available carrying the R-factor plasmid (pKM101) as TA98 and TA100 (McCann *et al.*, 1975), making the bacteria more sensitive to polycyclic aromatic hydrocarbons, experiments became possible with cyclopenta[a]phenanthrenes. It was soon found that the carcinogenic 11-methyl-17-ketone (**26**) was readily detected using TA100 and a standard homogenate obtained from the livers of rats induced with the chlorinated biphenyl mixture Aroclor 1254, but it was less readily detected with TA98. Thereafter, *Salmonella typhimurium* TA100 was used exclusively (Coombs *et al.*, 1976; Bhatt *et al.*, 1982; Hadfield *et al.*, 1984) in a standardized protocol. Each compound was first tested with three concentrations of the enzyme preparation (homogenate) to ascertain the concentration needed to give the highest mutation rate. As can be seen for the 7-methyl-17-ketone (**230**) in Fig. 57, $20\,\mu L$ or $50\,\mu L$ of homogenate give the same initial slope of the dose/response curve, but this slope is less steep with $100\,\mu L$, although the maximum number of revertant colonies is larger at a higher dose. The compound was then retested, at least in triplicate, using the optimum enzyme concentration and at 1, 5, 10, 50, and $100\,\mu g$/plate; the mutagenicity was expressed as the

Fig. 57. Induction of his⁺ mutations in *Salmonella typhimurium* TA100 with 15,16-dihydro-7-methylcyclopenta[a]phenanthren-17-one (**230**) at increasing doses and at three levels of enzyme (μL of homogenate).

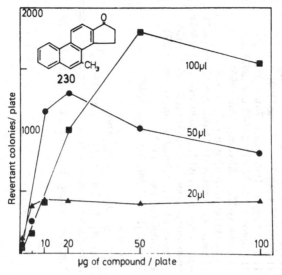

number of revertant colonies/nmol calculated from the initially straight part of the dose/response curve where cytotoxicity is minimal. Compounds exhibiting less than 0.2 colony/nmol were considered non-mutagenic; this number is approximately equivalent to the spontaneous mutation rate of these bacteria under these conditions. Also collected in this Table are Iball indices of carcinogenicity for skin tumours induced in T.O. mice under the standard repeated-application (120 nmol twice weekly) and two-stage (1600 nmol once, twice-weekly promotion with croton oil) procedures, as already outlined. Compounds for which this index is <1 were not carcinogenic in these tests, i.e., the tumour incidence was less than 5% (<1 in 20 animals) in 700 days.

In this study all the carcinogens were mutagenic with the possible exception of the 1-methyl-17-ketone (**302**) and the 11-*n*-butoxy-17-ketone (**393**); the former may possess marginal carcinogenicity whilst the latter appears to be a very weak carcinogen. However, the reverse was not true, for out of the 15 non-carcinogens six (marked with asterisks) were mutagenic. Also there was no consistent relationship between carcinogenic and mutagenic potency, although several strong carcinogens were also strong mutagens, giving dose/response curves similar to that shown in Fig. 58 for the 11-methyl-17-ketone (**26**). The dramatic

Fig. 58. Dose/response showing the effect of the increasing toxicity of the carcinogenic 11-methyl-17-ketone (**26**) above 10 μg/plate, and the inhibitory effect of a constant amount (30 μg) of 7,8-benzoflavone (BF) on mutation induction.

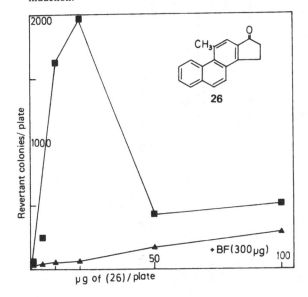

Table 22. Mutagenicity of 15,16-dihydrocyclopenta[a]phenanthren-17-one (**4**) and four related ketones in V79 cells mediated by HepG2 cells in vitro

Compound	Concentration (µg/mL)	Treatment time (h)	Percentage cloning efficiency[a]	Mutation frequency[b]
15,16-dihydrocyclopenta[a]phenanthren-17-one (**4**)	1.0	48	4.5	7.8
2-methyl-15,16-dihydrocyclopenta[a]phenanthren-17-one (**303**)	1.0	48	10.7	1.2
3-methyl-15,16-dihydrocyclopenta[a]phenanthren-17-one (**304**)	1.0	48	7.0	1.0
11-methyl-15,16-dihydrocyclopenta[a]phenanthren-17-one (**26**)	0.5	24	26.2	34.4
11-methyl-1,2,3,4-tetrahydrochrysen-1-one (**450**)	0.5	24	20.31	28.2

a Percentage of reduction in cloning efficiency compared with untreated control cells.
b Number of 6-TG-resistant mutants/10⁵ viable V79 cells at the end of a four-day expression period; the average mutation frequency in control cells was 0.37.

decrease in the number of mutant colonies observed with doses above 20 μg/plate probably reflects the considerable toxicity of this compound. This figure also demonstrates the effect of adding 7,8-benzoflavone (300 μg) to the plate; in agreement with its inhibitory effect on tumour induction, this flavone also considerably reduced the apparent mutagenicity of this compound, presumably by blocking metabolism. It is noticeable that of the six mutagenic non-carcinogens, five are parent unsubstituted compounds which become carcinogens upon 11-methyl substitution. Of these 15,16-dihydrocyclopenta[a]phenanthren-17-one (4) is of particular interest for it has been tested side-by-side with its 11-methyl homologue (26) on many occasions, but has never been found to give tumours.

In order to carry this investigation a little further, these two compounds were also tested for mutagenicity in a mammalian cell culture system (Bhatt *et al.*, 1983), using V79 Chinese hamster cells and scoring for mutations conferring 6-thioguanine resistance (Huberman and Sachs, 1974). It was unexpectedly discovered that hamster embryo cells, used by these authors metabolically to activate polycyclic aromatic hydrocarbon carcinogens, did not appear to activate the cyclopenta[a]phenanthrenone (26). The method of Diamond *et al.* (1980) was therefore employed, making use of human hepatoma cells (Hep G2) to cause activation. Under these conditions the 11-methyl-17-ketone (26) and its strongly carcinogenic chrysenone analogue (450) were both potent mutagens whilst the 2- and 3-methyl-17-ketones (303 and 304, respectively, both non-carcinogens) were inert. However, the non-carcinogenic parent ketone (4) was still moderately mutagenic in this system (Table 22). Again substantial toxicity was encountered with the carcinogen (26) in these cells, the cloning efficiency being reduced 50% at a dose of 1 μg/mL, at which the highest mutation frequency was observed (Fig. 59). These two cyclopenta[a]phenanthrenes (4) and (26) were also compared for their ability to increase the frequency of sister chromatid exchanges in human lymphocytes, again using Hep G2 cells to cause biological activation (Lindahl-Kiessling *et al.*, 1984). In this case it was found that the carcinogen (26) was able consistently to increase this frequency whereas the non-carcinogen (4) was not.

Several of these compounds have also been tested in yeast (Kelly, 1983; Kelly and Parry, 1983). Gene conversion at the *trp5* locus was measured in *Saccharomyces cerevisiae* strain JD1, whilst strain D6 was used to detect mitotic aneuploidy. The experiments were carried out in ignorance of the identities of the compounds until completion of the series. Results are summarized in Table 23 in which a positive response (+) denotes at least a two-fold increase over control levels in white, cycloheximide resistant, monosomic colonies in strain D6 or trp⁺ prototrophs in strain JD1. For reference carcinogenicity is displayed alongside, again either positive or negative, without any indication of potency. There is a remarkably good correlation between genetic activity and carcinogenicity in both strains of this yeast. Of the carcinogens only the 11-phenol (**206**) was not detected; this compound is almost insoluble in water and most organic solvents, so that a sufficient concentration was probably not achieved in the incubation medium. The 11-isopropoxy-17-ketone (**392**) was active in D6, but not in JD1 thus confirming its apparent very weak carcinogenicity, whereas the 11-*n*-butoxy-17-ketone, also a very weak carcinogen, was active in both, although it was not detected in the Ames' test. All the non-carcinogens were inactive in both D6 and JD1, including the unsubstituted parent ketone (**4**) which was mutagenic in both the Ames' test and in V79 cells in culture. The 1-methyl-17-ketone (**302**) was not mutagenic in any of these tests, thus throwing further doubt on its questionable carcinogenicity. Sensitivity for these compounds was poor,

Fig. 59. Toxicity (reduction in plating efficiency) and mutagenicity (induction of 6-thioguanine-resistant colonies) with the carcinogenic 11-methyl-17-ketone (**26**) in V79 cells mediated by human Hep G2 liver cells.

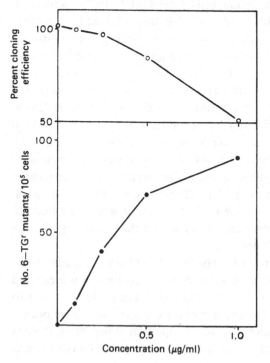

Table 23. *Induction of genetic activity in the yeast Saccharomyces cerevisiae strains D6 and JD1*

Compound	Strain D6 (mitotic aneuploidy)	Strain JD1 (gene conversion)	Carcinogenicity (see Table 20)
15,16-dihydrocyclopenta[a]phenanthren-17-one (**4**)	–	–	–
1-methyl-15,16-dihydrocyclopenta[a]phenanthren-17-one (**302**)	–	–	– (?)
2-methyl-15,16-dihydrocyclopenta[a]phenanthren-17-one (**303**)	–	–	–
3-methyl-15,16-dihydrocyclopenta[a]phenanthren-17-one (**304**)	–	–	–
7-methyl-15,16-dihydrocyclopenta[a]phenanthren-17-one (**230**)	+	+	+
11-methyl-15,16-dihydrocyclopenta[a]phenanthren-17-one (**26**)	+	+	+
11,12-dimethyl-15,16-dihydrocyclopenta[a]phenanthren-17-one (**131**)	+	+	+
1,11-methano-15-16-dihydrocyclopenta[a]phenanthren-17-one (**310**)	+	+	+
11-methoxy-15,16-dihydrocyclopenta[a]phenanthren-17-one (**132**)	+	+	+
11-ethoxy-15,16-dihydrocyclopenta[a]phenanthren-17-one (**390**)	+	+	+
11-*n*-propoxy-15,16-dihydrocyclopenta[a]phenanthren-17-one (**391**)	–	–	–
11-isopropoxy-15,16-dihydrocyclopenta[a]phenanthren-17-one (**392**)	+	–	+
11-*n*-butoxy-15,16-dihydrocyclopenta[a]phenanthren-17-one (**393**)	+	+	+
11-*n*-pentoxy-15,16-dihydrocyclopenta[a]phenanthren-17-one (**394**)	–	–	–
11-hydroxy-15,16-dihydrocyclopenta[a]phenanthren-17-one (**206**)	–	–	+
1,2,3,4-tetrahydro-11-methylchrysen-1-one (**450**)	+	+	+

the maximum increase in genetic activity over background never reaching more than three-fold, and there was little indication of potency. Addition of rat liver homogenate to the plates generally increased the observed frequency of mitogenic conversion and aneuploidy events, but the yeasts were to some extent capable of activating these compounds themselves, especially when they had been grown on low glucose (0.5%) to the exponential phase and then transferred to high glucose (20%) to suppress mitochondrial function. Under these conditions a marked increase in the P450/448 content of the yeast could be demonstrated.

Of these methods for measuring genetic toxicity the Ames' test is to be preferred on grounds of operational simplicity as well as sensitivity. In this cyclopenta[a]phenanthrene series the test is capable of detecting virtually all the carcinogens, but suffers chiefly from being too sensitive in that it also detects some non-carcinogens as mutagens. This is of little consequence when the test is used to distinguish the biologically active metabolites of these compounds among the many separable by hplc, as is described in Chapter 7.

6.4   References

Abbott, P. J. (1983). Strain-specific tumorigenesis in mouse skin induced by the carcinogen, 15,16-dihydro-11-methylcyclopenta[a]phenanthren-17-one, and its relation to DNA adduct formation and persistence. *Cancer Res.*, **43**, 2261–6.

Ames, B. N., Durston, W. E., Yamaski, E. & Lee, F. D. (1973). Carcinogens are mutagens: a simple test system combining liver homogenates for activation and bacteria for detection. *Proc. Nat. Acad. Sci. U.S.A.*, **70**, 2281–5.

Berenblum, I. (1969). A re-evaluation of the concept of co-carcinogenesis. *Prog. Exp. Tumor Res.*, **11**, 21–30.

Berry, D. L., Slaga, T. J., Viaje, A., Wilson, N. M., DiGiovanni, J., Juchau, M. R. & Selkirk, J. K. (1977). Effect of trichloropropene oxide on the ability of polyaromatic hydrocarbons and their 'K-region' oxides to initiate skin tumours in mice and to bind to DNA *in vitro*. *J.N.C.I.*, **58**, 1051–5.

Bhatt, T. S., Coombs, M., DiGiovanni, J. & Diamond, L. (1983). Mutagenesis in Chinese hamster cells by cyclopenta[a]phenanthrenes activated by a human hepatoma cell line. *Cancer Res.*, **43**, 984–6.

Bhatt, T., Coombs, M. & O'Neill, C. (1984). Biogenic silica fibre promotes carcinogenesis in mouse skin. *Int. J. Cancer*, **34**, 519–28.

Bhatt, T. S. (1986). The effect of 15,16-dihydro-11-methylcyclopenta[a]-phenanthren-17-one and biogenic silica fibre on Sprague-Dawley rats. *Carcinogenesis*, in press.

Bhatt, T. S., Hadfield, S. T. & Coombs, M. M. (1982). Carcinogenicity and mutagenicity of some alkoxy cyclopenta[a]phenanthren-17-ones: effect of obstructing the bay region. *Carcinogenesis*, **3**, 677–80.

Bryan, W. R. & Shimkin, M. B. (1941). Quantitative analysis of dose-response data obtained with carcinogenic hydrocarbons. *J.N.C.I.*, **1**, 807–33.

Burki, K., Wheeler, J. E., Akamatsu, Y., Scribner, J. E., Candelas, G. & Bresnick, E. (1974). Early differential effects of 3-methylcholanthrene and its 'K-region' epoxide on mouse skin. Possible implication in the two stage mechanism of tumorigenesis. *J.N.C.I.*, **53**, 967–76.

Butenandt, A. & Suranyi, L. A. (1942). Uberfuhrung von Steroidhormonen in methylhomloge des cyclopenta[a]phenanthrenes. *Ber.*, **75B**, 597–606.

Butenandt, A. & Dannenberg, H. (1953). Untersuchungen über die krebserzengende Wirksamkeit der Methylhomlogen des 1,2-Cyclopentenophenathrenes. *Arch. Geschwulstforsch.*, **6**, 1–7.

Coombs, M. M. & Bhatt, T. S. (1978). Lack of initiating activity in mutagens which are not carcinogenic. *Br. J. Cancer*, **38**, 148–50.

Coombs, M. M. & Bhatt, T. S. (1982). High skin tumour initiating activity of the metabolically derived *trans*-3,4-dihydro-3,4-diol of the carcinogen 15,16-dihydro-11-methylcyclopenta[a]phenanthren-17-one. *Carcinogenesis*, **3**, 449–51.

Coombs, M. M., Bhatt, T. S. & Croft, C. J. (1973). Correlation between carcinogenicity and chemical structure in cyclopenta[a]phenanthrenes. *Cancer Res.*, **33**, 832–7.

Coombs, M. M., Bhatt, T. S., Hall, M. & Croft, C. J. (1974). The relative carcinogenic activities of a series of 5-methylchrysene derivatives. *Cancer Rès.*, **34**, 1315–18.

Coombs, M. M., Bhatt, T. S. & Vose, C. W. (1975). The relationship between metabolism, DNA binding, and carcinogenicity of 15,16-dihydro-11-methylcyclopenta[a]phenanthren-17-one in the presence of a microsomal enzyme inhibitor. *Cancer Res.*, **35**, 305–9.

Coombs, M. M., Bhatt, T. S. & Young, S. (1979). The carcinogenicity of 15,16-dihydro-11-methylcyclopenta[a]phenanthren-17-one. *Br. J. Cancer*, **40**, 914–21.

Coombs, M. M. & Croft, C. J. (1966). Carcinogenic derivatives of cyclopenta[a]phenanthrene. *Nature (London)*, **210**, 1281–2.

Coombs, M. M. & Croft, C. J. (1969). Carcinogenic cyclopenta[a]phenanthrenes. *Prog. Exp. Tumor Res.*, **11**, 69–85.

Coombs, M. M., Dixon, C. & Kissonerghis, A.-M. (1976). Evaluation of the mutagenicity of compounds of known carcinogenicity belonging to the benz[a]anthracene, chrysene, and cyclopenta[a]phenanthrene series using Ames' test. *Cancer Res.*, **36**, 4525–9.

Coombs, M. M., Hadfield, S. T. & Bhatt, T. S. (1982). 15,16-Dihydro-1,11-methanocyclopenta[a]phenanthren-17-one: a carcinogen with a bridged bay region. In *Polynuclear Aromatic Hydrocarbons: formation, metabolism and measurement*, ed. Cooke, M. W. & Dennis, A. J., pp. 351–63. Columbus: Battelle Press.

Craciun, E. C., Zugravesco, I. & Stefu, L. (1939). Carcinogenic action of well-defined chemical substances. *Acta Unio Int. Cancrum*, **4**, 675–8.

Diamond, L., Kruszewski, F., Aden, D. P., Knowles, B. B. & Baird, W. M. (1980). Metabolic activation of benzo[a]pyrene by a human hepatoma cell line. *Carcinogenesis*, **1**, 871–5.

Dannenberg, H. (1960). Uber Beziehungen zwischen Steroiden und krebserzeugenden Kohlenwasserstoffen. II. Mitteilung. 1:2-Cyclopentadienophenanthrene. *Z. Krebsforsch.*, **63**, 523–31.

Dannenberg, H., Scheurlen, H. & Dannenberg-von Dresler, D. (1956). Notiz zur Dehydrierung von Cholesterin mit chloranil. *Z. Physiol. Chem.*, **303**, 282–5.

168   *Carcinogenicity and mutagenicity*

Fisher, R. A. (1954). *Statistical Methods for Research Workers*, 12th Ed., p. 96. Edinburgh: Oliver & Boyd.

Flesher, J. N., Harvey, R. G. & Sydnor, K. L. (1976). Oncogenicity of K-region epoxides of benzo[a]pyrene and 7,12-dimethylbenz[a]anthracene. *Int. J. Cancer*, **18**, 351–3.

Hadfield, S. T., Bhatt, T. S. & Coombs, M. M. (1984). The biological activity and activation of 15,16-dihydro-1,11-methanocyclopenta[a]phenanthren-17-one, a carcinogen with an obstructed bay region. *Carcinogenesis*, **5**, 1485–91.

Hartnell, J. L. (1951). *Survey of Compounds which have been tested for Carcinogenic Activity*. US Public Health Service Publ. No. 149, p. 184.

Huberman, E. & Sachs, L. (1974). Cell mediated mutagenesis of mammalian cells with chemical carcinogens. *Int. J. Cancer*, **13**, 326–33.

Huggins, G. (1961). Rapid induction of mammary cancer and their suppression. *Science*, **133**, 1366.

Huggins, C. B., Ueda, N. & Russo, A. (1978). Azo dyes prevent hydrocarbon induced leukaemia in the rat. *Proc. Nat. Acad. Sci. U.S.A.*, **75**, 4524–7.

Kashino, S., Zacharias, D. E., Peck, R. M., Glusker, J. P., Bhatt, T. S. & Coombs, M. M. (1966). Bay region distortions in cyclopenta[a]phenanthrenes. *Cancer Res.*, **46**, 1817–29.

Kaufmann, C., Muller, M. A., Butenandt, A. & Friedrich-Freksa, H. (1949). Experimentelle Beitrage zur Bedeutung des Follikelhomous für die Carcinomentstehung. *Z. Krebsforsch.*, **56**, 482–542.

Kelly, D. E. (1983). *The Genotoxic Potential of Carcinogens in Yeast*. Ph.D. thesis, University College of Swansea.

Kelly, D. & Parry, J. M. (1983). Metabolic activation of cytochrome P.450/P–448 in the yeast Saccharomyces cerevisiae. *Mutation Res.*, **108**, 147–59.

Kinoshita, N. & Gelboin, H. V. (1972). The role of aryl hydrocarbon hydroxylase in 7,12-dimethylbenz[a]anthracene skin tumorigenesis: on the mechanisms of 7,8-benzoflavone inhibition of tumorigenesis. *Cancer Res.*, **32**, 1329–39.

Lindahl-Keissling, K., Bhatt, T. S., Karlberg, I. & Coombs, M. M. (1984). Frequency of sister chromatid exchanges in human lymphocytes cultivated with a human hepatoma cell line as an indicator of the carcinogenic potency of two cyclopenta[a]phenanthrenes. *Carcinogenesis*, **5**, 11–14.

McCann, J., Springarn, W. E., Kobori, J. & Ames, B. N. (1975). The detection of carcinogens as mutagens: bacterial tester strains with R factor plasmids. *Proc. Nat. Acad. Sci. U.S.A.*, **72**, 979–83.

Purchase, I. F. H., Longstaff, E., Asby, J., Styles, J. A., Anderson, D., Lefevre, P. A. & Westwood, F. R. (1976). Evaluation of six short term tests for detecting organic chemical carcinogens, and recommendations for their use. *Nature*, **264**, 624–7.

Selkirk, J. K., Croy, R. G., Roller, P. P. & Gelboin, H. V. (1974). High pressure liquid chromatographic analysis of benzo[a]pyrene metabolism and covalent binding and the mechanism of the action of 7,8-benzoflavone and 1,2-epoxy-3,3,3-trichloropropane. *Cancer Res.*, **34**, 3474–80.

Shay, H., Aegerter, E. A., Gruenstein, M. & Komarov, S. A. (1949). Development of adenocarcinoma of the breast in the Wistar rat following gastric instillation of methylcholanthrene. *J.N.C.I.*, **10**, 255–66.

Vose, C. W., Coombs, M. M. & Bhatt, T. S. (1981). Co-carcinogenicity of promoting agents. *Carcinogenesis*, **2**, 687–9.

Wood, A. W., Wislocki, P. G., Chang, R. L., Yagi, H., Hernanez, O.,

Jerina, D. M. & Conney, A. H. (1976). Mutagenicity and cytotoxicity of benzo[a]pyrene benzo-ring epoxides. *Cancer Res.*, **36**, 3358–66.

Yang, N. C., Castro, A. J., Lewis M. & Wong, T. W. (1961). Polynuclear hydrocarbons, steroids, and carcinogenesis. *Science*, **134**, 386–7.

Metabolic activation of cyclopenta[a]-phenanthrenes and their interaction with DNA

7.1   Activation of 15,16-dihydro-11-methylcyclopenta[a]phenanthren-17-one

In the various mutation tests described in the last chapter, without exception none of the cyclopenta[a]phenanthrenes was active in the absence of an added source of metabolism. Since there is a good parallelism between mutagenicity and carcinogenicity in this series, it seemed reasonable to suppose that metabolism was required before these compounds could act to cause tumours in animals. Dannenberg (1960) found that introduction of a double bond between C-16 and C-17 in Diels' hydrocarbon (7) to give 17-methyl-15H-cyclopenta[a]phenanthrene (133) led to weak carcinogenicity (see Table 9). He noted that this double bond was the most chemically reactive in the molecule, adding, for example, to osmium tetroxide to give the 16,17-cis-diol in preference to the K-region 6,7-double bond, and he suggested that the carcinogenicity of this hydrocarbon and its 15-methyl-17H-isomer (128) might be due to the reactivity of these double bonds in the five-membered ring-D. It has already been shown that some of the 17-ketones of this series, lacking a carbon–carbon double bond in the ring-D, are more active than the corresponding unsaturated ring-D hydrocarbons (see Tables 10 and 11), and in these ketones the most chemically reactive double bond is between C-6 and C-7 (i.e., in the K-region). Metabolism of cyclopenta[a]-phenanthrene hydrocarbons such as (128) and (133) does not appear to have been studied yet, although structure/activity relationships established since Dannenberg's suggestion do indicate interesting differences between the two series (see Table 24). Thus comparing the Iball indices obtained under the same standard conditions for several identically substituted pairs of 17-methyl-16,17-enes and 15,16-dihydro-17-ketones it is clear that carcinogenicity among the latter is confined to 11-

substituted derivatives, whereas all the hydrocarbons appear to be active to some extent. Analogously substituted 17-ketones are more active than the corresponding hydrocarbons, particularly in the case of the 11-methoxy derivatives.

At the outset the 11-methyl-17-ketone (**26**) was chosen for metabolic study because it was at that time the most carcinogenic cyclopenta[a]phenanthrene known; in many experiments the inactive unsubstituted parent 17-ketone (**4**) was examined alongside. An indication that simple metabolic experiments employing the microsomal fraction from rat liver in incubations in phosphate buffer containing an excess of NADPH in air would yield meaningful results came from an early experiment (Coombs *et al.*, 1975). In this it was established that the aryl hydrocarbon hydroxylase inhibitor 7,8-benzoflavone not only inhibited tumour production with this 11-methyl ketone (**26**), but also considerably diminished the binding of this ^{3}H-labelled carcinogen to calf thymus DNA under these *in vitro* metabolic conditions (Table 25). The carcinogen administered twice weekly at a total dose of 60 µg/week gave the expected skin tumour incidence (85%) and mean latent period (29 weeks). At one-tenth of this weekly dose, in two identical experiments the tumour incidence was approximately halved, and the mean latent period increased about 50%; these results illustrate the good reproducibility achievable in this type of tumour-induction experiment. No skin tumours were produced at one-hundredth of the original weekly dose. When a mixture of the carcinogen at the highest weekly dose was painted together with 7,8-benzoflavone at three times this dose, tumour incidence was reduced to 70% and the mean latent period was prolonged by almost 30%, but when both were repeatedly administered together at one-tenth

Table 24. *Comparison of Iball indices (T.O. mice, repeated application) of 17-methyl-15H-cyclopenta[a]phenanthrene hydrocarbons with the corresponding 15,16-dihydrocyclopenta[a]phenanthren-17-ones*

Substitution	Iball index (see Table 21)			
	17-methyl-16,17-ene		17-ketone	
unsubstituted	(133)	6	(4)	<1
11-methyl	(135)	27	(26)	46
12-methyl	(136)	7	(130)	<1
11,12-dimethyl	(137)	23	(131)	30
11-methoxy	(138)	11	(132)	25
3-methoxy	(134)	2	(24)	<1

Table 25. *Effect of the aryl hydrocarbon hydroxylase inhibitor 7,8-benzoflavone on tumour induction* (A), *and on in vitro binding* (B) *of the carcinogen 15,16-dihydro-11-methyl-cyclopenta[a]phenanthren-17-one* (26) *to DNA*

(A) Tumour induction (T.O. mice in groups of 20, painted twice weekly)

Treatment	Percentage skin tumour incidence	Mean latent period (weeks)
(26) 60 μg/week	85	29
(26) 6 μg/week	45	43
(26) 6 μg/week	42	46
(26) 0.6 μg/week	0	—
(26) 60 μg/week plus 7,8/benzoflavone (180 μg/week)	70	37
(26) 6 μg/week plus 7,8-benzoflavone (18 μg/week)	0	—
(26) 6 μg/week plus 15,16-dihydrocyclopenta[a]phenanthren-17-one (54 μg/week)	50	45

(B) DNA binding (covalent binding to calf thymus DNA added to the *in vitro* incubation)

Substrate	Microsomal preparation	DNA binding index (μmol ketone/mol DNA phosphorus)[a]
Preparation 1		
(26)	active	46.5 ± 2.5
(26)	heat-inactivated	0
(26) + 3 molar equiv. of 7,8-benzoflavone	active	0
Preparation 2		
(26)	active	18.1 ± 2.0
(26)	absent	0
(26) + 3 molar equiv. of 7,8-benzoflavone	active	0.87

a, average of 5 replicate determinations ± s.d.

of these amounts no skin tumours were observed. Thus this inhibitor is relatively more active at lower doses of the carcinogen as has been noted already. Administration of a nine-fold quantity of the non-carcinogenic parent ketone (4) together with the carcinogen (26) had no effect on the tumour induction by the latter. This carcinogen (26) bound covalently to calf thymus DNA added to the *in vitro* metabolic incubation, but this was largely prevented by inclusion of the inhibitor in the incubation mixture. No DNA binding occurred in the absence of the microsomal preparation, or if the enzyme was deactivated by heat treatment (2 min at 100°C) prior to incubation with the substrate and DNA. This whole experiment clearly supports the view that metabolism is involved in tumour induction with this carcinogen, and that this simple metabolic system is a valid model for its study.

Under similar *in vitro* metabolic conditions in the absence of added DNA and using microsomes isolated from the livers of uninduced Sprague-Dawley rats (Coombs *et al.*, 1976), the main metabolites extracted from the incubation mixture with ethyl acetate appeared to be mono-ols on examination by thin-layer chromatography (tlc). These were readily identified as the 15-ols (369 and 370) and 16-ols (345 and 346), from the unsubstituted -17-ketone (4) and its carcinogenic 11-methyl homologue (26), respectively, by direct comparison of R_F values and ultraviolet spectra of material recovered from the plates with those of the synthetic compounds. When ^{3}H-labelled compounds were used these identities were confirmed by dilution analysis of the derived acetates. The carcinogen also gave a small amount of its 11-hydroxy-methyl derivative (215) identified in the same way, and by the fact that as expected it retained only about 65% of the radioactivity of the original compound when the latter was labelled with tritium in the 11-methyl group. Other more polar metabolites were also detected by tlc, and these were increased relative to the mono-ols when the rats were induced by injection with 3-methylcholanthrene or phenobarbitone before sacrifice. While tlc gave a good separation of these metabolites and the overall structures of some could be tentatively deduced from their relative R_F values and their ultraviolet spectra, particularly after *in situ* reduction of the carbonyl group with sodium borohydride, not enough could be obtained in this way for further examination. Moreover, it was difficult to avoid aerial oxidation using this technique.

Rapid progress was made when high-pressure liquid chromatography (hplc) was introduced because it overcame both of these difficulties. Also developments in high-field Fourier transform nuclear magnetic resonance (nmr) spectroscopy at this time greatly increased the sensitivity of this analytical technique so that it became applicable to the amounts of metabolites obtainable by hplc. Finally, the renewed interest in the metabolism of polycyclic aromatic hydrocarbons had led to the identification of a bay-region diol-epoxide as the active form of benzo[a]pyrene (Sims *et al.*, 1974), and it was subsequently demonstrated that a number of other phenanthrene-derived hydrocarbons followed a similar activation route (Jerina *et al.*, 1978). It seemed probable that the carcinogenic 15,16-dihydro-11-methylcyclopenta[a]phenanthren-17-one (26) might undergo analogous metabolism, and this was reinvestigated using these new techniques with this in mind.

Figure 60 shows a typical hplc separation of *in vitro* metabolites of this compound (26) extracted with ethyl acetate after incubation with NADPH and a microsomal preparation obtained from the livers of male Sprague-Dawley rats previously injected with 3-methylcholanthrene (Coombs *et al.*, 1980). Under these conditions most of the conjugating enzymes normally present in the supernatant are absent, thus largely preserving the products of primary metabolism. After being shaken in the presence of atmospheric oxygen for 30 min at 37°C, extraction with ethyl acetate routinely led to recovery of about 80% of the material incubated, as determined by recovered radioactivity when a labelled substrate was metabolized. A reverse-phase column was employed to separate the complex mixture formed using a gradient of aqueous methanol increasing in methanol concentration, so that the more polar metabolites eluted first and last peak to emerge was the unreacted substrate (26). The profile shown in the figure was monitored continuously at 254 nm, but the profile of eluted radioactivity was very similar. The properties and the structures

Fig. 60. Profile of *in vitro* metabolites of the carcinogen (26) separated by reverse-phase hplc and monitored by their ultraviolet absorption at 254 nm; the first peak m is of microsomal origin, and the last is the unchanged substrate (26).

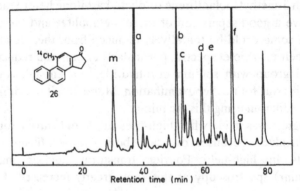

deduced for the main metabolites (**a–g**) are listed in Table 26 (Coombs *et al.*, 1980). The peak denoted M, of microsomal origin, was always present and acted as a useful chromatographic marker. Molecular formulae were based on molecular weights obtained from mass spectrometry; the patterns of fragment ions were in all cases those expected from previous work with synthetic compounds (see Chapter 5). With the

Table 26. *Structures and properties of the main metabolites* **a–g** *(Fig. 60) of the carcinogen 15,16-dihydro-11-methylcyclopenta[a]phenanthren-17-one* (**26**)

Metabolite	Structure
(**a**)	11-methyl-1,2,15,16-tetrahydro-1,2,15-trihydroxycyclopenta[a]phenanthren-17-one (**454**) $C_{18}H_{16}O_4$ Found: M^+ 296.1043; Calculated 296.1049 λ_{max} 265 (4.60), 322 (4.10), 334 (4.14), 354 (3.71), 373 (3.68) nm λ_{max} (reduced) 259 (4.65), 267 (4.69), 320 (3.80) nm
(**b**)	11-methyl-3,4,15,16-tetrahydro-3,4,15-trihydroxycyclopenta[a]phenanthren-17-one (**455**) $C_{18}H_{16}O_4$ Found: M^+ 296; Calculated 296 λ_{max} 273 (4.70), 327sh (3.83), 335 (3.84), 370sh (3.54) nm λ_{max} (reduced) 248 (4.74), 327 (3.97), 347 (3.85) nm
(**c**)	11-methyl-3,4,15,16-tetrahydro-3,4,16-trihydroxycyclopenta[a]phenanthren-17-one (**456**) $C_{18}H_{16}O_4$ Found: M^+ 296; Calculated 296 λ_{max} 272 (4.70), 327sh (3.89), 333 (3.90), 370sh (3.61) nm λ_{max} (reduced) 248 (4.76), 326 (4.03), 347 (3.90) nm
(**d**)	15,16-dihydro-15-hydroxy-11-hydroxymethylcyclopenta[a]phenanthren-17-one $C_{18}H_{14}O_3$ Found: M^+ 278.0948; Calculated 278.0943 λ_{max} 269 (4.78), 300 (4.27), 358 (3.26), 376 (3.24) nm λ_{max} (reduced) 255 (4.82), 279 (4.09), 290 (4.05), 301 (4.09), 334 (4.06), 350 (2.93) nm
(**e**)	3,4-dihydroxy-11-methyl-3,4,15,16-tetrahydrocyclopenta[a]phenanthren-17-one (**457**) $C_{18}H_{16}O_3$ Found: M^+ 280.1109; Calculated 280.1100 λ_{max} 273 (4.71), 332sh (3.84), 357 (3.57), 371 (3.55) nm λ_{max} (reduced) 250 (4.70), 306 (3.58), 330 (3.63), 349 (3.59) nm
(**f**)	15,16-dihydro-15-hydroxy-11-methylcyclopenta[a]phenanthren-17-one (**370**) Identified by reference to the synthetic compound (see Chapter 5 for physical data)
(**g**)	15,16-dihydro-16-hydroxy-11-methylcyclopenta[a]phenanthren-17-one (**346**) Identified by reference to the synthetic compound (see Chapter 5 for physical data)

vicinal *trans*-dihydro diols the molecular ions were weak, but the M^+-18 ions (loss of water) were prominent, and ions due to the ready loss of carbon monoxide (28 mass units) from ring-D confirmed the retention of this double-bonded oxygen atom in these metabolites. The ultraviolet spectra of these cyclopenta[a]phenanthrene derivatives after mild reduction of this conjugated double bond with sodium borohydride resembled those of the corresponding known phenanthrene derivatives, and allowed assignment of the points of saturation and hence the position of the *trans*-dihydrodiol systems. This was further checked by dehydration of these diols by heating them with 50% sulphuric acid for 30 min, and examining the resulting phenols (Table 27). Metabolites (b), (c), and (e) gave 4-phenols with almost identical ultraviolet spectra, similar to those of synthetic 15,16-dihydro-4-hydroxy-1-methylcyclopenta[a]phenanthren-17-one (458), whereas the 2-phenol from metabolite a resembled synthetic 15,16-dihydro-2-hydroxycyclopenta[a]phenanthren-17-one (396). The inter-relationships between these various metabolites are shown in Fig. 61. The mono-ols (215), (346, g), (370, f), and the A-ring diols (459) and (457, e) suffer further conversion into the triols (454, a), (455, b) (456, c), and the diol (d). This was confirmed by similar metabolism of the synthetic mono-ols which gave rise to these further-hydroxylated derivatives as expected. The minor

Table 27. *Ultraviolet spectra of phenols obtained by acid-catalysed dehydration of the metabolites* (a), (b), (c), *and* (e) *in comparison with those of two synthetic phenols*

Phenol	λ_{max} ($\log_{10} \varepsilon$)	
	Neutral	Alkaline
Derived from (a)	278 (4.71)	250 (4.53), 301 (4.55)
15,16-dihydro-2-hydroxycyclopenta[a]phenanthren-17-one (396)	274.5 (4.74)	245 (4.59), 296 (4.62)
Derived from (b)	269 (4.61), 274 (4.62), 301.5 (4.48)	261 (4.70), 327 (4.37)
Derived from (c)	269 (4.68), 274 (4.67), 301 (4.57)	262 (4.76), 328 (4.46)
Derived from (e)	271 (4.66), 301 (4.45)	261 (4.64), 325 (4.32)
15,16-dihydro-4-hydroxy-1-methylcyclopenta[a]phenanthren-17-one (458)	270, 305	260, 325

metabolites (215) and (459) were not resolved with a 10-μm reverse-phase column, but using a similar 5-μm column the 11-hydroxymethyl-17-ketone (215) ran as a small peak just ahead of the 15-ol (370), whilst the 1,2-diol (459) appeared just before the 3,4,15-triol (455) and possessed ultraviolet characteristics almost identical with those of the 1,2,15-triol (454). Thus the 1,2-diols are noticeably more polar than the corresponding 3,4-diols; it later appeared that this was due to the fact that the 1,2-diols were diaxial, whereas the 3,4-diols were diequatorial. It therefore seems that this ketone (26) suffered oxidative metabolic attack at rings -A and -D and at the methyl group, but not elsewhere in the molecule. In particular the 6,7-double bond, the most reactive chemically, was unaffected.

The kinetics of the formation of certain of these various metabolites were investigated, chiefly in order to optimize the amount of the 3,4-dihydrodiol since this was required for further study. Aliquots were withdrawn from an *in vitro* incubation of the ^{14}C-labelled carcinogen at intervals, immediately cooled in ice and extracted with ethyl acetate. Separation of the metabolites by hplc and quantitation were carried out

Fig. 61. Structures proposed for the main metabolites formed *in vitro* from the carcinogen (26).

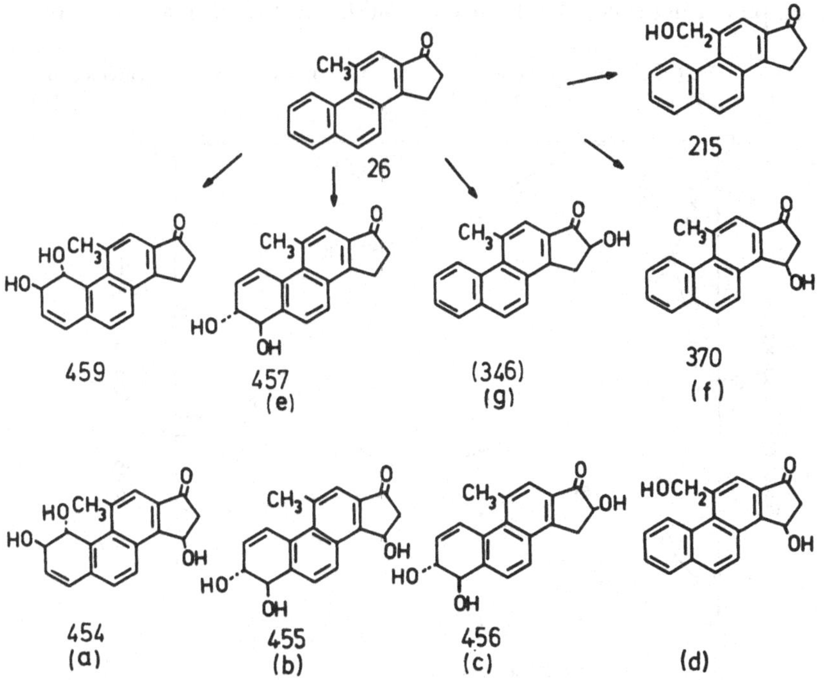

as usual to generate the curves shown in Fig. 62. About 75% of the substrate was consumed, but at a decreasing rate during 45 min, by shaking in air at 37°C. The 3,4-dihydrodiol increased in amount up to about 15 min and then remained fairly constant, decreasing somewhat only at times after 30 min. Presumably this plateau resulted from the rate of its formation just matching its loss by further metabolism until the amount of substrate was diminished substantially. The 15-ol, on the other hand, increased rapidly in amount at first, reaching a maximum accounting for about 25% of the substrate at 10 min, but thereafter decreased sharply. Conversely, the 1,2,15-triol after a sluggish start increased in amount roughly linearly up to about 30 min, confirming that it was formed largely from the 15-ol by further metabolic attack in ring-A. Subsequently, incubations were generally maintained for 30 min to allow consumption of about 70% of the substrate and to maximize the quantity of the 3,4-dihydrodiol under these conditions of substrate and enzyme concentration.

Identification of the biologically active metabolite(s) of this carcinogen (**26**) was tackled in two ways – by measuring the ability of metabolite fractions (**a–g**) to bind to calf thymus DNA *in vitro* after further metabolism, and by investigating their mutagenicity in the Ames' test. It has already been mentioned (Table 25) that after metabolism this compound binds covalently to DNA added to the incubation mixture.

Fig. 62. Kinetics of the formation of certain metabolites of the carcinogen (**26**) on *in vitro* incubation.

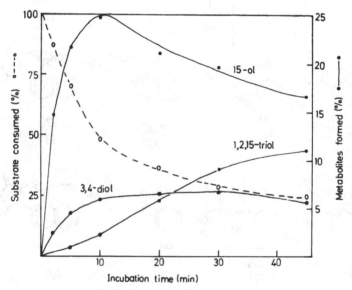

When DNA exposed in this way to the ^{14}C-labelled 11-methyl-17-ketone (**26**) was isolated, purified, hydrolysed enzymatically to its constituent nucleosides, and the latter were separated by chromatography on a column of Sephadex LH20 (hydroxypropyl cellulose) using a water–methanol gradient, two radioactive peaks A and B eluted following the natural nucleosides (detected by their ultraviolet absorption) as shown in Fig. 63. This carcinogen, generally labelled with tritium at very high specific activity (13.9 Ci/mmol), was also applied to mouse skin *in vivo* as in a tumour-initiation experiment; 24 h later the mice were killed and the treated skin was removed. Isolation of the DNA was achieved by initial digestion of the skin with proteinase K according to the method of Blin and Stafford (1976). After purification and enzymatic hydrolysis, the constituent nucleosides were separated as before by LH20 chromatography to give radioactive peaks A and B with the same retention times as those obtained from calf thymus DNA *in vitro*. In this experiment the amount of peak A relative to peak B was less, and owing to the lability of the tritium due to metabolism, the normal nucleosides also became

Fig. 63. Sephadex LH20 profiles of DNA hydrolysates: (a) profile from calf thymus DNA treated *in vitro* with the ^{14}C-labelled carcinogen (**26**) (the dotted line represents ultraviolet absorption of the eluate continuously monitored at 254 nm and the solid line radioactivity); (b) similar profile from DNA isolated from the skin of mice treated topically *in vivo* with the ^{3}H-labelled carcinogen (**26**); (c) co-chromatography of the *in vitro* ^{14}C-adduct B and *in vivo* ^{3}H-adduct B, establishing their identity.

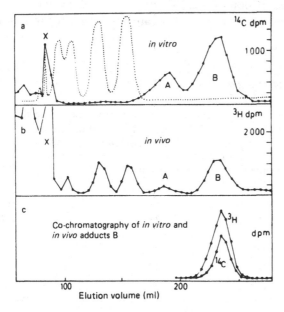

labelled to some extent. When the main adduct peak B, labelled with ^{14}C from the first *in vitro* experiment, was co-chromatographed on LH20 with the ^{3}H-labelled adduct peak B from the *in vivo* experiment they co-eluted together precisely. Thus it seemed that the simple *in vitro* model adequately represented the *in vivo* situation in mouse skin. The binding of the ^{14}C-labelled metabolic fractions (a–f) to DNA was next studied *in vitro* using hepatic microsomes and calf thymus DNA as before. In each case the recovered DNA was degraded to its constituent nucleosides which were separated by LH20 chromatography, and the radioactivity in peaks A and B from each was measured. The results obtained from this experiment are displayed in Table 28 which also lists the mutagenicity of these fractions a–f in the Ames' test. In both tests the metabolite (e) (3,4-dihydrodiol) was by far the most active, being two and a half times more mutagenic and binding to DNA nearly four times as much as the original carcinogen (26). It was also the only metabolite to yield adduct B; the fact that it also gave some adduct A proved that it underwent further hydroxylation to metabolites (b) or (c). Adduct A is formed from the 3,4,15- and 3,4,16-triols (b and c); the mono-ols (g) and (f) also gave this adduct, no doubt after their conversion into (b) and (c). The 1,2,15-triol (a) and the 11-hydroxymethyl-15-ol (d) were inactive in both tests. Thus the primary metabolite responsible for the biological activity of the carcinogen (26) is its 3,4-dihydrodiol (457, e). That this was also mainly responsible for its carcinogenicity was investigated in a direct, straight-forward manner (Coombs and Bhatt, 1982). Repeated large-scale (10 μmol) *in vitro* incubation of this carcinogen and separation of the

Table 28. *Mutagenicity and* in vitro *DNA binding of metabolites* a–g *(Fig. 60) of the carcinogen 15,16-dihydro-11-methylcyclopenta[a]-phenanthren-17-one* (26)

Metabolite	Mutagenicity (revertants/ nmol)	DNA-binding index (μmol of metabolite/mol of DNA phosphorus)		
		Adduct A	Adduct B	Total
(a)	0	0	0	0
(b)	8.9	347	0	347
(c)	14.8	74	0	74
(d)	0	0	0	0
(e)	45.6	56	541	597
(f)	6.6	58	0	58
(g)	13.6	31	0	31
Carcinogen (26)	17.5	30	127	157

metabolites produced by hplc gave enough of these main metabolites (**a–g**) for them to be tested for carcinogenicity in the standard two-stage initiation/promotion experiment with T.O. mice. Groups of 20 mice were employed as usual, and each received a topical dose of 100 nmol [in toluene–acetone (1:1 v/v) because this solvent was known to enhance the carcinogenicity of (**26**)]; twice-weekly promotion with 1% croton oil in toluene then led to the result illustrated in Fig. 64. Again the 3,4-diol (**457**) was more active than the original carcinogen both in respect to higher skin tumour incidence and to a shorter mean latent period. The 3,4,15- and 3,4,16-triols (**455** and **456**) were much less active as tumour initiators, and the 1,2,15-triol (**454**) and 11-hydroxymethyl-15-ol were inactive. This firmly established that 3,4-dihydroxy-11-methyl-3,4,15,16-tetrahydrocyclopenta[a]phenanthren-17-one is the main proximate form of the carcinogen (**26**).

The nature of the adduct peaks A and B was further investigated by hplc (Abbott and Coombs, 1981). When the total radioactive DNA adducts (peaks A and B) derived from mouse skin treated *in vivo* with the carcinogen (**26**) as already described were chromatographed on a 10-μm reverse-phase column in water–methanol (9:1 v/v) six discrete peaks were seen (Fig. 65). By chromatographing peaks A and B separately it

Fig. 64. First appearance of skin tumours in groups of 20 mice after a single topical (100 nmol) application of the carcinogen (**26**) and its metabolites (**455**)-(**457**), followed by twice-weekly promotion with croton oil.

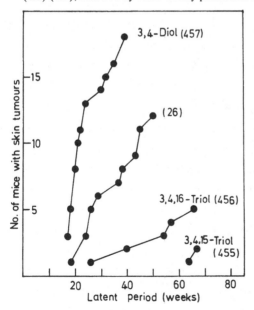

was found that A gave rise to I, II, and III, while peak B separated into IV, V, and VI. The DNA recovered from an *in vitro* binding experiment gave a similar result, and the origin of the individual peaks was determined by incubating each of the main metabolites (**b, c, e, g**) and (**f**) with DNA in the presence of rat liver microsomes *in vitro*. In this way it became clear that the proximate carcinogen (metabolite **e**) gave rise to the main adduct V accounting for over 80% of the total adducts, as well as the minor adduct IV, while the other peaks arose from the triols (**b**) and (**c**). By incubating DNA labelled with tritiated deoxyguanosine with the ^{14}C-labelled carcinogen (**26**) it was readily established that the major adduct V as well as II (probably the 16-hydroxy derivative of V) both involved binding to this base. By using poly(deoxyadenosine-thymidine) labelled with tritiated deoxyadenosine it was likewise shown that adduct VI (and possibly I) involved binding to adenosine. Thus it appears that

Fig. 65. hplc Profile of DNA adducts derived from the skin of mice treated topically with the ^{3}H-labelled carcinogen.

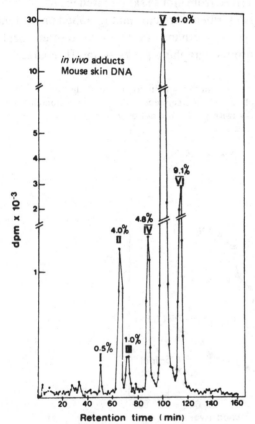

over 85% of the DNA binding observed with this carcinogen is to deoxyguanosine. Thus in this respect, as well as its activation via the 3,4-dihydrodiol, this 11-methyl-17-ketone closely resembled benzo[a]pyrene.

Since further metabolism was required before the 3,4-dihydrodiol (**457, e**) bound to DNA *in vitro* or caused mutations in bacteria it was tempting to assume that this, like benzo[a]pyrene, was mediated *via* a bay-region diol-epoxide. However, this was difficult to prove in the absence of the synthetic diol epoxide, although two separate pieces of evidence pointed in this direction. As has already been discussed in Chapter 5, a detailed and extensive mass spectral study of DNA treated *in vitro* with the carcinogen (**26**) established that a 2,3,4-trihydroxy derivative was bound to deoxyguanosine via its exocyclic N^2-amino group (Wiebers *et al.*, 1981). The other evidence comes from LH20 elution volume data with the nucleoside peak B, which as we have seen, consists mainly (>80%) of this deoxyguanosine adduct. In Tris buffer at pH 8.7 this adduct has an elution volume of about 250 mL, whereas in borate buffer of the same pH and ionic strength it elutes earlier, with an elution volume of about 200 mL (Coombs *et al.*, 1979). This is consistent only with an intermediate *anti*-1,2-epoxy-*trans*-3,4-dihydrodiol, nucleophilic opening of which would yield a 2,3,4-trihydroxy derivative in which the vicinal C-2 and C-3 hydroxy groups are *cis* with respect to one another, and therefore are able to complex with the borate. A *syn*-1,2-epoxy-*trans*-3,4-dihydrodiol would give rise to an all-*trans* arrangement unable to form a complex, and thus elute earlier (Fig. 66). The absolute stereochemistry was based on an nmr and circular dichroism study of the 3,4-diol (**457, e**) (Hadfield *et al.*, 1984*b*). Chemical shifts (δ values) and coupling constants for the ring-A protons in this 11-methyl-3,4-dihydroxy-3,4-dihydro-17-ketone and its unsubstituted homologue, both obtained from metabolism of (**26**) and (**4**) *in vitro*, together with the borohydride reduction product of the latter diol are shown in Table 29. From the large coupling constants between H-3 and H-4 in these com-

Fig. 66. Nucleophilic opening of 3,4-dihydro-3,4-dihydroxy-*anti*- and *syn*-1,2-oxides at C-1; only the *anti*-oxide can give a vicinal *cis*-diol which can complex with borate.

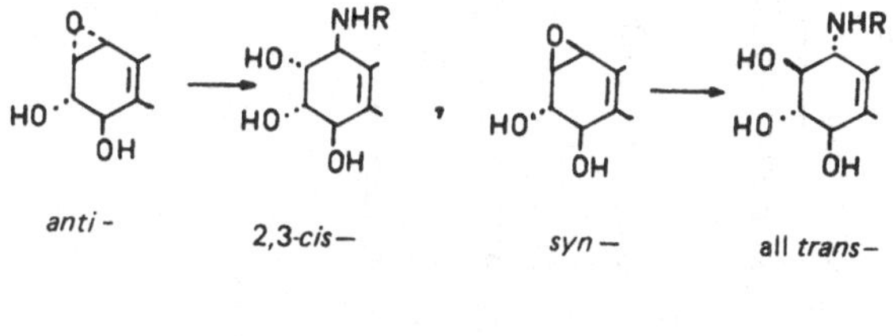

Table 29. *Chemical shifts (ppm) and coupling constants (Hz) of the A-ring protons in the metabolically derived 3,4-diol (457), its unsubstituted homologue and the borohydride reduction product of the latter*

Compound	H-1	H-2	H-3	H-4
11-methyl-3,4-dihydroxy-17-ketone (**457**)	7.58 double doublet $J_{1,2} = 10.5$ $J_{1,3} = 2$	6.32 double doublet $J_{1,2} = 10.5$ $J_{2,3} = 2$	4.6 multiplet $J_{3,4} = 12$	4.9 doublet $J_{3,4} = 12$
unsubstituted-3,4-dihydroxy-17-ketone	7.3 doublet (broad) $J_{1,2} = 10$	6.19 double doublet $J_{1,2} = 10$ $J_{2,3} = 2$	4.35 multiplet $J_{3,4} = 10$	4.75 doublet $J_{3,4} = 10$
unsubstituted-3,4,17-triol	7.24 double doublet $J_{1,2} = 10$ $J_{1,3} = 2$	6.12 double doublet $J_{1,2} = 10$ $J_{2,3} = 2$	4.30 multiplet $J_{3,4} = 11$	4.69 doublet $J_{3,4} = 11$

pounds it is clear that the 3,4-diol system is *trans* and diequatorial. Both 3,4-dihydroxy-17-ketones had similar circular dichroism curves of the same sign; the unsubstituted 3,4,17-triol had a circular dichroism curve similar to and of the same sign as that of *trans*-1R,2R-dihydroxy-1,2-dihydrophenanthrene. Taken together these findings point to [3R,4R]-dihydroxy-3,4,15,16-tetrahydrocyclopenta[a]phenanthren-17-one as the structure of the proximate carcinogen (**457**) which is further oxidized at C-1, C-2 and then interacts with DNA mainly as illustrated in Fig. 67.

The *in vitro* metabolism of this carcinogen (**26**) has also been studied with the human hepatoma cell line HepG2 (Bhatt, 1986) in connection with the ability of these cells to activate this compound to a mutagen in the V79 Chinese hamster cell system as described in Chapter 6. These cells are highly induceable (Dawson *et al.*, 1985) and after pretreatment with benzanthracene or Arochlor microsomes prepared from them gave the range of metabolites seen with rat liver microsomes, including a large amount of the proximate carcinogen (**457**). However, in addition products from enzymatic reduction of the 17-ketone function were also observed. Thus with uninduced microsomes the major metabolite was the 17-alcohol (16,17-dihydro-11-methyl-15*H*-cyclopenta[a]phenanthren-17-ol, **448**), while with induced microsomes the 16,17-diol and a phenol, probably the 4,15,17-triol, were also identified. The reductase responsible for 17-ketone reduction appeared to be largely present in the supernatant for when the microsomes were carefully washed these products were minimized. After exposure to these cells the carcinogen (**26**) bound to added DNA to give the adduct peaks A and B on LH20 chromatography, apparently identical with those found after activation with rat liver preparations. Little metabolism was seen when hamster embryo cells were used, whether they were induced or not, and this

Fig. 67. Proposed metabolic route leading to the ultimate carcinogen and its main deoxyguanosine adduct.

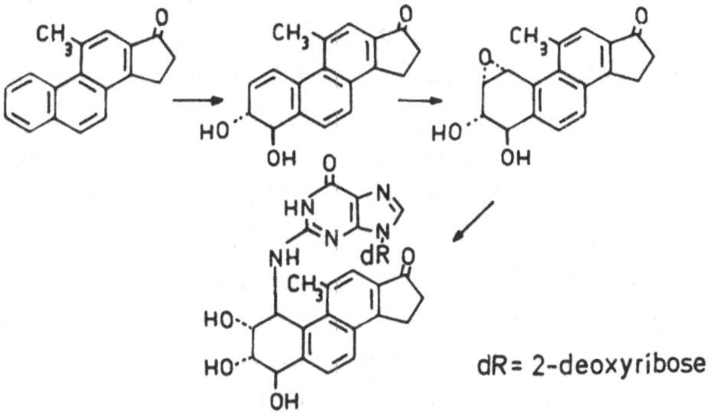

dR = 2-deoxyribose

explains why these cells fail to activate this carcinogen to a mutagen in V79 cells. In this respect this carcinogenic cyclopenta[a]phenanthrenone appears to differ from hydrocarbons such as benzo[a]pyrene, but the reason for this is not clear at present.

Mouse embryo cells derived from T.O. mice also activate this carcinogen (**26**). In a study of the binding of a number of polycyclic hydrocarbon carcinogens to nuclear and mitochondrial DNA (Allen, 1979; Allen and Coombs, 1980) in these cells, the familiar patterns of adduct peaks were again observed. However, the mitochondrial DNA binding index (μmol of compound bound per mol of DNA phosphorus) was over 500 times higher than was this index for the nuclear DNA. This was found to be common also for the other carcinogens, where the ratio ranged between 50-fold and 250-fold.

7.2   *In vivo* metabolism of 15,16-dihydro-11-methylcyclopenta[a]-phenanthren-17-one in the rat

Prior to the work on *in vitro* metabolism just described urinary metabolites of this carcinogen (**26**) and its inactive parent ketone (15,16-dihydrocyclopenta[a]phenanthren-17-one (**4**) were investigated in the rat. Adult Sprague-Dawley males were injected (100 mg/animal) intraperitoneally with these compounds, labelled with ^{14}C or tritium, and urine was collected for three days when excretion of radioactivity was largely completed. It was found advantageous to extract the metabolites from the crude urine by first absorbing them on to neutral charcoal, from which they could be recovered by elution with methanol containing ammonia. The extract was then evaporated to a syrup which was mixed with water and re-extracted with ethyl acetate. This work was, of course, carried out before the advent of hplc, and the metabolites obtained in this way were compared by careful semiquantitative tlc on silica gel-coated glass plates. Each compound gave over a dozen metabolites which formed discrete bands on the plate, and could be located by their radioactivity (after autoradiography on X-ray film), their fluorescence, and by various colour reactions. By removal of the material comprising these bands from the plate, and eluting it with ethanol ultraviolet spectra could be obtained. The result of this survey is shown in Table 30. The most noticeable feature is the remarkable similarity between the patterns of urinary metabolites of these two ketones. In most cases this similarity extended to a number of colour reactions (not shown) carried out by spraying the plates. The amounts in the bands, as judged by their radioactivity, were also similar for each pair with the exceptions shown in the second column. With the two pairs of phenols (bands 4 and 5) in each

Table 30. *Properties of urinary metabolites of ketones (4) and (26) separated by tlc*

Radioactive band derived from ketone (4) or (26)	Percentage of total radioactivity	R_F	Fluorescence	Ultraviolet spectra		
				Neutral [λ_{max} (nm)]	Anion	After reduction (neutral)
1 (4)	—	0.80	purple	265, 286, 297	unchanged	255, 284, 296
(26)	—	0.79	blue–purple	264, 286, 297	unchanged	256, 283, 294
2 (4)	—	0.64	yellow	262	unchanged	256
(26)	—	0.64	yellow	262	unchanged	256
3 (26)	—	0.61	purple	267, 288, 299	unchanged	255
4 (4)	15–20	0.53	yellow	266, 296	280	260
(26)	5	0.52	yellow	267, 300	281	259
5 (4)	15–20	0.50	green	263	276	259
(26)	5	0.50	green	264	278	259
6 (4)	—	0.45	yellow	262	unchanged	—
(26)	—	0.44	yellow	276	255, 296	259
7 (26)	—	0.40	purple	268, 288, 301	unchanged	—
8 (4)	—	0.32	yellow	261, 269	—	—
(26)	—	0.34	yellow	261, 269	—	—
9 (4)	—	0.20	purple	254, 260	unchanged	—
(26)	—	0.23	blue	254, 260	unchanged	—
10 (4)	~2	0.17	purple	263, 320, 333, 350, 368	unchanged	269, 269, 315
(26)	50	0.15	purple	264, 320, 332, 351, 370	unchanged	261, 269, 316
11 (4)	—	0.12	purple	256, 266, 278	unchanged	—
(26)	—	0.11	purple	260	282	—
12 (4)	—	0.09	purple	270	—	—
(26)	—	0.09	purple	261	—	—
13 (4)	—	0.05	yellow	270, 279	—	—
(26)	—	0.05	yellow	270	—	—

case 3–4 times as much was obtained from the parent ketone (**4**) as from its 11-methyl homologue (**26**), accounting for 30–40% of the total radioactivity for the former. By contrast the amounts of the similar metabolites in band 10 differed greatly; only a trace was obtained from (**4**), whereas it was a major metabolite from (**26**), accounting for about 50% of the total. The structure of this metabolite was therefore determined since this difference between the carcinogen and its inactive parent seemed possibly of significance.

To this end a total of 20 g of the 11-methyl-17-ketone (**26**) labelled with tracer amounts of tritium were injected into rats, and metabolites were isolated from their urine as already described. The mixture was then chromatographed on silica gel columns, finally to give the band-10 metabolite, after further purification by recrystallization, as 120 mg of pale fawn needles, mp 120°C decomp. It was optically active, $[\alpha]\,_D^{26°}-214°$ (*c*. 0.134, ethanol), and its ultraviolet characteristics, λ_{max} 267 (4.57), 320 (4.03), 332 (4.04), 352 (3.67), 370 (3.61) nm, were very similar to those of 11-methyl-1,2,15,16-tetrahydro-1,2,15-trihydroxy-cyclo-penta[a]phenanthren-17-one (**454**, metabolite **a**, Table 26) later isolated from *in vitro* metabolism of (**26**). Combustion analysis established the formula $C_{18}H_{16}O_5$ (see Fig. 68); the mass spectrum was informative, although the molecular ion was absent:

	m/z	% abundance	Derivation
$C_{18}H_{14}O_4$ requires	294.0892	—	—
Found	294.0893	6	M^+-H_2O
	278	34	M^+-H_2O-O
	260	21	M^+-2H_2O-O
	232	50	$M^+-2H_2O-O-CO$

Fig. 68. The structure (**460**) of the main urinary metabolite of the carcinogen (**26**) in the rat, and some of its chemically derived products.

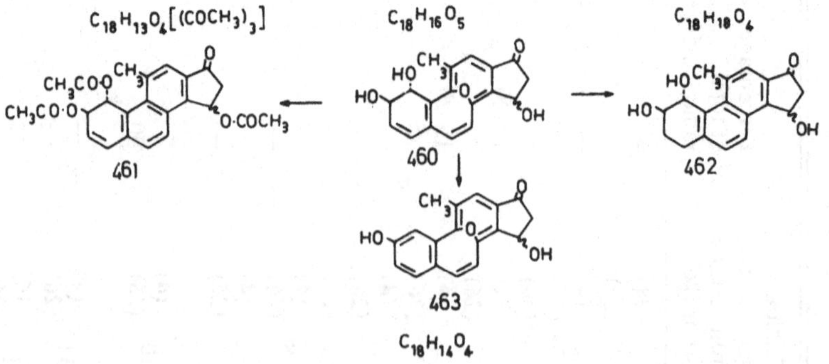

The fifth 'non-functional' oxygen atom was therefore thermally labile; it was also eliminated on acetylation with acetic anhydride in pyridine at room temperature, giving the triacetate $C_{24}H_{22}O_7$ (**461**) and on mild hydrogenation yielding the dihydro-deoxy derivative $C_{18}H_{18}O_4$ (**462**). Surprisingly, it was, however, retained when the metabolite was submitted to acid-catalysed dehydration (2.5-M sulphuric acid at 100°C for 1 h) to give the phenol $C_{18}H_{14}O_4$ (**463**). A full nmr study finally established the structures shown in Fig. 68 for these compounds (Coombs and Crawley, 1974, 1975) (see Chapter 5 under the appropriate molecular formula for details). Precedents exist in the chemical literature both for loss of the bridge oxygen in oxepins of this type (**460**) both thermally and on hydrogenation as well as its retention in strongly acidic media, but not for its loss on mild acetylation; the mechanism by which this occurs remains a mystery. The occurrence of a structure such as (**460**) as a metabolite of a polycyclic aromatic compound is, to the best of our knowledge, unique. Its structure is closely related to that of the major metabolite (**454**) encountered during *in vitro* metabolism with hepatic preparations, and it is tempting to postulate that it is formed from this metabolite by further microbiological oxidation in the gut. It has not been tested for carcinogenicity, but in view of its close relationship to (**454**) which is itself inactive, and the fact that the epoxide–oxepin structure appears to be stable enough to withstand the long and complicated extraction and purification procedures used in its isolation, it seems unlikely that it would prove to be active.

7.3 Biological activation of 15,16-dihydro-1,11-methanocyclopenta[a]phenanthren-17-one

It has been known for 40 years that nearly all carcinogenic polycyclic aromatic hydrocarbons are related to the angular hydrocarbon phenanthrene rather than the linear hydrocarbon anthracene, but the reason for this has become apparent only recently. It now seems that for activity the hydrocarbon needs a 'bay region' (the extramolecular area bounded by C-1, C-10, C-9, and C-11 in a cyclopenta[a]phenanthrene) in order to allow metabolic formation of a bay-region diol-epoxide of the type already discussed. This is the ultimate carcinogenic species and it is perhaps hardly surprising that the 1-, 2-, 3-, and 4-methyl derivatives are inactive, because these A-ring substituents would be expected to interfere with the formation of the 3,4-diol-1,2-oxide. However, on these grounds it is less clear why the unsubstituted structure is inactive and becomes carcinogenic only on substitution at C-7 or C-11; an analogous situation also exists in the related chrysene and benz[a]anthracene series.

It was reasoned that the 1,11-methano compound (**310**), in which C-1 is joined covalently to C-11 by a methylene group, should not be carcinogenic for although it has a small substituent at C-11 favouring activity, the substituent at C-1 was expected to obstruct the formation of a bay-region diol-epoxide. The first indication that this reasoning was not sound came when it was discovered that this compound was weakly mutagenic towards *Salmonella typhimurium* TA100. It was therefore tested more thoroughly than usual for carcinogenicity, and in two identical initiation/ promotion experiments appeared to possess initiating activity approaching that of its 11-methyl-17-ketone analogue (**26**), although it proved to be only moderately active as a complete carcinogen in two repeated-application experiments. An investigation into the metabolism of this compound (**310**) was therefore undertaken in an attempt to account for this unexpected result (Coombs *et al.*, 1982; Hadfield *et al.*, 1984*a*). The same strategy and tactics were employed as those that successfully unravelled the activation of the 11-methyl-17-ketone (**26**). After *in vitro* metabolism of the generally labelled [³H]-1,11-methano-17-ketone (**310**) metabolites were separated by hplc (Fig. 69) and the fractions (i)–(x) were assayed for mutagenicity in the Ames' test. This ketone is only weakly active in this test with TA100, giving under optimum conditions from two to three times the background number of revertants; nevertheless, the results of this comparison were clear (Table 31). Only fraction (iv) elicited a higher reversion rate than the starting material which was

Fig. 69. hplc Separation of *in vitro* metabolites of 15,16-dihydro-1,11-methanocyclopenta[a]phenanthren-17-one (**310**); equimolar amounts of fractions (i)–(x) were tested for mutagenicity (see Table 31).

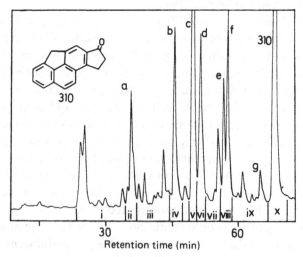

eluted in fraction (x). The structure of metabolite (**b**) contained in this fraction and purified to homogeneity by hplc was therefore studied, as were those of the other metabolites (**a–g**) obtained pure in sufficient quantity. Molecular formulae based on their mass spectra are shown in Table 32 together with selected ions of diagnostic value. All metabolites gave molecular ions except metabolite (**b**) which was, however, known to be a vicinal diol from other evidence (see below), and gave an abundant [M$^+$-H$_2$O] ion; the analogous ion was in fact the base peak in the spectrum of the diol (**a**). Both metabolites also gave abundant ions due to

Table 31. *Relative mutagenic response from equimolar amounts*[(a)] *of metabolites contained in fractions (i)–(x)* *(Fig. 69)*

Fraction	Relative mutagenicity (as percentage of fraction x)
(i)	18
(ii)	24
(iii)	23
(iv)	160
(v)	44
(vi)	28
(vii)	80
(viii)	59
(ix)	43
(x) (**310**)	100

a, based on radioactivity.

Table 32. *Molecular formulae of metabolites* (**a–g**) *and selected mass spectral ions of diagnostic value*

Metabolite	Selected diagnostic ions [observed (calculated) (relative abundance, %)]
(**a**) C$_{18}$H$_{14}$O$_3$	M$^+$ 278.0954 (278.0943) (69.2%); M-H$_2$O (100%); M$^+$-H$_2$O-C$_2$H$_2$O (80.7%)
(**b**) C$_{18}$H$_{14}$O$_3$	M$^+$-H$_2$O 260.0711 (260.0837) (58.6%); M$^+$-H$_2$O-C$_2$H$_2$O (58.6%)
(**c**) C$_{18}$H$_{12}$O$_3$	M$^+$ 276.07940 (276.07864) (62%); M$^+$-H$_2$O (100%)
(**d**) C$_{18}$H$_{10}$O$_2$	M$^+$ 258 (33%); M$^+$-CHO (17%)
(**e**) C$_{18}$H$_{12}$O$_2$	M$^+$ 260 (100%); M$^+$-C$_2$H$_2$O (70%)
(**f**) C$_{18}$H$_{12}$O$_2$	M$^+$ 260 (100%)
(**g**) C$_{18}$H$_{10}$O$_2$	M$^+$ 258.06808 (258.06770) (100%); M$^+$-CO (28%), M$^+$-2(CO) (91%)
(**310**) C$_{18}$H$_{12}$O	M$^+$ 244 (57.3%); M$^+$-C$_2$H$_2$O (100%)

Table 33. nmr Spectra of ring-A protons of metabolites (**a**) and (**b**) of the 1,11-methano-17-ketone (**310**)

Metabolite			
(a)	4.48 doublet ($J_{2,3} = 5.5$)	6.46 double doublet ($J_{3,4} = 9.5$; $J_{2,3} = 5.5$)	7.00 doublet ($J_{3,4} = 9.5$)	4.18 broad singlet
(b)	6.14 multiplet ($J_{2,3} = 3.5$; $J_{2,18} = 2.0$)	4.78 multiplet ($J_{3,4} = 5.5$; $J_{2,3} = 3.5$)	6.02 doublet ($J_{3,4} = 5.5$)	4.15 unresolved doublet

further loss of 42 mass units, as did the original 1,11-methano-17-ketone (**310**). This is not a common degradative pathway in 17-ketocyclopenta[a]phenanthrenes, nor was it seen with 4,5-methylenephenanthrene itself. The loss seems to be due to the formal elimination of ketene from the five-membered ring, and appears to be characteristic of this ring lacking further substitution in these 1,11-methano compounds. Although the ultraviolet spectrum of the 1,11-methano-17-ketone (**310**) [λ_{max} 266.5 (4.77), 277 (4.76) nm] differs appreciably from that of (say) the 11-methyl-17-ketone (**26**) [λ_{max} 264 (4.83) nm], the spectra of metabolites (**a**) and (**b**) strongly resembled those of, respectively, the 1,2- and 3,4-dihydrodiols of the latter, and this was fully confirmed by their nmr spectra listed in Table 33. The structures of the other metabolites were deduced from similar combinations of mass and ultraviolet spectral information. For example, the mono-ol (**e**) had a strong M^+-42 ion (unsubstituted 17-keto D-ring) and ultraviolet spectrum similar to that of the original ketone (**310**); after borohydride reduction the spectra of (**e**) and the diketone (**g**) were identical. These are therefore both 18-substituted-17-ketones. The ultraviolet spectrum of (**d**) differed from all the others in that it was altered on addition of alkali (enolizable β-diketone). The two hydroxyl groups in the diol (**c**) (ultraviolet spectrum similar to the original ketone) were at C-15 and C-18 because this diol had an intense M^+-H_2O ion, a characteristic of the 15-hydroxy-, but not 16-hydroxy-11-methyl-17-ketone. The proposed structures of all these metabolites are illustrated in Fig. 70. Thus again with this compound (**310**) the most mutagenic metabolite was a *trans*-3,4-dihydrodiol, but here the coupling constant, 5.5 Hz, was smaller than that associated with *trans*-3,4-dihydrodiols from other cyclopenta[a]phenanthren-17-ones (10–12 Hz) indicating that it possessed a conformation mid-way between diaxial and diequatorial. After metabolic activation *in vitro* (rat liver microsomes) the 1,11-methano-17-ketone (**310**) bound to added DNA which, after isolation and enzymatic hydrolysis, gave essentially a single nucleoside adduct. An identical result was obtained with DNA isolated from the skin of mice treated topically with this compound *in vivo*. As with the main adduct from the 11-methyl-17-ketone (**26**), this eluted from an LH20 column after the common nucleosides, and appeared significantly earlier in the presence of borate. This strongly suggests that the 3,4-dihydrodiol (metabolite **b**) is the proximate carcinogen, and that it is further converted by metabolism into an *anti*-3,4-dihydroxy-1,2-oxide. That the 1,2-double bond in (**310**) is capable of metabolism via a 1,2-oxide is proved by the isolation of the 1,2-dihydrodiol (metabolite **a**).

The bay region in the 1,11-methano-17-ketone (**310**) is obstructed mainly within the plane of the molecule. The bridge methylene protons are magnetically equivalent because they resonate as a singlet, and this part of the molecule is therefore essentially flat (as will be described later, this was also proved by X-ray crystallography). It therefore seems that the active oxygen species is inserted into the 1,2-double bond of this molecule from either above or below this plane in the active site of the oxidase. This helps to account for the rapid fall-off in carcinogenic activity with chain length at C-11 observed in both the alkyl and alkoxy series because these substituents would not be confined to this plane. The carcinogenicity of (310) further emphasizes the role of small substituents at C-11 in endowing cyclopenta[a]phenanthrenes with biological activity. In retrospect it is not entirely surprising that this compound is a carcinogen because as long ago as 1946 it was shown that the corresponding bridged analogue of 7,12-dimethylbenz[a]anthracene, namely 1,12-methano-7-methylbenz[a]anthracene, yielded tumours in mice after injection (Dunlap and Warren, 1946). Much more recently metabolic oxidation at methyl-substituted double bonds in both 7-methyl-benzo[a]pyrene (Kinoshita *et al.*, 1982) and 8-methylbenz[a]anthracene (Yang *et al.*, 1981) has been reported.

Fig. 70. Structures proposed for the *in vitro* metabolites of the 1,11-methano-17-ketone (310).

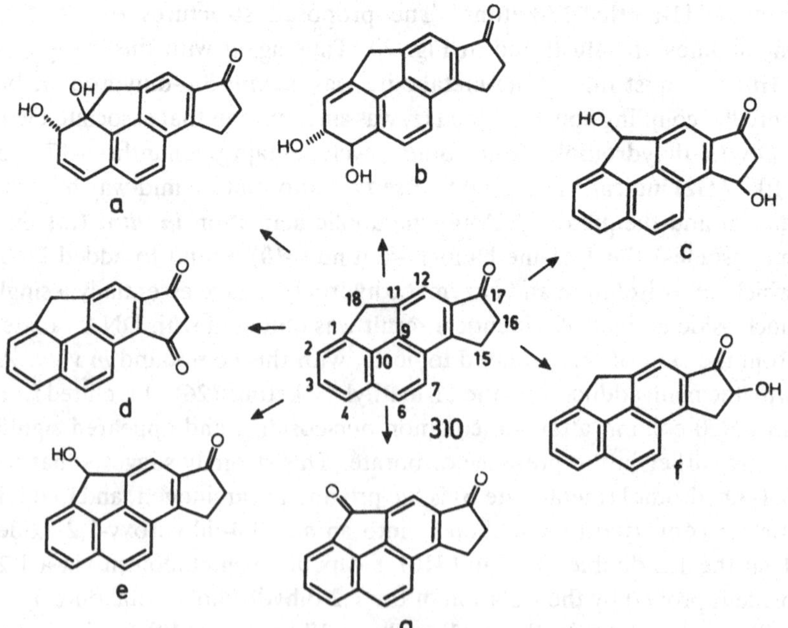

**7.4   Comparative *in vitro* metabolism of 15,16-dihydrocyclo-
penta[a]phenanthren-17-one and some of its methyl homologues**
The marked structure/biological activity relationships among
cyclopenta[a]phenanthrenes are, of course, mirrored in other polycyclic
aromatic systems. For example, in both the chrysene and benz[a]anthra-
cene series methyl substitution at the bay region in the position other than
on the terminal benzo ring leads to a considerable enhancement in
carcinogenicity, but there does not yet seem to be any general agreement
on the reason for this. In the series of 17-keto-cyclopenta[a]-
phenanthrenes the isomers are very similar to one another in most of
their physical properties, including solubility which is likely to be of
importance in their pharmacodynamics. Unlike polycyclic aromatic
hydrocarbons these polycyclic ketones are not appreciably soluble in
hexane; they are, however, reasonably soluble in aromatic hydrocarbons
and in alcohols, and are readily soluble in dipolar solvents such as
chloroform and dimethylsulphoxide. Their solubility in water is less than
$0.5\,\mu\text{g/mL}$, but is increased somewhat by the presence of protein as, for
example, in tissue culture media. No quantitative comparison of their
solubility has been made, but the virtual identity of their chromatographic properties in a number of solvent systems suggests that this is
closely similar for the isomeric members of this series, and probably their
tissue distribution in animals will not therefore be dissimilar. In their
chemistry, too, the inactive 15,16-dihydrocyclopenta[a]phenanthren-17-
one (4) and its carcinogenic 11-methyl homologue show close similarity
(see Chapter 4). However, an apparent major difference in the urinary
metabolites of these two ketones has already been noted, and made a
comparative study of the *in vitro* metabolism of compounds of this series
imperative since it was evident that metabolism was intimately connected
with the expression of their biological effects. In contemplating this it
seemed initially that the 1-, 2-, 3-, and 4-methyl derivatives could be
excluded, for it appeared likely that these ring-A substituents would
block diol-epoxide formation. However, when it was discovered that
the C-1 methylene group in 15,16-dihydro-1,11-methanocyclopenta[a]-
phenanthren-17-one (310) was unable to do this it was decided to include
in the study the 1-methyl-17-ketone (302), especially as the cancer tests
with this compound were not convincingly negative. The unsubstituted
parent ketone (4) and its 6- and 12-methyl derivatives (306 and 130), all
non-carcinogens, and the carcinogenic 7- and 11-methyl-17-ketones (230
and 26) and the 11,12-dimethyl-17-ketone (131) have also been investigated using the *in vitro* method with hepatic microsomes from 3-methyl-
cholanthrene-induced rats as already described.

Table 34. *Ultraviolet maxima of the main in vitro metabolites of the unsubstituted -17-ketone (4), and its 11-methyl (26), 12-methyl (130), and 11,12-dimethyl (131) derivatives separated by hplc as shown in Fig. 71*

Metabolite	unsubstituted -17-ketone (4)	11-methyl-17-ketone (26)	12-methyl-17-ketone (130)	11,12-dimethyl-17-ketone (131)
(a)	266, 320, 332, 336 (255, 264, 310, 347)	265, 322, 334, 373 (259, 267, 305)	268, 321, 333, 375 (257, 266, 310)	273, 323, 336, 366, 386 (261, 270, 328)
(b)	266, 316, 328, 365 (257, 265)	262, 306, 319, 332 (259, 267, 305)	261, 303, 315, 327 (257, 266)	—
(c)	267, 317, 327, 365 (243, 264, 320)	273, 327, 333, 370 (248, 327, 347)	269, 325, 360, 372 (245, 308, 322)	276, 320, 338, 372 (252, 332, 349)
(d)	278, 330, 360, 376 (253, 312, 328)	272, 327, 333, 370 (250, 326, 347)	268, 362, 374 (246, 322)	275, 320, 338, 372 (254, 320, 334, 350)
(e)	269, 350, 368 (243, 300, 309, 321, 341)	273, 332, 357, 371 (250, 306, 330, 349)	270, 355, 375 (248, 310, 323, 342)	275, 321, 336, 370 (256, 274, 321, 337)
(f)	268, 280, 297, 352, 369 (256, 278, 281, 298)	265, 300, 359, 374 (256, 280, 291, 303, 337, 352)	270, 308, 358, 375 (259, 281, 303)	268, 291, 303, 363, 383 (259, 296, 332, 356)

λ_{max} (nm); peaks of highest intensity are underlined and spectra in parentheses were obtained following *in situ* reduction of the carbonyl group to the secondary alcohol.

As was anticipated from earlier tlc work it was found (Hadfield *et al.*, 1984*a*) that the main metabolites of the unsubstituted ketone (**4**) were analogous to those of its 11-methyl derivative already described. Lacking the methyl group they were somewhat more polar, eluting about five minutes earlier from the reverse-phase hplc column than their 11-methyl counterparts. They were readily identified by their ultraviolet spectra (Table 34) which were very similar to those of the metabolites derived from the carcinogen (**26**). The most polar (Fig. 71) was again the 1,2,15-trihydroxy-17-ketone (**a**) followed by the 1,2-diol (**b**); the latter was formed in larger amount from this compound (**4**) than from its 11-methyl derivative (**26**), possibly because the methyl group in the latter partially hinders approach of the active site in the enzyme to the 1,2-double bond. After removal of the extra conjugation by reduction of the ketone to the secondary alcohol, the circular dichroism spectrum of the product had the same sign as phenanthrene-[1R,2R]-diol (Fig. 72); the absolute stereochemistry of this metabolite is therefore also [1R,2R] or 1α,2β as

Fig. 71. hplc Profiles of the *in vitro* metabolites formed from the unsubstituted 17-ketone (**4**) and its 11-methyl (**26**) and 12-methyl (**130**) derivatives.

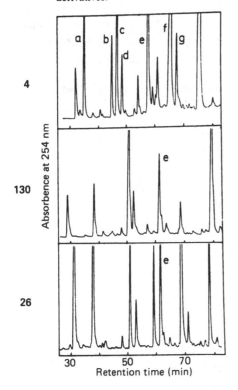

shown. Next in order of decreasing polarity were the two 3,4,15- and 3,4,16-triols (**c** and **d**), followed by the 3,4-dihydrodiol (**e**) shown by its nmr spectrum (Table 29) to be diequatorial and by its circular dichroism spectrum (after borohydride reduction) to be [3R,4R] or $3\alpha,4\beta$. It was further characterized by its mass spectrum which showed a molecular ion (M$^+$ found 266.09379; $C_{17}H_{14}O_3$ requires 266.09429) (81.4%), and *inter alia* ions at 248 (M$^+$-H$_2$O, 100%), 200 (M$^+$-H$_2$O-CO, 72.8%). Finally a large amount of the 15-ol (**f, 369**) and a smaller quantity of the 16-ol (**g, 345**) were eluted, and characterized by comparison with the synthetic materials.

The 12-methyl-17-ketone (**130**) yielded a similar range of *in vitro* metabolites (Fig. 71), and the 3,4-dihydrodiol (**e**) was again conspicuous. It was characterized by its ultraviolet spectrum and elution time (both virtually identical to those of its 11-methyl isomer) and its mass spectrum (M$^+$ found 280.10949; $C_{18}H_{16}O_3$ requires 280.10994, 8.6%; M$^+$-H$_2$O, 100%; M$^+$-H$_2$O-CO, 16.5%). Its nmr spectrum shown in Table 35 demonstrated that this diol was *trans*-diequatorial, and again the circular dichroism spectrum showed that it was [3R,4R] or $3\alpha,4\beta$. The additional methyl group in the 11,12-dimethyl-17-ketone (**131**) led to further retention on the reverse-phase column so that this ketone and its metabolites were eluted about five minutes later than the 11- or 12-methyl-17-ketone and their analogous metabolites. The range of major metabolites formed was the same as those (**a–f**) obtained from the other compounds, but the

Fig. 72. Circular dichroism spectra of phenanthrene-[1R,2R]-dihydrodiol and of the borohydride reduction product of the 1,2-dihydro-1,2-dihydroxy metabolite of (**4**).

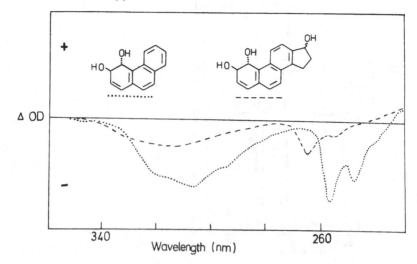

Wavelength (nm)

Table 35. *Chemical shifts (ppm) and coupling constants (Hz) of A-ring protons in trans-3,4-dihydrodiols derived from the 6-methyl- and 12-methyl-17-ketones by metabolism*

3,4-diol from:	H-1	H-2	H-3	H-4
6-methyl-17-ketone (**306**)	7.68 double doublet $J_{1,2} = 9$; $J_{1,3} = 0.5$	6.52 double doublet $J_{1,2} = 9$; $J_{2,3} = 4$	4.46 double doublet $J_{2,3} = 4$; $J_{1,3} = 0.5$	5.06 singlet
12-methyl-17-ketone (**130**)	7.29 double doublet $J_{1,2} = 10$; $J_{1,3} = 2$	6.21 double doublet $J_{1,2} = 10$; $J_{2,3} = 2.5$	4.46 multiplet $J_{3,4} = 11$; $J_{2,3} = 2.5$; $J_{1,3} = 2$	— (obscured by methyl signal)

extra methyl group also caused the expected bathochromic shift in the ultraviolet maxima observed (see Table 34). From its elution time the 3,4-dihydrodiol formed from the 11,12-dimethyl compound (i.e., metabolite **e**) was *trans*-diequatorial, and its absolute stereochemistry was in all probability [3R,4R] like all the others. Under identical conditions of incubation, extraction, and chromatographic separation, the four 17-ketones gave these metabolites in the relative amounts shown in Table 36. Thus at very similar total percentage conversion, all four compounds (two carcinogens, and two non-carcinogens) yielded commensurate amounts of 3,4-dihydrodiols, which appeared to be *trans* and of the same conformation and absolute stereochemistry. Thus metabolism cannot account for the lack of carcinogenicity of the ketones (**4**) and (**130**).

The 6- and 7-methyl-17-ketones (**306** and **230**, respectively) have not been studied in such detail (Coombs *et al.*, 1981), but examination of the hplc profiles of their *in vitro* metabolites showed a marked difference. Whereas the 6-methyl compound gave just three main metabolites, the 7-methyl ketone yielded many metabolites, all in small amounts. Amongst these was a *trans*-3,4-dihydrodiol with retention time and ultraviolet characteristics similar to those of the analogous 11-methyl-17-ketone-3,4-diol. It was further characterized by its mass spectrum: M^+, 280 (31.5%); M^+-H_2O, 262 (100%); M^+-H_2O-CO, 234 (14%). After metabolic activation *in vitro* the 7-methyl-17-ketone (**230**) bound to calf thymus DNA added to the incubation to about half the extent of the 11-methyl isomer; this seems to account satisfactorily for its weaker carcinogenicity. The 6-methyl-17-ketone (**306**), on the other hand, failed to exhibit appreciable binding to DNA *in vitro* or *in vivo* (mouse skin) in line with its failure to

Table 36. *Relative amounts of major metabolites formed from the unsubstituted -17-ketone* (**4**), *its 11-methyl* (**26**), *12-methyl* (**130**), *and 11,12-dimethyl* (**131**) *derivatives under identical incubation conditions in vitro*

Metabolite	(Compound) amount of metabolite as percentage of the total ethyl acetate extractable radioactivity			
	(**4**)	(**26**)	(**130**)	(**131**)
(**a**)	11.2	8.0	5.2	0.9
(**c**)	9.2	5.7	12.1	6.3
(**d**)	4.2	4.0	6.6	5.3
(**e**)	11.6	9.2	7.7	11.1
(**f**)	4.3	10.8	1.7	9.2
Other metabolites	35.7	38.1	39.1	42.1
Unchanged compound	23.8	24.2	27.6	25.1

evoke tumours in mice. Nevertheless, the major metabolite of this ketone, accounting for about 30% of the material in the extract, was a *trans*-3,4-dihydrodiol, λ_{max} 271.5, 309, 322.5, 358, 373 nm. However, the total lack of magnetic coupling between H-3 and H-4 in its nmr spectrum (Table 35; see also Fig. 73) demonstrated that the bonds connecting these protons to C-3 and C-4 in this metabolite were at right angles to one another, and consequently the diol hydroxyl groups were diaxial. This was also confirmed by the polarity of this diol which eluted about 10 minutes earlier than the diequatorial 3,4-dihydrodiols formed by the other compounds. Further microsomal metabolism of this diol led to several more polar metabolites with ultraviolet spectra characteristic of 1,2,3,4-tetrahydro derivatives. However, if a 3,4-diol-1,2-epoxide was involved its half-life must have been exceedingly short because the 6-methyl-17-ketone did not bind significantly to DNA added to the incubation medium. Introduction of a methoxy group at C-6 in the 11-methyl-17-ketone (**26**) to yield (**468**) diminished its carcinogenicity drastically (Iball indices 46 and 14, respectively – see Table 12), again demonstrating the inhibitory effect of a *peri* substituent. In the hydrocarbon series 16,17-dihydro-7-methylcyclopenta[a]phenanthrene (**94**) is a weak carcinogen, but its 6,7-dimethyl analogue (**105**) is inactive (see Table 7). Also 5,12-dimethylchrysene (which has methyl groups in the bay region and the *peri*

Fig. 73. nmr Signals due to H-3 and H-4 of the metabolically derived 3,4-dihydrodiol of 15,16-dihydro-6-methylcyclopenta[a]phenanthren-17-one (**306**).

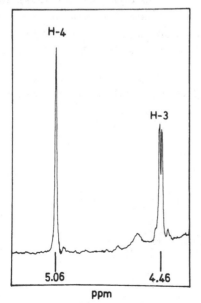

positions equivalent to C-11 and C-6 in a cyclopenta[a]phenanthrene) is much less carcinogenic than 5-methylchrysene itself (Hecht *et al.*, 1979). Probably any bulky group at the *peri* position (C-6 in cyclopenta[a]phenanthrenes) would force an adjacent 3,4-diol into the diaxial conformation, and this appears to have a deleterious effect on carcinogenicity.

The *in vitro* metabolism of the 1-methyl-17-ketone (302) has also been examined recently (Coombs *et al.*, 1985) for the reasons already given. The profiles of metabolites (Fig. 74) obtained in the usual way, although not separated in quite the same way as shown in Fig. 71, did not bear much resemblance to those of the other isomers. In particular no less than six metabolites (hatched in the figure) were phenolic, whereas only traces of phenols were found before. Phenolic metabolites, even if their structure is unknown, are easy to identify because addition of a little alkali to the methanolic solution in the cuvette generates the anion with its own characteristic ultraviolet absorption spectrum. As can be seen from Table 37 three of these phenols (q, r, and x) were extremely similar, and the latter (x) was positively identified as 15,16-dihydro-4-hydroxy-1-methylcyclopenta[a]phenanthren-17-one (458) by comparison of its elution time and ultraviolet spectra (neutral, anion, and reduced) with those of the synthetic compound which had been completely characterized. The spectra of the other phenolic metabolites (n, s, and t) also shared some similarities with this compound. It therefore appears that a major pathway in the metabolism of the 1-methyl-17-ketone (302) involves epoxidation of the 3,4-double bond followed by rapid isomerization of 3,4-epoxide to the 4-phenol (metabolite x), rather than enzymatic opening to give a 3,4-dihydrodiol as observed with all the other compounds.

Fig. 74. hplc Profile of the *in vitro* metabolites of 15,16-dihydro-1-methylcyclopenta[a]phenanthren-17-one (302); the hatched peaks are phenolic.

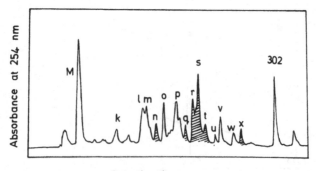

Retention time

Table 37. *Ultraviolet maxima of metabolites* (**k–x**) *formed from the 1-methyl-17-ketone* (**302**) (Fig. 74) (λ_{max}, *nm; peaks of highest intensity underlined*)

Metabolite	Neutral	Anion	Reduced	Assignment
(**k**)	259, 277, 290, 301	—	236, 259	1,2,3,4-tetraol
(**l**)	269, 331, 337, 368	—	258, 267, 305	1,2,15(or 16)triol
(**m**)	269, 279, 298	258, 293	257, 266, 282, 294, 303	cpp-triol[a]
(**n**)	264, 297	—	248, 267, 273, 284, 293	phenol
(**o**)	270, 302, 359, 367	—	259, 282, 292, 304	cpp-diol[a]
(**p**)	268, 302, 369	—	259, 303, 363	cpp-diol[a]
(**q**)	254, 278, 303	261, 290, 324	249, 282, 296, 318, 346, 365	phenol
(**r**)	253, 277, 301	262, 291, 325	249, 255, 281, 344, 361	phenol
(**s**)	243, 267, 293	262, 291	248, 258, 281, 291	phenol
(**t**)	252, 276, 299	268, 290, 301	247, 258, 266, 292	phenol
(**u**)	266, 284, 302, 357, 375	—	258, 281, 292, 304	cpp-ol[a]
(**v**)	270, 285, 303, 358, 375	—	256, 281, 292, 303	cpp-ol[a]
(**w**)	268, 290, 303	—	256, 282, 292, 305	cpp-ol[a]
(**x**)	270, 305	260, 284, 324	250, 285, 300, 320	4-phenol
(**302**)	266, 288, 303, 359, 375	—	256, 282, 293, 305, 338, 353	1-methyl-17-ketone

a cpp indicates that the metabolite has a typical 15,16-dihydrocyclopenta[a]phenanthrene chromophore.

Further hydroxylation of this metabolite then leads to the other, more polar, phenols. Presumably isomerization is promoted by electron release by the *p*-methyl group for the reverse, stabilization of epoxides towards isomerization, is known to be favoured by electron withdrawal (Chiasson and Berchtold, 1977). Another six metabolites (designated ccp-diol, etc. in the Table) appeared to be hydroxylated derivatives retaining the intact phenanthrene chromophore; their extents of hydroxylation can be guessed from their relative elution times, but an extensive nmr and mass spectral investigation would be needed to establish their exact structures. Only two metabolites, (**k**) and (**l**), had spectra suggesting partial unsaturation. Metabolite (**l**) was obviously a 1,2-dihydrodiol from the characteristic splitting of the ultraviolet maximum into two peaks of similar intensity (λ_{max} 258, 267 nm) on borohydride reduction; from its polarity it was probably further hydroxylated at C-15, C-16, or at the methyl group. Thus again there is evidence for enzymatic attack at the carbon-substituted double bond at C-1,2. The spectra of metabolite (**k**) were those typical of a 1,2,3,4-tetrahydro-17-ketone; this compound may therefore be a 1,2,3,4-tetrahydro-tetraol formed either by further hydroxylation of 1,2-diol or of a 3,4-diol. The former seems the more likely because there is no evidence of a 3,4-dihydro-diol, and this seems to account adequately for the 1-methyl-17-ketone (**302**) being essentially inactive as a carcinogen and mutagen.

Thus to summarize, metabolic studies have shown that the carcinogenic 11-methyl-, 7-methyl-, and 11,12-dimethyl-17-ketones all yield *trans*-diequatorial 3,4-dihydrodiols, presumably capable of further transformation to diol-epoxides since they bind to DNA after metabolism. The 1-methyl and 6-methyl-17-ketones are non-carcinogens because, for different reasons, they do not form diol-epoxides of this sort. This leaves the unsubstituted and 12-methyl-17-ketones which are anomalous because they form *trans*-[3R,4R]diequatorial diols and yet are not carcinogens.

7.5   Formation of DNA adducts, and their persistence

Further progress in understanding these structure/activity relationships came from examining the binding of some of these compounds to DNA. The unsubstituted-17-ketone (**4**) is a bacterial mutagen although it is not carcinogenic. After *in vitro* metabolic activation it bound to added DNA, albeit to a lesser extent than the 11-methyl ketone. The pattern of nucleoside adducts separated by Sephadex chromatography was similar to those given by the latter (see Fig. 63). Originally (Table 21) the 12-methyl-17-ketone was classed as a non-mutagen; however, a more recent study (Hadfield, 1983) disclosed weak activity with *Salmonella typhimurium* TA100. After metabolic activation *in vitro* this compound also bound to added DNA, but to only about 15% of the extent of the 11-methyl isomer (Russell *et al.*, 1985). It yielded the familiar pattern of nucleosides except that peak A was almost the same size as peak B. When the binding of these compounds to mouse skin DNA was measured *in vivo* as before the following results were obtained, where DNA binding is quoted as nmol of compound/mol of DNA phosphorus in peaks A and B:

	DNA binding
unsubstituted-17-ketone (**4**)	19
11-methyl-17-ketone (**26**)	458
12-methyl-17-ketone (**130**)	155
11,12-dimethyl-17-ketone (**131**)	974

Thus the unsubstituted-17-ketone essentially failed to bind covalently to DNA *in vivo* in the target tissue, and this seems to explain its failure to act as a carcinogen. The 12-methyl-17-ketone, however, bound to DNA *in vivo* to about one-third of the extent of the 11-methyl isomer, i.e., to a greater extent than it did *in vitro*. When in each case the major adduct B was chromatographed on Sephadex LH20 using borate buffer (Hadfield *et al.*, 1984*a*), the 12-methyl adduct showed the usual early elution expected if it were derived from an *anti*-diol-epoxide. By contrast the adduct from the unsubstituted ketone showed no such effect (Fig. 75). This experiment was repeated several times, always with the same result, and on the face of it seems to indicate that this adduct is derived from a *syn*-diol-epoxide as outlined in Fig. 66. However, further experiments are needed to confirm this surprising result. By analogy with benzo[a]pyrene only the *anti*-diol-epoxides might be expected to exhibit carcinogenicity (Levin *et al.*, 1977; Buening *et al.*, 1978) although *syn*-diol-epoxides are mutagenic to bacteria (Wood *et al.*, 1977).

This still left the lack of carcinogenicity of the 12-methyl-17-ketone unexplained for at the topical dose of 1000 nmol on mouse skin this compound gave a DNA binding ratio equivalent to that given by about 340 nmol of its 11-methyl isomer, and at this dose on mouse skin the latter is strongly carcinogenic (Russell *et al.*, 1985). However, an interesting result was obtained when the persistence of these DNA adducts was investigated.

The rate of formation and persistence of DNA adducts of the carcinogenic 11-methyl-17-ketone was studied by Abbott and Crew (1981). They found that after topical application (400 μg per mouse, to the dorsal skin) or intramuscular injection (3 μg per mouse, into the shoulder) binding to the DNA of skin, lung, and liver reached a maximum at 1–2 days, and then declined. The half-life in skin and lung, targets for this carcinogen, was about 7 days, whereas it was only 2.5 days for liver which is not a target (Fig. 76). By labelling the skin with tritiated thymidine it was shown that labelled DNA was lost from this tissue with a half-life of about 6 days. Hence there is little evidence for active repair of the 11-methyl lesions in skin whereas they are rapidly eliminated from liver. When this type of experiment was extended to the 12-methyl- (Russell *et al.*, 1985) and 11,12-dimethyl-17-ketones (Furn, personal communication, 1985) (1000 nmol/mouse, topical), maximum binding was again found at about 2 days, but loss of adducts from the skin occurred with a half-life of 3.5

Fig. 75. Elution of the main DNA adducts formed by the unsubstituted (4) and 12-methyl-17-ketones (130) from Sephadex LH20 columns with Tris and borate buffers of the same pH and molarity.

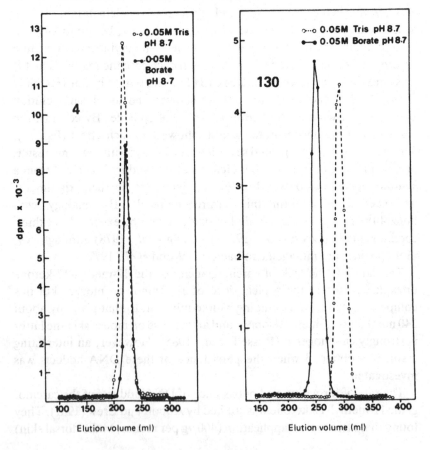

days for the former while it was about 7 days for the latter, like the result for the 11-methyl-17-ketone. Thus it appears the 12-methyl-17-ketone is not carcinogenic because the DNA damage it causes in skin is largely repaired before cell division occurs. This is another unexpected result that needs confirmation.

7.6   Summary

Carcinogens of the 17-oxocyclopenta[a]phenanthrene series are not mutagenic in the absence of prior metabolism. This suggests that the observed carcinogenicity/chemical structure relationships might, at least in part, be related to the correct metabolic activation of these molecules and, as has been outlined above, this indeed proves to be the case. These compounds are biologically activated like polycyclic aromatic hydrocarbons, through benzo-ring oxidation. Specifically, epoxidation of the 3,4-double bond followed by enzyme-induced hydrolylic ring opening to give a diequatorial *trans*-3α,4β-dihydrodiol is required. This metabolite must then be further oxidized at C-1,2 to an *anti*-3α,4β-diol-1α,2α-epoxide, which must be stable enough to avoid reaction with the nucleophiles such as water present in the environment in which it is

Fig. 76. Loss of ^{3}H-labelled DNA adducts of the carcinogen (**26**) from mouse skin, lung, and liver; total amounts of the adducts were estimated from the adduct peaks A and B eluting from Sephadex columns (see Fig. 63). The half lives ($t_\frac{1}{2}$) were not adjusted for the rate of DNA turnover in these tissues, about six days for skin and lung, and much longer for liver (Abbott and Crew, 1981).

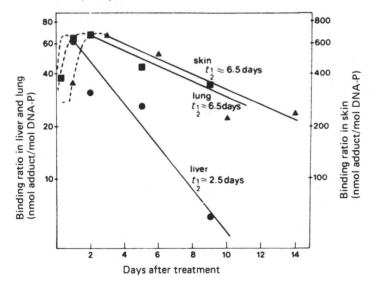

produced. It must also survive transport through the nuclear membrane and into the cell's genetic material in the nucleus. There it must be capable of reacting covalently with specific nucleoside bases to give adducts that resist removal by the efficient DNA repair enzymes, and be able to cause mutations that ultimately lead to abnormal and uncontrolled cell division, possibly by activation of a cellular oncogene. All these requirements must be met in turn, and it is consequently clear why most of the methyl isomers (for instance) are inactive. On the other hand, this information does not help us to understand why 7- and 11-methyl substitution are uniquely able to lead to diol-epoxides which fulfil all these requirements. This problem, which applies also to other polycyclic aromatic systems and has recently been discussed (DiGiovanni *et al.*, 1983), will be mentioned again in Chapter 8.

7.7   References

Abbott, P. J. & Coombs, M. M. (1981). DNA adducts of the carcinogen 15,16-dihydro-11-methylcyclopenta[a]phenanthren-17-one, *in vivo* and *in vitro*: high pressure liquid chromatographic separation and partial characterisation. *Carcinogenesis*, **2**, 629–36.

Abbott, P. J. & Crew, F. (1981). Repair of DNA adducts of the carcinogen 15,16-dihydro-11-methylcyclopenta[a]phenanthren-17-one in mouse tissue and its relation to tumour induction. *Cancer Res.*, **41**, 4115–20.

Allen, J. A. (1979). *The Binding of a Number of Potentially Carcinogenic Polycyclic Aromatic Compounds to Mitochondrial and Nuclear DNA.* Ph.D. Thesis, University of Surrey.

Allen, J. A. & Coombs, M. M. (1980). Covalent binding of polycyclic aromatic compounds to mitochondrial and nuclear DNA. *Nature (London)*, **287**, 244–5.

Bhatt, T. S. (1986). Comparison of the metabolism and DNA binding of the carcinogen 15,16-dihydro-11-methylcyclopenta[a]phenanthren-17-one by hamster embryo cells and the human hepatoma cell line HepG2. *Carcinogenesis*, **7**, 143–8.

Blin, N. & Stafford, W. D. A. (1976). A general method of isolation of high molecular weight DNA from eukaryotes. *Nucleic Acids Res.*, **3**, 2302–8.

Buening, M. K., Wislocki, P. G., Levin, W., Yagi, H., Thakker, D. R., Akagi, H., Koreeda, M., Jerina, D. M. & Conney, A. H. (1978). Tumorigenicity of the optical enantiomers of the diastereomeric benzo[a]pyrene 7,8-diol-9,10-epoxides in newborn mice: exceptional activity of (+)−7β-8α-dihydroxy-9α,10α-epoxy-7,8,9,10-tetrahydrobenzo[a]pyrene. *Proc. Nat. Acad. Sci. U.S.A.*, **75**, 5358–61.

Chiasson, B. A. & Berchtold, G. A. (1977). 3-Carbo-*tert*-butoxybenzene oxide. *J. Org. Chem.*, **42**, 2008–9.

Coombs, M. M. & Bhatt, T. S. (1982). High skin tumour initiating activity of the metabolically derived *trans*-3,4-diol of the carcinogen 15,16-dihydro-11-methylcyclopenta[a]phenanthren-17-one. *Carcinogenesis*, **3**, 449–51.

Coombs, M. M., Bhatt, T. S., Kissonerghis, A.-M. & Vose, C. W. (1980). Mutagenic and carcinogenic metabolites of the carcinogen 15,16-dihydro-11-cyclopenta[a]phenanthren-17-one. *Cancer Res.*, **40**, 882–6.

Coombs, M. M., Bhatt, T. S., Livingston, D. C., Fisher, S. W. & Abbott, P. J. (1981). Chemical structure, metabolism, and carcinogenicity in the cyclopenta[a]phenanthrene series. In *Polynuclear Aromatic Hydrocarbons: Chemical Analysis and Biological Fate*, ed. M. Cooke & A. J. Dennis, pp. 63–73. Battelle Press: Columbus.

Coombs, M. M., Bhatt, T. S. & Vose, C. W. (1975). The relationship between metabolism, DNA binding, and carcinogenicity of 15,16-dihydro-11-methylcyclopenta[a]phenanthren-17-one in the presence of a microsomal enzyme inhibitor. *Cancer Res.*, **35**, 305–9.

Coombs, M. M. & Crawley, F. E. H. (1974). Potentially carcinogenic cyclopenta[a]phenanthrenes, Part IX. Characterisation of a 5,10-epoxybenzocydodecene as a major urinary metabolite of the carcinogen 15,16-dihydro-11-methylcyclopenta[a]phenanthren-17-one. *J. Chem. Soc. Perkin Trans.* I, 2330–5.

Coombs, M. M. & Crawley, F. E. H. (1975). An important difference in the urinary metabolites formed from 15,16-dihydrocyclopenta[a]phenanthren-17-one and its 11-methyl homologue in the rat. *Cancer Biochem. Biophys.*, **1**, 157–62.

Coombs, M. M., Hadfield, S. T. & Bhatt, T. S. (1982). 15,16-Dihydro-1,11-methanocyclopenta[a]phenanthren-17-one: a carcinogen with a bridged bay-region. In *Polynuclear Aromatic Hydrocarbons; Seventh International Symposium on Formation, Metabolism, and Measurement*, ed. M. W. Cooke and A. J. Dennis, pp. 351–63. Battelle Press: Columbus, Ohio.

Coombs, M. M., Hall, M., Siddle, V. A. & Vose, C. W. (1976). Identification of monohydroxy metabolites of 15,16-dihydro-cyclopenta[a]phenanthren-17-one and its carcinogenic 11-methyl homolog produced by rat liver preparations *in vitro*. *Archives Biochem. Biophys.*, **172**, 434–8.

Coombs, M. M., Kissonerghis, A.-M., Allen, J. A. & Vose, C. W. (1979). Identification of the proximate and ultimate forms of the carcinogen 15,16-dihydro-11-methylcyclopenta[a]phenanthren-17-one. *Cancer Res.*, **39**, 4160–5.

Coombs, M. M., Russell, J. C., Jones, J. R. & Ribeiro, O. (1985). A comparative examination of the *in vitro* metabolism of five cyclopenta[a]phenanthrenes of varying carcinogenic potential. *Carcinogenesis*, **6**, 1217–22.

Dunlap, C. E. & Warren, S. (1946). The carcinogenic activity of some new derivatives of aromatic hydrocarbons. *Cancer Res.*, **6**, 454–65.

Dannenberg, H. (1960). Uber Beziehungen zwischen Steroiden und krebserzeugenden Kohlenwasserstoffen. II. Mitteilung, 1:2-Cyclopentadienophenanthrene. *Z. Krebsforsch.*, **63**, 523–31.

Dawson, J. R., Adams, D. J. & Wolf, C. R. (1985). Induction of drug metabolising enzymes in human liver cell line HepG2. *FEBS Lett.*, **183**, 219–22.

DiGiovanni, J., Diamond, L., Harvey, R. G. & Slaga, T. J. (1983). Enhancement of skin tumor-initiating activity of polycyclic aromatic hydrocarbons by methyl substitution at non-benzo 'bay region' positions. *Carcinogenesis*, **4**, 403–7.

Hadfield, S. T. (1983). *The Influence of Chemical Structure on the Metabolism of Cyclopenta[a]phenanthren-17-ones*. Ph.D. Thesis, University of London, p. 69.

Hadfield, S. T., Abbott, P. J., Coombs, M. M. & Drake, A. F. (1984a). The effect of methyl substituents on the *in vitro* metabolism of cyclopenta[a]-phenanthren-17-ones: implications for biological activity. *Carcinogenesis*, **5**, 1395–9.

Hadfield, S. T., Bhatt, T. S. & Coombs, M. M. (1984b). The biological activity and activation of 15,16-dihydro-1,11-methanocyclopenta[a]-phenanthren-17-one, a carcinogen with an obstructed bay region. *Carcinogenesis*, **5**, 1485–91.

Hecht, S. S., Amin, S., Rivenson, A. & Hoffman, D. (1979). Tumor initiating activity of 5,11-dimethylchrysene and the structural requirements favouring carcinogenicity of methylated polynuclear aromatic hydrocarbons. *Cancer Lett.*, **8**, 65–70.

Jerina, D. M., Yagi, H., Lehr, R. E., Thakker, D. R., Schaefer-Ridder, M., Karle, J. M., Levin, W., Wood, A. W., Chang, R. L. & Conney, A. H. (1978) The bay-region theory of carcinogenesis by polycyclic aromatic hydrocarbons. In *Polycyclic Hydrocarbons and Cancer*, vol. 1, ed. H. V. Gelboin & P. O. P. Ts'o, pp. 173–88. Academic Press: New York.

Kinoshita, T., Konieczny, M., Santella, R. & Jeffrey, A. M. (1982). Metabolism and covalent binding to DNA of 7-methylbenzo[a]pyrene. *Cancer Res.*, **42**, 4032–8.

Levin, W., Wood, A. W., Wislocki, P. G., Kapitulnik, J., Yagi, H., Jerina, D. M. & Conney, A. H. (1977). Carcinogenicity of benzo-ring derivatives of benzo[a]pyrene on mouse skin. *Cancer Res.*, **37**, 3356–61.

Russell, J. C., Bhatt, T. S., Jones, J. R. & Coombs, M. M. (1985). Comparison of the binding of some carcinogenic and non-carcinogenic cyclopenta[a]phenanthrenes to DNA *in vitro* and *in vivo*. *Carcinogenesis*, **6**, 1223–5.

Sims, P., Grover, P. L., Swaisland, A., Pal, K. & Hewer, A. (1974). Metabolic activity of benzo[a]pyrene proceeds by a diol-epoxide. *Nature (London)*, **254**, 326–8.

Wiebers, J. L., Abbott, P. J., Coombs, M. M. & Livingston, D. C. (1981). Mass spectral characterisation of the major DNA-carcinogen adduct formed from the metabolically activated carcinogen 15,16-dihydro-11-methylcyclopenta[a]phenanthren-17-one. *Carcinogenesis*, **2**, 637–43.

Wood, A. W., Chang, R. L., Levin, W., Yagi, H., Thakker, D. R., Jerina, D. M. & Conney, A. H. (1977). Differences in mutagenicity of the optical enantiomers of the diastereomeric benzo[a]pyrene 7,8-diol-9,10-epoxides. *Biochem. Biophys. Res. Commun.*, **77**, 1389–96.

Yang, S. K., Chou, M. W. & Fu, P. P. (1981). Microsomal oxidations of methyl-substituted and unsubstituted aromatic hydrocarbons of monomethylbenz[a]anthracenes. In *Polynuclear Aromatic Hydrocarbons*, ed. M. Cook & A. J. Dennis, pp. 253–64. Battelle Press: Columbus.

8

X-ray crystallography of some cyclopenta[a]-
phenanthrenes: an apparent correlation
between molecular strain and carcinogenicity

8.1 Early work

We usually think of X-ray crystallography as being a technique which has been developed to its present high state of sophistication over the last 25 years. However, its origins go back much further, and in fact one of its earliest uses was to help establish the structure of sterols. In 1932 Bernal studied the X-ray diffraction patterns of crystals of several sterols, and from their experimentally established cell dimensions deduced that these molecules were 17–20 Å long, 7–8 Å wide, and 5 Å thick. The original Windaus formula (Chapter 1, Fig. 3) would have required these dimensions to be approximately $18.0 \times 7.0 \times 8.5$ Å, making the molecules too thick to fit into the unit cell derived from the X-ray diffraction data. The same conclusion was also reached from a study of the molecular cross-section sizes derived from the surface area of monolayer films by Adam (1930). Diels' hydrocarbon had, of course, previously been isolated from the products of selenium dehydrogenation of cholesterol and other sterols and its identification as a cyclopenta[a]phenanthrene had strengthened this evidence for a revised steroid structure. However, at that time uncertainty still existed as to whether this hydrocarbon was 16,17-dihydro-15H-cyclopenta[a]phenanthrene (1) or its 17-methyl homologue (7) (Fig. 77), and Bernal set out to examine

Fig. 77. The two cyclopenta[a]phenanthrene hydrocarbons studied by X-ray crystallography in 1935.

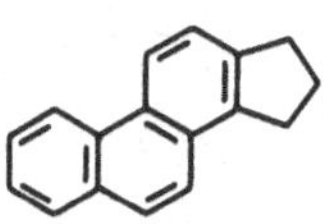

16,17-Dihydro—15H-cyclopenta-
[a] phenanthrene (1)

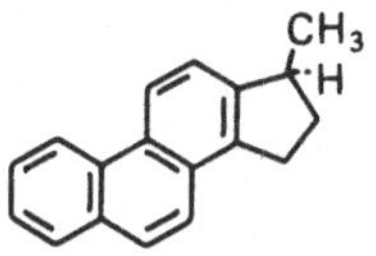

Diels' hydrocarbon (7)

this question by X-ray crystallography (Bernal and Crowfoot, 1935). For comparison the synthetic parent hydrocarbon (1) and Diels' hydrocarbon prepared by dehydrogenation of cholesterol (Diels *et al.*, 1927), as well as the two specimens of the 17-methyl hydrocarbon synthesized by different methods by Bergmann and Hillemann (1933) and by Harper *et al.* (1934) were available. Suitable crystals were obtained by crystallization from the melt by the hot-wire method (Bernal and Crowfoot, 1933) because in many cases the crystals which separated from solution were too small and imperfect for X-ray examination.

All four crystal samples were found to consist of 'lath-shaped molecules of width approximately 6 Å and thickness 4 Å packed together in parallel bundles'. Two characteristic crystalline forms were observed: monoclinic in which the planes of the rings were inclined to the basal plane, and orthorhombic with them approximately parallel to it. The parent hydrocarbon (1) crystallized in both forms and both were examined, while all three samples of the 17-methyl homologue formed only monoclinic crystals and appeared to be crystallographically identical with one another within the limits of the experimental method (Table 38). It was therefore concluded that Diels' hydrocarbon was definitely not the parent compound (1), and it was observed (correctly) that the small differences in melting points and crystal habit found between the three samples of the 17-methyl derivative were probably due 'to the presence of impurities, possibly in very small quantities'. For this compound the unit cell had a density = 1.185 ± 0.005 g/cm^3 indicating that it contained four molecules of molecular weight 232 ± 3 ($C_{18}H_{16}$ requires 232); the molecules were arranged in the crystal as shown in Fig. 78.

The parent hydrocarbon (1) was also studied by Iball (1935) who pointed out that the X-ray intensities found were remarkably similar to those observed for crystals of chrysene, and proposed the structure of the

Table 38. *Crystal data for 16,17-dihydro-15H-cyclopenta[a]-phenanthrene* (1) *and Diels' hydrocarbon* (7)

Hydrocarbon	Space group	Cell dimensions (Å)			Probable molecular length (Å)
		a	b	c	
(1) $C_{17}H_{14}$ (stable)	B2$_1$/a	18.2	6.05	21.2	11.6
(1) $C_{17}H_{14}$ (metastable)	Aba	8.10	6.4	22.8	11.4
(7) $C_{18}H_{16}$	Aba	8.50	6.25	24.3	12.1

former on this basis. However, it was not until 20 years later that the positions of the carbon atoms could be located in this structure using the Fourier transformation (Entwhistle *et al.*, 1954) which, because of the extensive computation required, became practicable only after the introduction of electronic digital computers. The definitive paper did not appear for another seven years (Entwhistle and Iball, 1961) and in the meantime another X-ray structure for this compound had been published (Basak and Basak, 1959). Iball's structure was based on Fourier synthesis with 50 terms and subsequent refinement of the atomic co-ordinates by four cycles of least-squares calculations, reducing the reliability factor finally to $R = 0.108$. The reliability factor (discrepancy index) is an estimate of the agreement between the measured diffraction pattern intensities and those calculated for a particular model of arrangement of atoms in the repeat unit; values of 0.06–0.02 are considered good for present-day structural determinations (Glusker and Trueblood, 1985). Basaks' results were obtained from a study restricted to Fourier synthesis

Fig. 78. Arrangement of the molecules of 16,17-dihydro-15*H*-cyclopenta[a]phenanthrene (1) in the orthorhombic and monoclinic crystals (Bernal and Crowfoot, 1935).

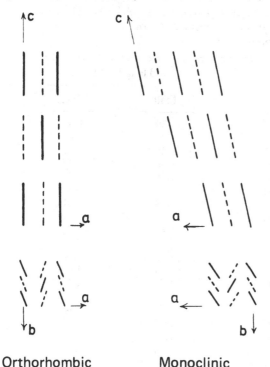

Orthorhombic   Monoclinic

in two zones with no refinement of the co-ordinates ($R = 0.28$) and in many instances the bond lengths differed appreciably from those of Iball, although the overall structure was the same (see Table 39). The K-region C–C bond C(6)–C(7) was short, as found for other aromatic compounds containing a phenanthrene nucleus. The bonds joining the five-membered ring to the aromatic system C(14)–C(15) and C(17)–C(13) were intermediate in length between a single aliphatic single bond and an aromatic bond, whereas the other cyclopentene bonds C(15)–C(16) and C(16)–C(17) were rather longer than a normal aliphatic single bond. The aromatic rings in this molecule were essentially flat, but carbon atoms C(15) and C(17) bonded to them were 0.1 Å below the plane while C(16) was 0.18 Å above. Bond angles are shown in Table 40. The exocyclic angle at C(9) is unusually large, no doubt relieving the interaction between the protons H(1) and H(11) in the bay region. No other X-ray crystallographic studies of cyclopenta[a]phenanthrenes seem to have been published since 1961 until the recent work on the 17-ketones described below.

Table 39. *Carbon–carbon bond lengths for 16,17-dihydro-15H-cyclopenta[a]phenanthrene* (**1**) *obtained from X-ray crystallography measurements*

Bond	Bond length (Å)	
	Iball	Basak
C(1)–C(2)	1.39	1.38
C(2)–C(3)	1.34	1.40
C(3)–C(4)	1.40	1.42
C(4)–C(5)	1.40	1.37
C(5)–C(6)	1.45	1.42
C(6)–C(7)	1.36	1.39
C(7)–C(8)	1.44	1.41
C(8)–C(9)	1.45	—
C(9)–C(10)	1.43	1.40
C(10)–C(5)	1.45	—
C(9)–C(11)	1.41	1.40
C(11)–C(12)	1.41	1.41
C(12)–C(13)	1.44	1.42
C(13)–C(14)	1.36	—
C(14)–C(15)	1.52	1.48
C(15)–C(16)	1.55	1.52
C(16)–C(17)	1.57	1.53
C(17)–C(13)	1.51	1.46

Table 40. *Carbon–carbon bond angles (°) in 16,17-dihydro-15H-cyclopenta[a]phenanthrene* (1)

Endocyclic angles	
C(10)–C(1)–C(2)	120
C(1)–C(2)–C(3)	121
C(2)–C(3)–C(4)	122
C(3)–C(4)–C(5)	120
C(4)–C(5)–C(10)	118
C(5)–C(6)–C(7)	118
C(6)–C(5)–C(10)	121
C(6)–C(7)–C(8)	124
C(7)–C(8)–C(9)	118
C(8)–C(9)–C(10)	118
C(8)–C(9)–C(11)	119
C(9)–C(11)–C(12)	124
C(11)–C(12)–C(13)	116
C(12)–C(13)–C(14)	123
C(13)–C(14)–C(8)	121
C(13)–C(14)–C(15)	112
C(14)–C(15)–C(16)	102
C(15)–C(16)–C(17)	101
C(16)–C(17)–C(13)	101
C(17)–C(13)–C(14)	113
Exocyclic angles	
C(4)–C(5)–C(6)	121
C(7)–C(8)–C(14)	123
C(8)–C(14)–C(15)	127
C(1)–C(10)–C(9)	121
C(10)–C(9)–C(11)	124
C(12)–C(13)–C(17)	124

8.2   The molecular structures of thirteen 15,16-dihydro-17-ketones derived from X-ray crystallography: the shapes of the molecules

As part of an in-depth study of 15,16-dihydrocyclopenta[a]phenanthren-17-one and its isomeric methyl homologues aimed at improving understanding of the structure/carcinogenicity relationships found among them, thirteen 17-ketones have been studied by X-ray crystallography. The compounds, chosen to cover the widest possible range of biological activities from inactive compounds to the strongest carcinogen, are shown in Fig. 79. Two quite separate investigations have been made; in the first (Clayton *et al.*, 1983) the 11-methyl-17-ketone (**26**) and the six ketones shown in the top half of the figure were studied at the Northern Polytechnic, London, under the supervision of Dr Mary McPartlin using Cu-Kα radiation for (**4**) and Mo-Kα radiation for the rest. The six compounds shown in the bottom half of this figure, together with ketone (**26**), were later investigated in the laboratory of Dr Jenny Glusker at the Institute for Cancer Research, Fox Chase, Philadelphia, using Mo-Kα radiation for the 11,12-dihydro compound (**252**) and Cu-Kα radiation for all the rest (Kashino *et al.*, 1986). The carcinogen (**26**) (15,16-dihydro-11-methylcyclopenta[a]phenanthren-17-one) was therefore common to both groups and was studied using both types of radiation. The sample used at Fox Chase was synthesized there by a variation of the published method, and the structure of the compound was solved independently in the two laboratories without prior knowledge of one another's results. It is satisfying to observe close agreement between the two sets of data; for example, the average differences between C–C distances and angles were within ±0.002 Å and ±0.11°, less than the quoted experimental errors. For this reason the two sets of

Fig. 79. The 13 cyclopenta[a]phenanthrenes studied by X-ray crystallography (Clayton *et al.*, 1983; Kashino *et al.*, 1986).

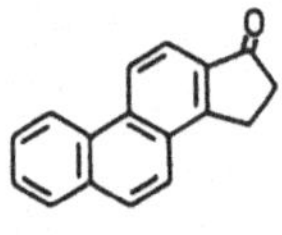
4

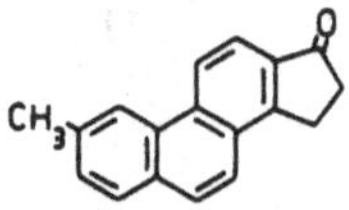

303

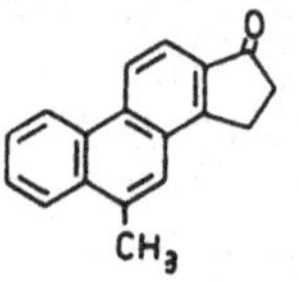

306

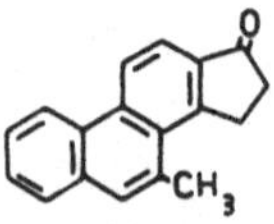

230

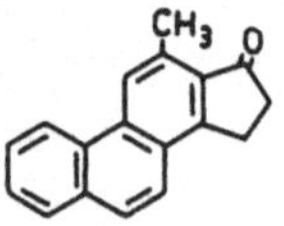

130

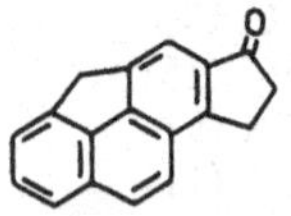
310

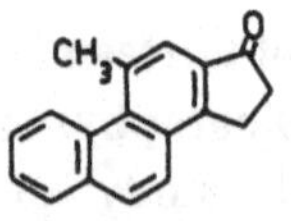

26

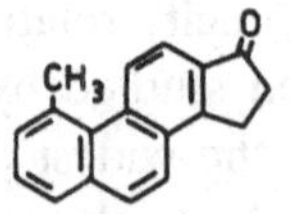

302

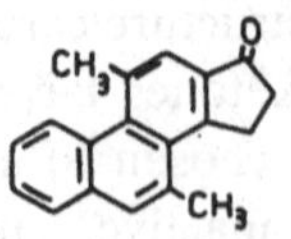

309

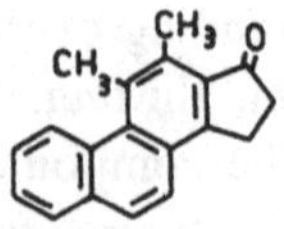

131

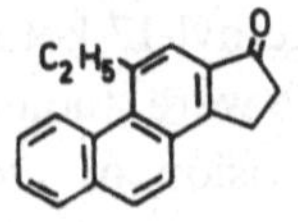

211

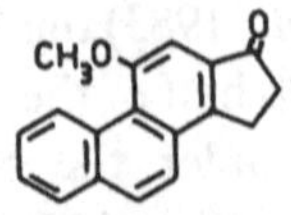

132

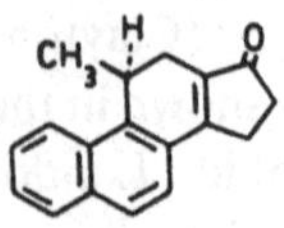

252

Table 41. *Crystal data for the thirteen cyclopenta[a]phenanthrenes shown in Fig. 79*

Compound	Unsubst. (4)	1-Me (302)	2-Me (303)	6-Me (306)	7-Me (230)	11-Me (26)	12-Me (130)	7,11-diMe (309)	11,12-diMe (131)	11-Et (211)	11-OMe (132)	1,11-CH$_2$ (310)	11-Me-11,12-H$_2$ (252)
Formula	C$_{17}$H$_{12}$O	C$_{18}$H$_{14}$O	C$_{18}$H$_{14}$O	C$_{18}$H$_{14}$O	C$_{18}$H$_{14}$O	C$_{18}$H$_{14}$O	C$_{18}$H$_{14}$O	C$_{19}$H$_{16}$O	C$_{19}$H$_{16}$O	C$_{19}$H$_{16}$O	C$_{18}$H$_{14}$O$_2$	C$_{18}$H$_{12}$O	C$_{18}$H$_{16}$O
Mol. wt	232.25	246.31	246.31	246.31	246.31	246.31	246.31	260.33	260.33	260.33	262.31	244.30	248.32
mp (°C)	203–204	189–190	221–222	210.5–212	198–199	171–172	233	208–210	149–150	129–130	179	195	177–178
Space group	P2$_1$/c	Pbca	P2$_1$/c	P2$_1$/c	P2$_1$/c	Pcab	Pbca	P2$_1$cn	P2$_1$/n	Pnaa	Fddd	Pbca	P2$_1$/n
a (Å)	10.243	14.344	11.965	7.587	7.562	14.355	9.746	11.640	20.368	17.820	21.567	7.504	12.743
b (Å)	20.642	23.121	10.749	21.122	13.490	23.153	20.882	15.131	5.751	20.365	35.192	21.869	8.781
c (Å)	5.445	7.571	9.867	7.777	12.532	7.526	12.231	7.531	11.494	7.584	13.823	15.093	11.721
β (°)	109.20	—	93.71	100.98	92.97	—	—	—	90.68	—	—	—	95.92
Calc. density (g cm^{-3})	1.146	1.303	1.294	1.337	1.282	1.308	1.314	1.304	1.284	1.257	1.329	1.316	1.264
Volume (Å^3)	1089.2	2510.9	1263.6	1223.4	1275.8	2488.5	2489.2	1326.3	1346.5	2752.3	10.491	1304.5	2464.3
Z	4	8	4	4	4	8	8	4	4	8	32	4	8
Final R (%)	8.3	5.2	8.4	5.8	8.1	5.1	7.1	5.6	5.9	7.0	6.6	6.3	8.1

The angle β (°) is the angle between the a and c crystal axes; where it is not quoted it is 90.0° and the crystals are orthorhombic.

results are considered together for the purpose of the discussion which follows. Some fundamental crystal data for the thirteen 17-ketones shown in Fig. 79 are presented in Table 41. The structures were refined by full matrix least squares, and in all cases the final reliability factors were between 0.051 and 0.084. These, and the complete agreement between the two structures independently derived for the 11-methyl-17-ketone (26), give us reason to believe that the differences in bond lengths and angles calculated from the X-ray data are meaningful. They lead to an interesting correlation.

Carbon–carbon and carbon–oxygen bond lengths for the 13 compounds are listed in Table 42 together with estimated standard deviations in parentheses; Table 43 similarly displays the bond angles. It is noticeable that equivalent C–C bonds in these molecules differ from the average values by not more than 0.03 Å. This applies equally to the 1,11-methano compound (310) although it is obviously strained owing to the five-membered ring fused in the bay region. All have long (1.418–1.470 Å) C(9)–C(10) bay-region bonds, and short (1.320–1.371 Å) K-region bonds, very similar to those observed in the hydrocarbon (1), 1.433 and 1.355 Å (Entwhistle and Iball, 1961) and in phenanthrene itself, 1.460 and 1.352 Å, respectively (Kay *et al.*, 1971). In the 11,12-dihydro derivative (252) C(11)–C(12) is a single bond (1.538 Å) while C(9)–C(11) and C(13)–C(14) fall within the range of the aryl–methyl bond lengths (1.503–1.531 Å). The aryl–methylene C(1)–C(18) and C(11)–C(18) bond lengths in the 1,11-methylene compound (310) are similar. In contrast to the bond lengths, the bond angles show more variability among these 17-oxocyclopenta[a]phenanthrenes. For example, the endocyclic angles in six-membered rings (120.0° for a regular hexagon) vary between 115.8° and 128.1°. With two exceptions (the 7-methyl and 1,11-methano compounds, 230 and 310) the exocyclic bay-region angles C(1)–C(10)–C(9) and C(10)–C(9)–C(11) are greater than 120° (range 120.5–126.0°); this is particularly marked in compounds with substituents at C-1 or C-11 in the bay region. The 1,11-bridged compound (310) is quite anomalous in that these two angles are only 110.7° and 109.9°, resulting in considerable distortion from the normal pattern. This can readily be seen by superimposing it upon the parent molecule 15,16-dihydrocyclopenta[a]phenanthren-17-one (4) as shown in Fig. 80. To compensate for these small bay-region angles, the angles at the other side of the molecule, C(4)–C(5)–C(6) and C(7)–C(8)–C(14), are exceptionally large, 129.5° and 131.2°. The perturbing effect this distortion has on the electronic distribution in this molecule is demonstrated by comparing their ultraviolet absorption spectra. That of the unsubstituted compound

Table 42. *Bond lengths (Å) with estimated standard deviations (in parentheses) for the thirteen cyclopenta[a]phenanthrenes shown in Fig. 79*

Bond	Unsubst. (4)	1-Me (302)	2-Me (303)	6-Me (306)	7-Me (230)	11-Me (26)	12-Me (130)	7,11-Me2 (309)	11,12-Me2 (131)	11-Et (211)	11-OMe (132)	1,11-CH2 (310)	11-Me-11,12-H2 (252)
C(1)-C(2)	1.366(8)	1.391(3)	1.404(10)	1.367(8)	1.371(12)	1.376(3)	1.375(7)	1.371(6)	1.383(3)	1.354(4)	1.390(4)	1.403(8)	1.363(2)
C(2)-C(3)	1.361(9)	1.378(3)	1.396(12)	1.384(8)	1.397(12)	1.386(3)	1.404(7)	1.388(8)	1.378(3)	1.403(5)	1.401(4)	1.408(9)	1.400(3)
C(3)-C(4)	1.323(8)	1.358(3)	1.340(12)	1.371(9)	1.378(12)	1.357(3)	1.373(7)	1.345(7)	1.353(3)	1.343(4)	1.347(4)	1.370(9)	1.362(3)
C(4)-C(5)	1.397(8)	1.414(2)	1.412(11)	1.417(8)	1.417(12)	1.412(3)	1.390(7)	1.419(7)	1.419(3)	1.423(4)	1.415(4)	1.440(8)	1.423(2)
C(5)-C(6)	1.410(8)	1.426(2)	1.430(12)	1.433(8)	1.400(11)	1.426(2)	1.420(7)	1.426(6)	1.423(9)	1.439(4)	1.414(4)	1.418(8)	1.414(2)
C(6)-C(7)	1.331(8)	1.334(3)	1.336(11)	1.348(7)	1.353(10)	1.337(2)	1.340(8)	1.331(7)	1.333(3)	1.320(4)	1.354(4)	1.371(8)	1.357(2)
C(7)-C(8)	1.412(8)	1.429(2)	1.424(12)	1.429(7)	1.464(11)	1.429(2)	1.435(7)	1.462(5)	1.436(2)	1.438(3)	1.440(3)	1.440(8)	1.420(2)
C(8)-C(9)	1.393(8)	1.425(2)	1.421(11)	1.405(8)	1.411(11)	1.425(2)	1.421(7)	1.438(5)	1.422(2)	1.414(4)	1.407(3)	1.387(8)	1.392(2)
C(9)-C(10)	1.445(8)	1.468(2)	1.454(10)	1.460(8)	1.454(11)	1.462(2)	1.443(7)	1.453(6)	1.471(2)	1.475(3)	1.470(3)	1.418(8)	1.433(2)
C(10)-C(5)	1.383(8)	1.431(2)	1.396(11)	1.417(7)	1.419(11)	1.425(2)	1.416(7)	1.415(6)	1.426(2)	1.402(4)	1.421(3)	1.393(8)	1.426(2)
C(10)-C(1)	1.391(8)	1.428(2)	1.421(11)	1.407(9)	1.419(11)	1.409(2)	1.409(7)	1.404(6)	1.411(3)	1.423(4)	1.407(3)	1.396(8)	1.429(2)
C(9)-C(11)	1.397(8)	1.423(2)	1.433(10)	1.413(7)	1.434(10)	1.442(2)	1.417(7)	1.446(5)	1.437(2)	1.441(4)	1.435(3)	1.413(8)	1.522(2)
C(11)-C(12)	1.355(8)	1.362(2)	1.380(10)	1.370(8)	1.350(11)	1.370(2)	1.369(7)	1.363(7)	1.392(2)	1.385(4)	1.358(3)	1.370(8)	1.538(2)
C(12)-C(13)	1.369(8)	1.395(2)	1.402(10)	1.395(8)	1.390(11)	1.395(2)	1.414(7)	1.394(6)	1.409(2)	1.404(4)	1.387(3)	1.422(8)	1.494(2)
C(13)-C(14)	1.338(8)	1.371(2)	1.357(11)	1.371(7)	1.382(11)	1.364(4)	1.377(7)	1.390(6)	1.373(2)	1.360(4)	1.370(3)	1.363(8)	1.343(3)
C(14)-C(15)	1.489(8)	1.513(2)	1.528(11)	1.519(9)	1.534(10)	1.513(2)	1.518(7)	1.530(7)	1.516(2)	1.530(3)	1.518(4)	1.528(8)	1.508(2)
C(14)-C(8)	1.402(8)	1.409(2)	1.391(10)	1.419(7)	1.426(11)	1.412(2)	1.386(7)	1.410(6)	1.401(2)	1.405(4)	1.415(3)	1.398(8)	1.460(2)
C(15)-C(16)	1.522(8)	1.533(3)	1.544(11)	1.553(7)	1.534(12)	1.527(2)	1.530(8)	1.537(8)	1.516(3)	1.558(4)	1.541(4)	1.529(8)	1.520(2)
C(16)-C(17)	1.473(9)	1.513(3)	1.461(13)	1.502(9)	1.509(12)	1.515(2)	1.508(8)	1.517(8)	1.505(3)	1.521(4)	1.521(4)	1.506(9)	1.510(2)
C(17)-C(13)	1.476(9)	1.465(3)	1.503(11)	1.487(8)	1.475(11)	1.472(2)	1.475(8)	1.460(7)	1.485(2)	1.468(4)	1.454(3)	1.484(8)	1.468(2)
C(17)-O	1.187(7)	1.222(2)	1.228(11)	1.219(7)	1.226(10)	1.215(2)	1.228(6)	1.209(7)	1.219(2)	1.211(4)	1.224(3)	1.228(8)	1.217(2)
C(2)-C(18)	—	—	1.503(12)	—	—	—	—	—	—	—	—	—	—
C(6)-C(18)	—	—	—	1.514(7)	—	—	—	—	—	—	—	—	—
C(7)-C(18)	—	—	—	—	1.513(11)	—	—	—	—	—	—	—	—
C(11)-C(18)	—	—	—	—	—	1.508(2)	—	1.510(7)	1.514(2)	1.537(4)	—	1.540(8)	1.526(6)
C(12)-C(18)	—	—	—	—	—	—	1.528(7)	—	—	—	—	—	—
C(1)-C(18)	—	1.504(3)	—	—	—	—	—	—	—	—	—	1.527(8)	—
C(7)-C(19)	—	—	—	—	—	—	—	1.531(7)	—	—	—	—	—
C(12)-C(19)	—	—	—	—	—	—	—	—	1.508(2)	—	—	—	—
C(18)-C(19)	—	—	—	—	—	—	—	—	—	1.460(4)	—	—	—
C(11)-O	—	—	—	—	—	—	—	—	—	—	1.368(3)	—	—
C(18)-O	—	—	—	—	—	—	—	—	—	—	1.419(3)	—	—

Table 43. *Bond angles (°) with estimated s.d. (in parentheses) for the non-hydrogen atoms in the thirteen cyclopenta[a]-phenanthrenes shown in Fig. 79*

Bond	Unsubst. (4)	1-Me (302)	2-Me (303)	6-Me (306)	7-Me (120)	11-Me (26)	12-Me (130)	7,11-Me$_2$ (309)	11,12-Me$_2$ (131)	11-Et (211)	11-OMe (132)	1,11-CH$_2$ (310)	11-Me-11,12-H$_2$ (252)
Endocyclic angles													
C(10)–C(1)–C(2)	120.2(7)	118.9(2)	120.2(10)	121.1(7)	121.3(10)	122.1(2)	121.0(6)	122.5(4)	121.9(2)	122.2(2)	121.1(2)	117.4(7)	121.0(2)
C(1)–C(2)–C(3)	121.6(7)	122.9(2)	118.1(10)	120.4(7)	120.5(10)	120.8(2)	120.6(7)	120.0(4)	121.0(2)	121.4(3)	121.2(2)	115.2(7)	120.6(20)
C(2)–C(3)–C(4)	119.8(7)	120.0(2)	122.3(10)	120.3(7)	119.9(11)	119.3(2)	119.2(7)	119.3(5)	119.2(2)	118.3(3)	117.9(2)	127.6(8)	120.7(1)
C(3)–C(4)–C(5)	120.6(7)	119.8(2)	121.1(11)	121.0(7)	120.8(10)	121.2(2)	121.1(6)	122.3(4)	122.1(2)	121.8(3)	123.2(2)	117.9(8)	120.7(2)
C(4)–C(5)–C(10)	120.8(7)	121.2(2)	118.7(10)	118.1(7)	119.3(9)	120.3(2)	120.3(6)	118.7(4)	119.3(2)	120.5(2)	119.0(2)	113.9(7)	119.0(1)
C(5)–C(10)–C(1)	117.2(6)	117.0(1)	119.5(9)	119.0(6)	118.1(9)	115.8(1)	117.7(5)	116.8(4)	116.4(2)	115.8(2)	117.3(2)	128.1(7)	118.1(1)
C(10)–C(5)–C(6)	118.5(6)	121.0(1)	120.8(9)	119.6(6)	119.1(9)	119.7(1)	119.5(6)	119.2(4)	120.2(2)	121.0(2)	120.9(2)	116.4(6)	119.7(1)
C(5)–C(6)–C(7)	121.0(7)	121.6(2)	120.2(11)	120.7(6)	124.3(9)	121.3(1)	121.9(7)	123.4(4)	121.4(2)	120.6(2)	121.5(2)	122.3(7)	120.5(1)
C(6)–C(7)–C(8)	122.4(7)	120.8(2)	122.3(10)	121.2(6)	119.0(8)	120.9(1)	120.9(6)	119.5(4)	121.2(2)	120.7(2)	119.6(2)	122.0(7)	120.8(1)
C(7)–C(8)–C(9)	119.1(5)	120.3(1)	118.8(8)	120.7(6)	118.4(8)	121.2(1)	119.3(5)	118.7(4)	120.6(1)	122.1(2)	121.5(2)	115.2(6)	120.6(1)
C(8)–C(9)–C(10)	117.9(6)	119.2(1)	119.2(9)	118.2(6)	120.9(7)	116.7(1)	119.2(5)	118.7(3)	117.4(1)	116.3(2)	118.1(2)	122.8(6)	119.0(1)
C(9)–C(10)–C(5)	121.1(6)	117.0(1)	118.7(9)	119.3(6)	118.4(8)	119.5(1)	118.4(5)	118.5(4)	118.7(1)	119.2(2)	118.3(2)	121.2(7)	119.2(1)
C(8)–C(9)–C(11)	118.3(6)	117.3(1)	118.4(8)	119.4(6)	120.1(8)	118.2(1)	122.7(6)	119.5(4)	118.3(1)	118.9(2)	117.1(2)	127.2(6)	120.3(1)
C(9)–C(11)–C(12)	123.0(6)	122.5(2)	121.7(9)	122.5(7)	121.3(8)	119.1(1)	117.8(6)	118.5(4)	120.6(1)	118.0(2)	121.8(2)	117.6(6)	113.6(1)
C(11)–C(12)–C(13)	117.9(7)	119.1(2)	117.4(9)	117.3(6)	117.9(9)	121.9(1)	120.5(6)	121.5(4)	118.7(1)	121.9(3)	119.9(2)	115.6(6)	111.8(1)
C(12)–C(13)–C(14)	121.2(6)	121.0(2)	122.4(8)	122.4(6)	124.2(9)	120.2(1)	122.2(5)	121.0(4)	121.3(1)	120.6(3)	121.1(2)	125.7(6)	123.1(1)
C(13)–C(14)–C(8)	122.3(6)	120.8(1)	121.6(9)	120.6(7)	118.4(8)	120.6(1)	118.3(6)	120.1(4)	121.0(1)	119.8(2)	119.8(2)	119.9(6)	121.7(1)
C(14)–C(8)–C(9)	117.3(6)	119.2(1)	118.4(9)	117.7(6)	118.0(7)	119.5(1)		117.9(3)	119.3(1)	120.7(2)	120.2(2)	114.0(6)	118.8(1)
C(13)–C(14)–C(15)	111.1(6)	111.3(1)	112.6(8)	112.7(6)	111.2(8)	111.6(1)	110.9(5)	108.7(4)	112.0(1)	111.6(2)	112.0(2)	112.1(6)	112.4(1)
C(14)–C(15)–C(16)	103.8(5)	104.4(1)	103.0(8)	103.6(5)	104.1(7)	104.5(1)	105.1(5)	105.4(4)	104.2(2)	103.1(2)	103.5(2)	103.7(6)	104.0(1)
C(15)–C(16)–C(17)	107.4(6)	106.1(1)	107.6(8)	106.2(6)	106.5(8)	106.2(1)	105.8(5)	106.2(4)	107.2(2)	106.4(2)	106.1(2)	106.9(6)	106.2(1)
C(16)–C(17)–C(13)	105.5(6)	107.6(2)	108.2(10)	108.4(6)	108.2(9)	107.3(1)	108.2(6)	106.9(4)	107.4(2)	107.9(3)	107.8(2)	107.7(6)	107.2(1)
C(17)–C(13)–C(14)	114.5(6)	110.5(2)	109.0(9)	109.1(6)	109.8(9)	110.3(1)	109.9(6)	112.5(4)	109.3(1)	110.8(3)	110.4(2)	109.6(6)	110.1(1)
Exocyclic angles													
C(4)–C(5)–C(6)	120.7(6)	117.8(2)	120.3(6)	122.0(6)	121.6(8)	119.9(2)	120.1(9)		122.0(4)	120.4(2)	118.5(2)	120.1(2)	**129.5(7)**
C(7)–C(8)–C(14)	123.7(6)	120.5(1)	122.4(10)	121.6(6)	123.7(8)	119.2(1)	122.3(9)		123.4(4)	120.1(1)	117.2(2)	118.3(2)	**130.2(6)**

	(1)	(2)	(3)	(4)	(5)	(6)	(7)	(8)	(9)	(10)	(11)	(12)	(13)
C(8)–C(14)–C(15)	—	127.9(1)	—	—	—	127.8(1)	—	122.2(8)	131.1(4)	127.0(1)	128.5(2)	128.1(2)	125.8(1)
C(1)–C(10)–C(9)	121.7(6)	126.0(1)	122.3(9)	121.7(6)	123.5(8)	124.6(1)	122.9(9)	129.5(9)	124.4(4)	124.7(1)	124.9(2)	124.4(2)	**120.7(6)**
C(3)–C(9)–C(11)	123.8(6)	123.5(1)	122.6(9)	123.3(6)	119.0(8)	125.0(1)	—	—	121.8(4)	124.3(1)	124.8(2)	124.8(2)	**109.9(6)**
C(12)–C(13)–C(17)	127.3(6)	128.5(2)	128.3(9)	128.5(6)	126.0(9)	129.4(1)	—	—	126.2(4)	129.4(1)	128.6(3)	128.4(2)	126.7(1)

Angles involving oxygen

	(1)	(2)	(3)	(4)	(5)	(6)	(7)	(8)	(9)	(10)	(11)	(12)	(13)
C(13)–C(17)–O(1)	—	126.2(2)	—	—	—	127.0(2)	—	126.6(5)	127.5(2)	126.9(2)	126.5(3)	—	126.9(1)
C(16)–C(17)–O(1)	—	126.2(2)	—	—	—	125.7(2)	—	126.5(4)	125.1(2)	125.1(2)	125.6(3)	—	125.9(1)
C(9)–C(11)–O(2)	—	—	—	—	—	—	—	—	—	—	116.2(2)	—	—
C(12)–C(11)–O(2)	—	—	—	—	—	—	—	—	—	—	122.0(2)	—	—
C(11)–O(2)–C(18)	—	—	—	—	—	—	—	—	—	—	119.0(2)	—	—

Angles involving methyl and methylene groups

	(1)	(2)	(3)	(4)	(5)	(6)	(7)	(8)	(9)	(10)	(11)	(12)	(13)
C(2)–C(1)–C(18)	—	115.1(2)	—	—	—	—	—	—	—	—	—	133.9(7)	—
C(10)–C(1)–C(18)	—	126.0(1)	—	—	—	—	—	—	—	—	—	108.7(6)	—
C(1)–C(2)–C(18)	—	—	119.6(10)	—	—	—	—	—	—	—	—	108.0(5)	—
C(3)–C(2)–C(18)	—	—	122.9(1)	—	—	—	—	—	—	—	—	134.3(6)	—
C(5)–C(6)–C(18)	—	—	—	118.9(6)	—	—	—	—	—	—	—	102.6(5)	—
C(7)–C(6)–C(18)	—	—	—	120.4(6)	—	—	—	—	—	—	—	—	—
C(6)–C(7)–C(18)	—	—	—	—	118.1(9)	—	—	—	—	—	—	—	—
C(8)–C(7)–C(18)	—	—	—	—	123.0(8)	—	—	—	—	—	—	—	—
C(12)–C(11)–C(18)	—	—	—	—	—	116.9(8)	—	—	—	—	—	—	—
C(9)–C(11)–C(18)	—	—	—	—	—	124.5(7)	—	—	—	—	—	—	—
C(11)–C(12)–C(18)	—	—	—	—	—	—	119.3(10)	—	—	—	—	—	—
C(13)–C(12)–C(18)	—	—	—	—	—	—	122.6(9)	—	—	—	—	—	—
C(2)–C(1)–C(18)	—	—	—	—	—	—	—	—	—	—	—	—	—
C(10)–C(1)–C(18)	—	—	—	—	—	—	—	—	—	—	—	—	—
C(9)–C(11)–C(18)	—	—	—	—	—	—	—	—	—	—	—	—	—
C(12)–C(11)–C(14)	—	—	—	—	—	—	—	—	—	—	—	—	—
C(1)–C(18)–C(11)	—	—	—	—	—	—	—	—	—	—	—	—	—
C(11)–C(12)–C(19)	—	—	—	—	—	—	—	—	121.3(1)	—	—	—	—
C(13)–C(12)–C(19)	—	—	—	—	—	—	—	—	119.9(1)	—	—	—	—
C(6)–C(7)–C(19)	—	—	—	—	—	—	—	118.1(4)	—	—	—	—	—
C(8)–C(7)–C(19)	—	—	—	—	—	—	—	122.3(4)	—	—	—	—	—
C(11)–C(18)–C(19)	—	—	—	—	—	—	—	—	—	117.1(3)	—	—	—

(**4**) (dotted line) is characteristic of all its methyl homologues, and different from that of the 1,11-methano-17-ketone (**310**) (solid line). In the compounds lacking substituents in the bay region the long C(9)–C(11) bond and large bay-region bond angles help to minimize the repulsive interaction between H(1) and H(11). However, this is still marked as can be seen from their proton magnetic resonance spectra in which these hydrogens are deshielded by about 1 ppm compared with the other aromatic protons in these molecules. As was previously found by Ent-

Fig. 80. Superimposed plan views of 15,16-dihydrocyclopenta[a]phenanthren-17-one (**4**) (dotted lines) and its 1,11-methano derivative (**310**) (solid lines) and their ultraviolet absorption spectra.

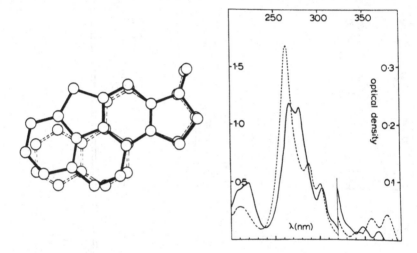

Table 44. *Dihedral angles between planes of rings*

Compound	Dihedral angle (°) between rings		
	A/B	B/C	A/C
unsubstituted (**4**)	1.5	1.1	2.6
1-methyl (**302**)	2.4	2.5	4.9
2-methyl (**303**)	2.2	3.3	4.2
6-methyl (**306**)	0.9	0.7	1.5
7-methyl (**230**)	2.5	1.4	3.9
11-methyl (**26**)	7.0	5.5	12.5
12-methyl (**130**)	1.0	1.3	2.6
7,11-dimethyl (**309**)	9.7	11.1	20.6
11,12-dimethyl (**131**)	7.9	5.7	13.6
11-ethyl (**211**)	4.0	3.8	7.3
11-methoxy (**132**)	1.3	1.9	1.9
1,11-methano (**310**)	1.3	2.7	3.9

whistle and Iball (1961) for the parent hydrocarbon 16,17-dihydro-15*H*-cyclopenta[a]phenanthrene (**1**), these 17-ketones are essentially planar. The exceptions are the compounds with methyl or ethyl groups in the bay-region, particularly at C-11. This is best demonstrated by consideration of the dihedral angles observed between the planes of the aryl rings listed in Table 44 [the dihydro derivative (**252**) is obviously not comparable and is omitted from this Table]. The angle between rings -A and -C is roughly the sum of those between rings -A and -B and rings -B and -C. Thus severe steric interactions in the bay region in those compounds bearing a methyl or ethyl group at C(11) are avoided by considerable out-of-plane deformation, as illustrated by side views of these molecules (Fig. 81). In the 11-methyl-11,12-dihydro-17-ketone (**252**) the methyl group is axial, with the bond joining it to C(11) at right angles to the plane of the rings (Fig. 82). This compound is not dehydrogenated by quinones which require the substrate to possess a *trans*-diaxial arrangement of the protons to be abstracted, and this axial methyl conformation had previously been correctly assigned to it (Coombs *et al.*, 1970) on these grounds. The approximate planarity of the 1,11-methano-17-ketone (**310**) was suggested by its nmr spectrum in which the bridge methylene protons are equivalent, resonating as a singlet (Ribeiro *et al.*, 1983).

The effects these factors have on the geometry of the bay region are summarized in Table 45, in which the distances are in Å and the interbond and torsion angles are given in degrees. The torsion angle C(1)–C(10)–C(9)–C(11) is defined as the angle between the bonds C(1)–C(10) and C(9)–C(11), looking along the central bond C(10)–C(9). A carbon substituent at C(11) causes the molecule to twist about the central ring so that this substituent and the proton at C(1) are not in the same plane, thus minimizing their interaction. When the substituent is a methyl group this leads to a bay-region torsion angle of 13.5–20.5° and all these 17-ketones are strong carcinogens. In the benz[a]anthracene and chrysene series 7,12-dimethylbenz[a]anthracene and 5,6-dimethylchrysene, both potent carcinogens, have torsion angles of this order. The weakly carcinogenic 11-ethyl-17-ketone (**211**) has a smaller torsion angle (8.9°) whilst the inactive compounds range between 6.8° (2-methyl) to 0.1° (12-methyl). Interestingly, a methyl group at the other bay-region position, at C(1), does not have this effect; the torsion angle is only 5.2°. However, the C(10)–C(1)–C(2) angle in this compound is narrowed by comparison with that in the other compounds, and the associated bonds C(1)–C(2) and C(1)–C(10) are longer than average. In plan view these molecules closely resemble steroids; for example, as is shown in Fig. 83 in which the 11-methyl-17-ketone (**26**) is superimposed on oestrone. However, this

Fig. 81 (i) and (ii). Views of structures of twelve 15,16-dihydrocyclopenta[a]phenanthren-17-ones calculated from X-ray crystallography data; all are shown as plan and side views, and tilted at 30°.

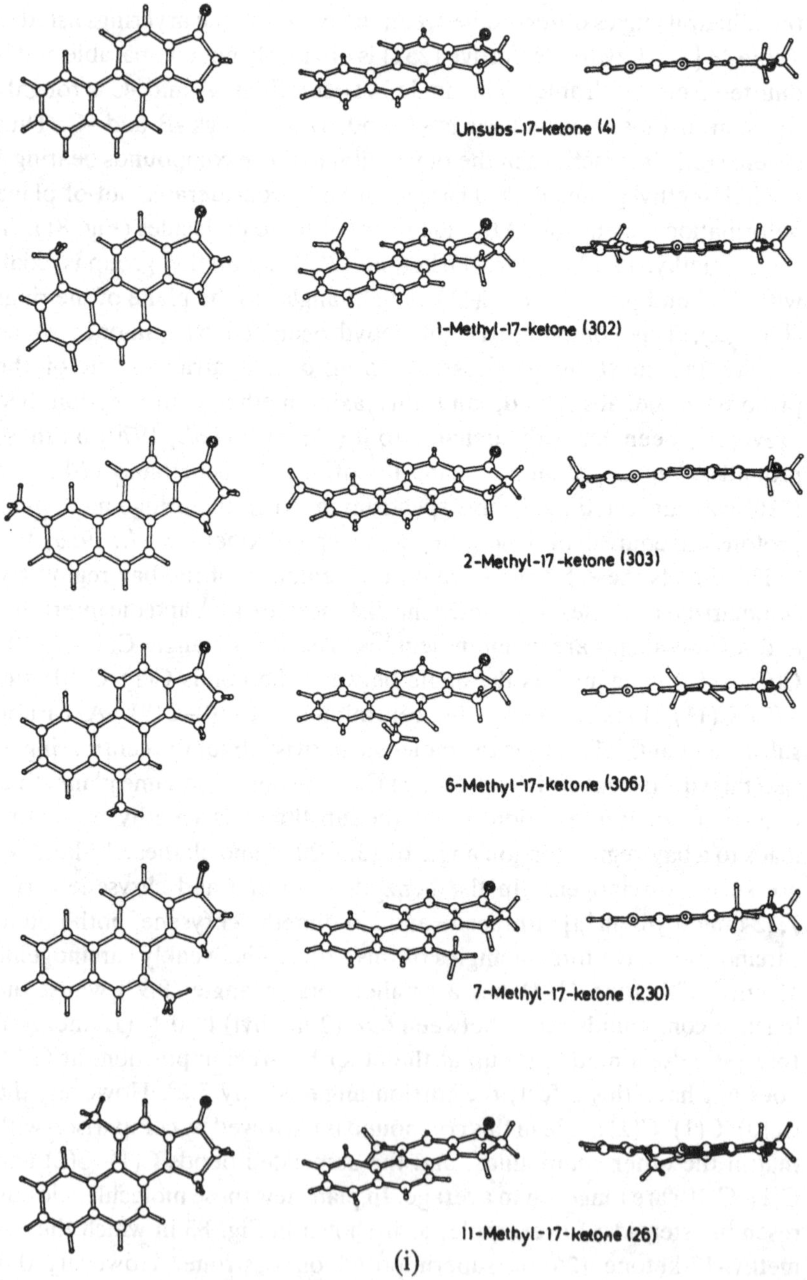

Unsubs-17-ketone (4)

1-Methyl-17-ketone (302)

2-Methyl-17-ketone (303)

6-Methyl-17-ketone (306)

7-Methyl-17-ketone (230)

11-Methyl-17-ketone (26)

(i)

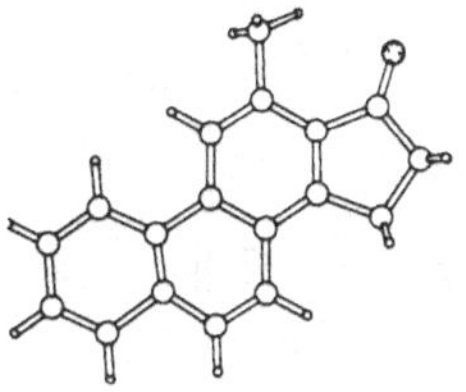

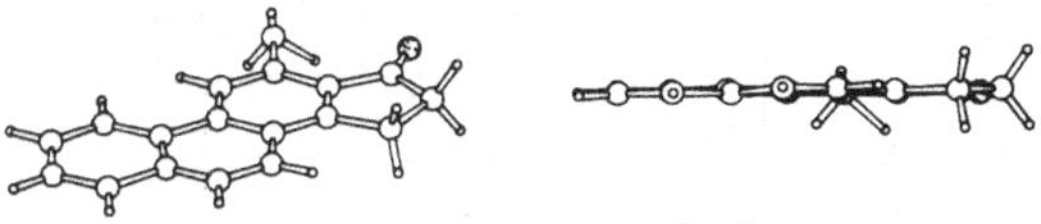

12-Methyl-17-ketone (130)

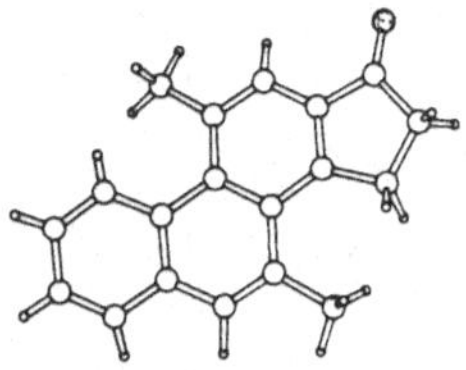

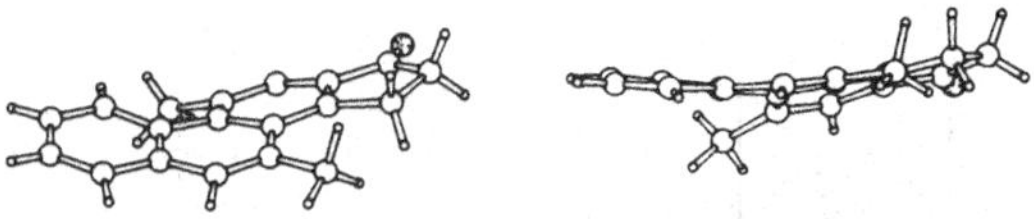

11,11-Dimethyl-17-ketone (309)

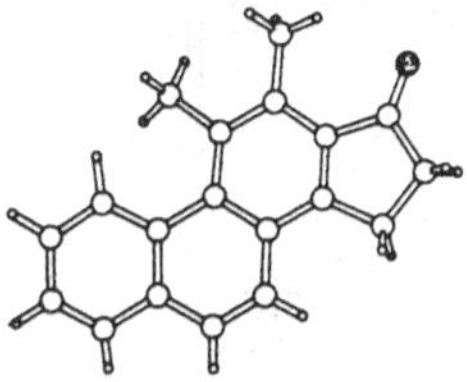

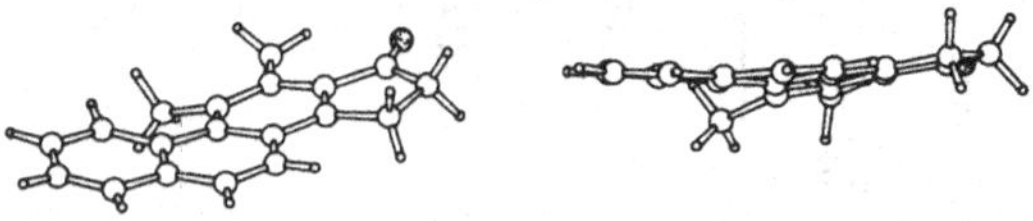

11,12-Dimethyl-17-ketone (131)

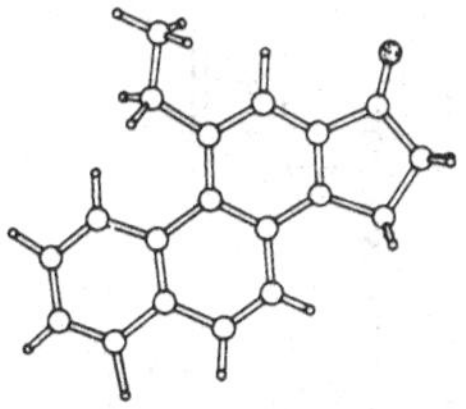

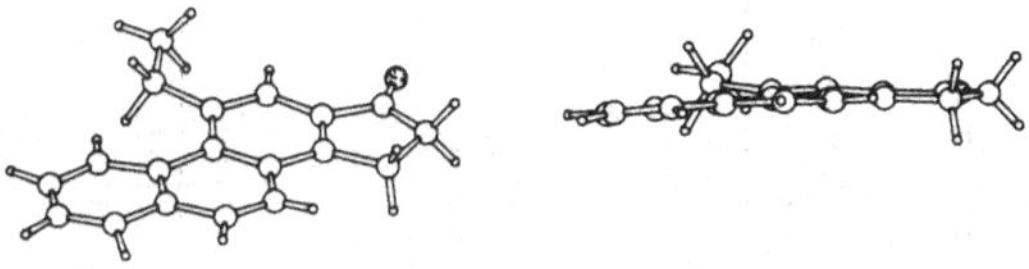

11-Ethyl-17-ketone (211)

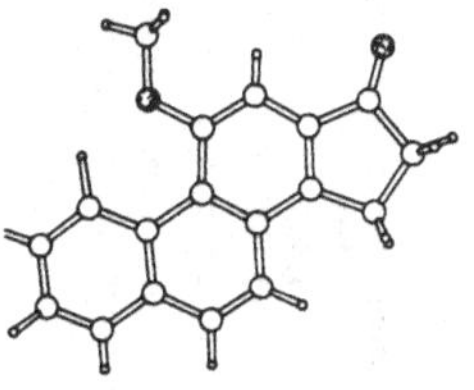

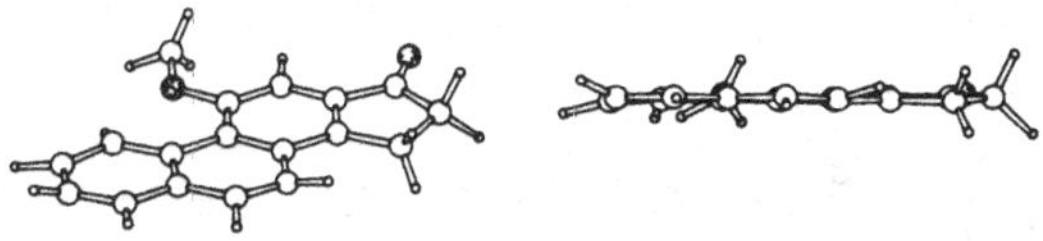

11-Methoxy-17-ketone (132)

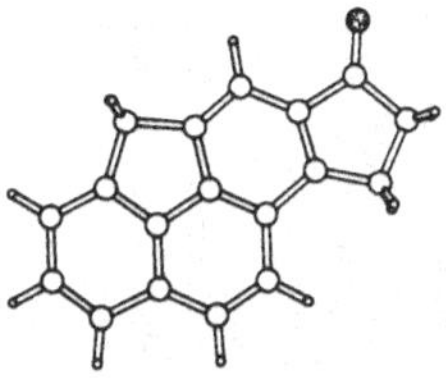

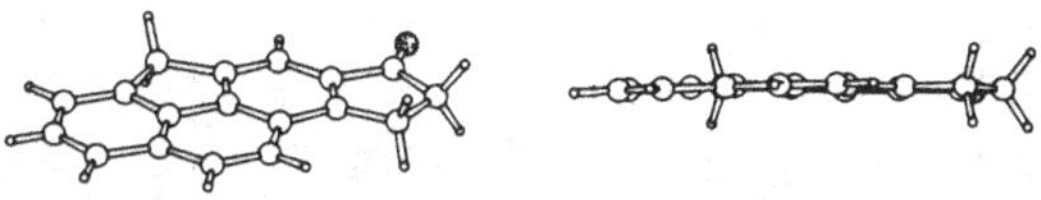

1,11-Methano-17-ketone (310)

(ii)

Table 45. *Bay-region geometry*

	Bond (Å) C(1)–C(10)	Bond (Å) C(9)–C(10)	Bond (Å) C(9)–C(11)	Angle (°) C(1)–C(10)–C(9)	Angle (°) C(10)–C(9)–C(11)	Torsion angle (°) C(1)–C(10)–C(9)–C(11)	Non-bonded distances (Å) C(1)...C(11)	C(1)...C(18)
H at C(1) and C(11)								
Unsubstituted (**4**)	1.392	1.445	1.395	123.4	123.8	2.6	2.988	—
2-Methyl (**303**)	1.395	1.454	1.434	124.2	122.5	6.8	3.012	—
6-Methyl (**306**)	1.407	1.459	1.414	121.6	122.3	2.7	2.953	—
7-Methyl (**230**)	1.419	1.455	1.434	123.5	119.0	2.0	2.935	—
12-Methyl (**130**)	1.409	1.455	1.417	122.9	122.4	0.1	2.970	—
(average)	(1.404)	(1.452)	(1.419)	(123.1)	(122.0)	(2.8)	(2.971)	—
CH$_3$ at C(1), H at C(11)								
1-Methyl (**302**)	1.428	1.469	1.423	126.0	123.5	5.2	3.095	—
H at C(1), CH$_3$ at C(11)								
11-Methyl (**26**)	1.409	1.462	1.442	124.6	125.0	13.5	3.102	2.997
7,11-Dimethyl (**309**)	1.410	1.449	1.446	124.6	121.8	20.5	3.042	2.953
11,12-Dimethyl (**131**)	1.411	1.470	1.437	124.7	124.3	13.8	3.096	2.959
(average)	(1.410)	(1.457)	(1.441)	(124.6)	(123.7)	(15.6)	(3.08)	(2.969)
H at C(1), CH$_2$CH$_3$ at C(11)								
11-Ethyl (**211**)	1.423	1.475	1.441	124.9	124.8	8.9	3.118	2.960
H at C(1), OCH$_3$ at C(11)								
11-Methoxy (**132**)	1.407	1.470	1.435	124.4	124.8	0.7	3.084	—
Carcinogenic hydrocarbons (using numbering analogous to that used above)								
DMBA[a]	1.410	1.470	1.402	123.0	123.5	22.1	3.044	2.971
5,6-DMC[b]	1.405	1.483	1.408	123.5	121.8	21.2	3.047	2.957
(average)	(1.408)	(1.477)	(1.405)	(123.3)	(122.7)	(21.7)	(3.045)	(2.964)

a, DMBA, 7,12-Dimethylbenz[a]anthracene (Glusker, 1981).
b, 5-6-DMC, 5,6-Dimethylchrysene (Zacharias *et al.*, 1984).

Fig. 82. Three views (as in Fig. 81) of 11-methyl-11,12,15,16-
tetrahydrocyclopenta[a]phenanthren-17-one (**252**).

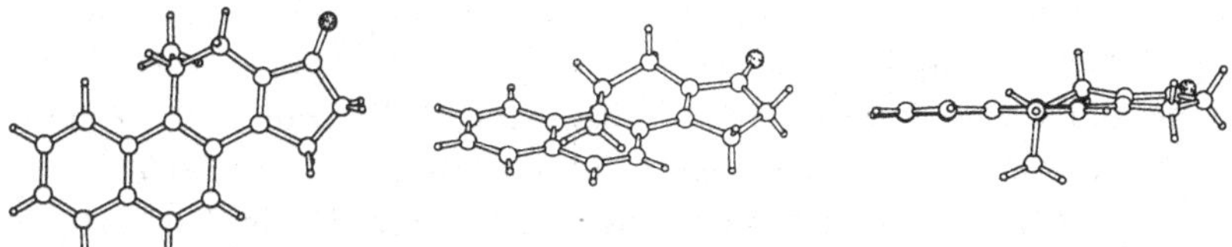

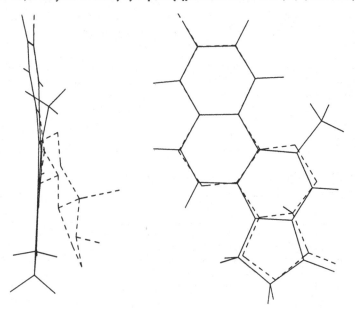

11,12-Dihydro-11-methyl-17-ketone (252)

Fig. 83. Plan and side views of oestrone (dotted lines) superimposed on
15,16-dihydro-11-methylcyclopenta[a]phenanthren-17-one (**26**) (solid lines).

similarity in two dimensions is lost in the third dimension because rings -C
and -D in the steroid are not *quasi* planar.

8.3   An apparent correlation between carcinogenicity and molecular strain

Thus there seems to be a rough correlation between out-of-plane
deformation and carcinogenicity, but in this respect the 7-methyl-17-
ketone (**230**) is anomalous since it is essentially flat. Molecular strain is,
however, introduced also into this structure by the 7-methyl group which
is locked in the plane of the ring system. Non-bonding distances between
the two C(15) hydrogen atoms and one of the 7-methyl hydrogens are
exceptionally short (1.82 and 1.84 Å), even shorter than those found for

the two hydrogen atoms in the bay region (1.94 Å). Moreover, movement of the methyl group out of the plane of the rings would further decrease one of these. This leads to several consequences; for example, the bay-region angle C(10)–C(9)–C(11) is 119.0°, 3° less than the average for the compounds lacking a bay-region substituent, and results in the H(1) to H(11) non-bonding distance being the shortest observed (Table 46). In the five-membered ring the protons at C(15) are deshielded by 0.42–0.46 ppm, and the rate of proton exchange at C(16) is approximately

Table 46. *Non-bonding H(1) ... H(11) distances, rate constants for detritiation at C(16), and nmr chemical shifts at C(15) for six 17-ketones*

Compound	H(1)...H(11) distance (Å)	Rate constant ($10^2 K_{OH}^T$– nmol^{-1} s^{-1})	Chemical shift (δ)
unsubstituted (4)	1.999	1.83 ± 0.14	3.28
2-methyl (303)	2.019	(not measured)	3.25
6-methyl (306)	1.973	1.15 ± 0.14	3.27
7-methyl (230)	1.942	3.17 ± 0.08	3.70
11-methyl (26)	—	1.47 ± 0.06	3.24
12-methyl (130)	2.004	0.67 ± 0.07	3.28

Table 47. *Molecular strain and carcinogenicity*

Compound	General state of molecule	Iball index[a]
unsubstituted (4)	planar, unstrained	<1
1-methyl (302)	essentially planar, some bond and angle distortion in ring-A	1
2-methyl (303)	essentially planar, unstrained	<1
6-methyl (306)	planar, unstrained	<1
7-methyl (230)	essentially planar, evidence of strain in bay region and ring-D	10
11-methyl (26)	out-of-plane deformation, bay-region torsion angle 13.5°	46
12-methyl (130)	planar, unstrained	<1
7,11-dimethyl (309)	out-of-plane deformation, bay-region torsion angle 20.5°	>49[b]
11,12-dimethyl (131)	out-of-plane deformation, bay-region torsion angle 13.8°	30
11-ethyl (211)	some out-of-plane deformation, bay-region torsion angle 8.9°	8
11-methoxy (132)	planar, unstrained	25
1,11-methano (310)	planar, but severe bond angle distortions	16

a, Figure for repeated application of the compound twice weekly for one year.
b, Twice-weekly applications for 10 weeks only.

doubled compared with the other five compounds. This strain built into the 7-methyl-17-ketone (**230**) was reflected originally in the difficulty experienced in the synthesis of this structure.

The general condition of 12 compounds examined by X-ray crystallography and shown in Fig. 79 (neglecting the 11,12-dihydro compound (**252**) which is not comparable) are summarized in Table 47 alongside their potencies as skin carcinogens in T.O. mice, as indicated by their Iball indices taken from Tables 11 and 12. It is evident that there is (with one exception) a direct correlation between molecular strain and carcinogenicity among these 17-oxocyclopenta[a]phenanthrenes. Newman (1983), of course, has also noted a similar relationship in the benz[a]anthracene series, but the way in which these two properties are connected is quite obscure at the present time. There is one exception to this general rule among the compounds studied by X-ray crystallography; the 11-methoxy-17-ketone (**132**) is a fairly strong carcinogen although it is planar and its bond angles are quite normal. Unlike the carbon substituents at C(11), the ether oxygen at C(11) is in the molecular plane and only 1.98 Å from the hydrogen at C(1), suggesting that this contact is attractive. This is reflected in its nmr spectrum in which H(1) is further deshielded, resonating at δ 9.8 compared with δ 8.8 for the 11-methyl-17-ketone (**26**) (Abraham and Loftus, 1978). There is a marked difference between the 11-alkoxy and 11-alkyl series in regard to their ability to induce skin tumours, summarized in Table 48. This comparison is

Table 48. *Comparison of Iball indices of 11-alkyl- and 11-alkoxy-15,16-dihydrocyclopenta[a]phenanthren-17-ones*

Compound	Iball index	
	Repeated application	Initiation/ promotion
11-Alkyl series		
11-methyl (**26**)	46	57
11-ethyl (**211**)	8	—
11-*n*-butyl (**212**)	>1	—
7,11-dimethyl (**309**)	49[a]	66
11-Alkoxy series		
11-methoxy (**132**)	25	38
11-ethoxy (**390**)	—	28
11-*n*-butoxy (**393**)	—	5
7-methyl-11-methoxy (**447**)	17	—

a, Incomplete treatment, see Table 47.

somewhat confused because two methods of skin painting have been employed, giving rise to two series of Iball indices (see Chapter 6 for a discussion of this), and not all the compounds have been tested by both methods. However, it is obvious that in the alkyl series carcinogenic activity falls off rapidly with increase in alkyl chain length so that the ethyl derivative is only weakly active and the butyl homologue is inactive. In the 11-alkoxy series, on the other hand, the ethoxy compound is not much less active than its methoxy homologue, and even the *n*-butoxy compound is a weak carcinogen. Moreover, whereas introduction of a 7-methyl group into the 11-methyl compound to give the 7,11-dimethyl-17-ketone (**309**) increases its potency so that this ketone is the most active so far encountered in this series, the 7-methyl-11-methoxy-17-ketone (**447**) is appreciably less carcinogenic than the 11-methoxy analogue (**132**). It therefore seems probable that the way in which 11-alkyl and 11-alkoxy groups endow the parent molecule with carcinogenic potential may be fundamentally different.

8.4   Investigation of the diol-epoxides of 15,16-dihydrocyclopenta[a]-phenanthren-17-ones by computer modelling

The enhancing effect of methyl substitution at the non-benzo bay-region position (the 'bay-region methyl effect') is, of course, well known among several polycyclic aromatic hydrocarbon systems, and has been noted by many authors (DiGiovanni *et al.*, 1983; Hecht *et al.*, 1979; Iyer *et al.*, 1980). However, no really satisfactory explanation for this effect has been advanced. With this large amount of exact X-ray data to hand it seemed worth while investigating the effects of the methyl group on the structures of the diol-epoxides of the strongly carcinogenic 11-methyl-17-ketone (**26**) by computer construction (Kashino *et al.*, 1986). These metabolites have not been synthesized, but they are known to be concerned in the expression of biological activity; it is probable that they are very reactive and this would further complicate their study by X-ray crystallography, although the diol-epoxides of benzo[a]pyrene have been studied in this way (Neidle *et al.*, 1980; Neidle and Cutbush, 1983).

An interesting result which follows from the dihedral angle of 12.5° between rings -A and -C in the 11-methyl-17-ketone (**26**) is that this molecule can exist in right- and left-handed mirror-image forms, and as normally prepared consists of the racemate. This can be seen in the crystal structure disclosed by X-ray analysis and is illustrated in Fig. 84, in which both forms are clearly visible. The energy required to flip one form to the other is not known and cannot be reliably calculated, so that it is unclear whether the two forms exist as stable conformers in solution. A study of the temperature factors from the X-ray structure (Table 49) indicates that the atoms having the lowest temperature factors, and hence least motion in the crystalline state, are those in the bay region. That is, there is no disorder of the 11-methyl group in the crystal, and no evidence for interconversion of the two forms in the crystalline state.

In constructing the diol-epoxides this has therefore been borne in mind, and the four structures, two *syn* and two *anti*, shown in Fig. 85 have been considered although as described in Chapter 7 the biologically derived diol-epoxide appears to be exclusively *anti*, with the diol system [3R,4R] (i.e., 3α, 4β). These four structures were obtained by superimposing the X-ray co-ordinates of the *syn*- and *anti*-diol-epoxides of benzo[a]pyrene on those of the two conformers of 15,16-dihydro-11-methylcyclopenta[a]phenanthren-17-one (26). Four further [3S,4S] optical isomers are possible, and are precise mirror images of those shown. The diol-epoxides of 15,16-dihydro-11-methoxycyclopenta[a]-phenanthren-17-one (132) were similarly constructed although here, of

Fig. 84. Mirror-image forms of the 11-methyl-17-ketone (26) disclosed by X-ray crystallography; the two forms have been superimposed with the bond joining C(13) to C(14) in common.

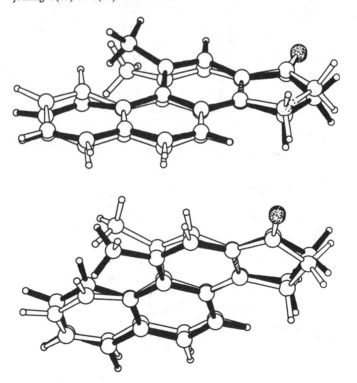

course, only one conformer exists because the oxygen at C(11) is in the plane of the flat aromatic rings. Selected interatomic distances measured from these computer-simulated diol-epoxides are shown in Table 50. Some of these distances are unacceptably short, as indicated, and this leads to the conclusion that the most likely structure for the diol-epoxide of the 11-methyl-17-ketone (26) is an *anti* structure with the epoxide oxygen and 11-methyl group on the same side of the molecular plane [(a) in Fig. 85]. Neither *syn* conformers would appear to be likely. This therefore confirms the same conclusion previously drawn from entirely different reasoning. In the absence of the 11-methyl group either diol-epoxide may be formed without generating unacceptably short non-bonding distances; in practice only the *syn*-diol-epoxide is observed for

Table 49. *Temperature factors (B) for the oxygen and carbon atoms in 15,16-dihydro-11-methylcyclopenta[a]phenanthren-17-one*

Atom	B	Atom	B
0	7.3	C(9)	4.0
C(1)	6.3	C(10)	4.6
C(2)	7.7	C(11)	4.1
C(3)	7.7	C(12)	4.4
C(4)	6.7	C(13)	4.3
C(5)	5.2	C(14)	4.2
C(6)	5.8	C(15)	5.4
C(7)	5.0	C(16)	6.3
C(8)	4.1	C(17)	5.3

Fig. 85. The two *anti-* and two *syn*-diol epoxides of the 11-methyl-17-ketone (26) studied by computer construction.

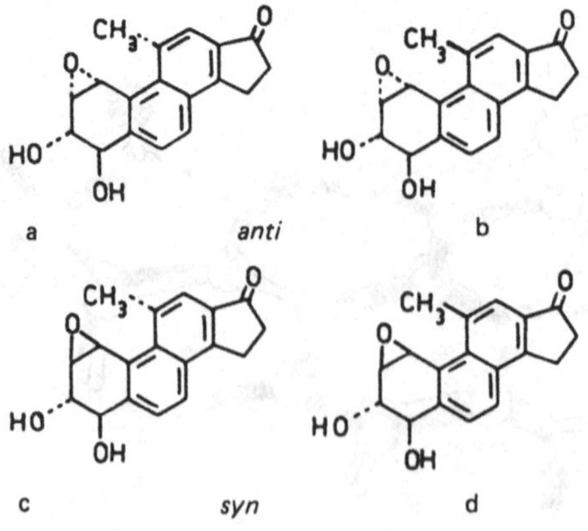

Table 50. *Interatomic distances (Å) in models of diol-epoxides*

Diol-epoxides of 15,16-dihydro-11-methylcyclopenta[a]phenanthren-17-one (**26**)		
O(epoxide)---H(11-methyl)	*anti*	(a) 3.06
		(b) 3.74
	syn	(c) 2.89
		(d) 2.38 (rather short)
H(1)(epoxide)----H(11-methyl)	*anti*	(a) 1.85
		(b) 1.56 (too short)
	syn	(c) 1.31 (too short)
		(d) 1.83
Diol-epoxides of 15,16-dihydro-11-methoxycyclopenta[a]phenanthren-17-one (**132**)		
O(epoxide)----O(methyl)	*anti*	3.81
	syn	3.07
H(1)(epoxide)----O(methyl)	*anti*	1.76
	syn	1.77

the parent unsubstituted 17-ketone (**4**) (Hadfield *et al.*, 1984). In the case of the 11-methoxy-17-ketone (**132**) the computer model indicates that there is little differentiation between *syn*- and *anti*-diol-epoxides except for a rather short O---O distance in the *syn*-isomer.

8.5 Molecular orbital calculations

Ground-state molecular orbital wave functions have been calculated by the CNDO/2 all valence approximation (Pople *et al.*, 1965; Pople and Segal, 1966) for the seven structures examined in London (Clayton, 1982). Bond indices, defined as the number of electrons statistically localized between a pair of atomic centres (Wiberg, 1968), are shown in Table 51. The values for aromatic C–C bonds vary considerably from that for benzene, 1.425e (Ibata *et al.*, 1975), from the highest values (1.660—1.720e) for C(6)–C(7) to the lowest (1.14–1.20e) for the adjacent C(5)–C(6) bond. The sum of the bond indices for each aromatic ring (Table 52) is less than that for benzene owing to migration of electronic charge to the carbon–oxygen dipole at C(17). As a consequence of this aromatic bromination, for example, occurs at C(15) and not at aromatic carbon in these ketones (see Chapter 4). There are three other notable features apparent in this Table. Firstly, the sum of bond indices for rings -A and -C are in all cases greater than for ring-B. Thus this ring acts as an electron donor towards the two outer aromatic rings; a similar pattern is also observed in phenanthrene (Dixon *et al.*, 1978). Secondly, the sum of the bond indices for ring-A is always greater than that for ring-C, emphasizing the electron-acceptor characteristics of the

Table 51. *Bond indices for seven 17-oxocyclopenta[a]phenanthrenes*

Bond	Unsubstit. (4)	2-Methyl (303)	6-Methyl (306)	7-Methyl (230)	11-Methyl (26)	12-Methyl (130)	1,11-Methano (310)
C(10)—C(1)	1.315	1.315	1.320	1.250	1.295	1.325	1.275
C(1)—C(2)	1.540	1.505	1.535	1.550	1.565	1.535	1.485
C(2)—C(3)	1.350	1.305	1.355	1.340	1.310	1.350	1.345
C(3)—C(4)	1.555	1.580	1.535	1.555	1.590	1.535	1.550
C(4)—C(5)	1.290	1.280	1.315	1.295	1.280	1.320	1.270
C(5)—C(6)	1.165	1.165	1.140	1.200	1.200	1.175	1.190
C(6)—C(7)	1.720	1.725	1.680	1.660	1.700	1.695	1.700
C(7)—C(8)	1.175	1.165	1.175	1.140	1.165	1.145	1.175
C(8)—C(9)	1.340	1.345	1.345	1.345	1.330	1.350	1.350
C(9)—C(10)	1.125	1.135	1.125	1.145	1.165	1.140	1.150
C(10)—C(5)	1.340	1.330	1.335	1.315	1.320	1.310	1.335
C(9)—C(11)	1.310	1.305	1.305	1.265	1.255	1.320	1.250
C(11)—C(12)	1.555	1.560	1.560	1.560	1.530	1.520	1.560
C(12)—C(13)	1.305	1.310	1.305	1.290	1.320	1.280	1.280
C(13)—C(14)	1.460	1.460	1.455	1.465	1.450	1.480	1.480
C(14)—C(8)	1.280	1.300	1.280	1.280	1.300	1.320	1.270
C(14)—C(15)	1.015	1.005	1.020	1.010	1.005	1.010	1.005
C(15)—C(16)	1.015	1.010	1.000	1.015	1.025	1.020	1.020
C(16)—C(17)	1.015	1.005	1.020	1.010	0.995	1.005	1.010
C(17)—C(13)	1.015	1.020	1.030	1.030	1.025	1.045	1.030
C(aryl)—C(18)	—	1.035	1.030	1.030	—	1.040	—
C(1)—C(18)	—	—	—	—	—	—	1.015
C(11)—C(18)	—	—	—	—	1.030	—	1.010

adjacent five-membered ring. Finally, the sum of the bond indices for any ring with a methyl or methano substituent is less than that for the corresponding unsubstituted ring. Thus the methyl groups show electron-acceptor character, and this is reflected in the aryl $C–CH_3$ bond indices which average 1.033 for these ketones. This somewhat surprising feature has been observed previously for benzene–toluene by Libit and Hoffmann (1974) who concluded that the 'classic' electron-donor character of the methyl group is realized through a polarization mechanism resulting in a decrease and increase in electron density at the *ipso* and *ortho* carbon atoms, respectively. The expected changes in charge distribution are evident in the molecular fragments surrounding the methyl group in these substituted ketones. For example, the bond indices for C(1)–C(2) and C(2)–C(3) in the 2-methyl-17-ketone (**303**) are less than those in the unsubstituted compound (**4**), whilst the reverse is true for C(3)–C(4).

Orbital energies of the three highest occupied molecular orbitals (HOMO) and three lowest unoccupied molecular orbitals (LUMO) of these seven ketones are listed in Table 53. Two important features are apparent. Firstly, LUMO and LUMO + 1 orbitals are energetically similar and well separated from the remaining unoccupied orbitals, with energy differences between LUMO + 1 and LUMO + 2 of 67.0–80.0 au × 10^{-3}. Energy differences between the highest occupied orbitals are smaller, the differences between HOMO and HOMO-1 varying between 22.5 and 31.0 au × 10^{-3}. Secondly, the introduction of a methyl or methano group slightly increases the energy of HOMO and decreases that of LUMO. This is consistent with the dual character of the methyl group, as an electron acceptor and as electron donor *via* an hyperconjugative mechanism. Pure electron donors increase the energy of both HOMO and LUMO, whereas pure conjugative groups increase the

Table 52. *Sum of bond indices for each aromatic ring in seven*
17-oxocyclopenta[a]phenanthrenes

Compound	Ring-A	Ring-B	Ring-C
unsubstituted (**4**)	8.390	7.865	8.250
2-methyl (**303**)	8.315	7.865	8.275
6-methyl (**306**)	8.395	7.805	8.255
7-methyl (**230**)	8.365	7.825	8.225
11-methyl (**26**)	8.365	7.880	8.185
12-methyl (**130**)	8.380	7.815	8.190
11,12-methano (**31**)	8.260	7.900	8.175

[benzene, 8.550e (Ibata *et al.*, 1975)].

Table 53. *Orbital energies (au × 10⁻³) of the three highest occupied (HOMO) and three lowest unoccupied (LUMO) orbitals for seven 17-oxo-cyclopenta[a]phenanthrenes*

Orbital	Unsubst. (4)	2-Methyl (303)	6-Methyl (306)	7-Methyl (230)	11-Methyl (26)	12-Methyl (130)	1,11-Methano (310)
LUMO + 2	161.5	150.5	154.5	154.5	159.0	153.0	142.5
LUMO + 1	81.5	78.0	74.5	76.0	79.0	73.0	75.5
LUMO	80.5	70.5	71.0	64.5	65.5	55.5	69.5
(LUMO–HOMO	489.5	472.0	474.0	460.5	462.0	451.0	468.5
HOMO	−409.5	−401.5	−403.0	−395.0	−396.5	−395.5	−399.0
HOMO-1	−432.0	−426.5	−426.5	−426.0	−425.5	−422.5	−417.0
HOMO-2	−439.5	−440.5	−439.5	−438.5	−436.0	−439.0	−442.5

au = atomic units.

energy of HOMO while they decrease the energy of LUMO (Fleming, 1976).

8.6 References

Abraham, J. R. & Loftus, P. (1978). *Proton and Carbon-13 nmr Spectroscopy; an Integrated Approach*, pp. 23–4. Heyden: London.

Adam, N. K. (1930). *The Physics and Chemistry of Surfaces*. Oxford University Press: London.

Basak, B. S. & Basak, M. G. (1959). Crystal structure of 1,2-cyclopenteno-phenanthrene. *Indian J. Phys.*, **33**, 107–10.

Bergmann, E. & Hillemann, H. (1933). γ-Methyl-1,2-cyclopentenophenan-threne. *Ber.*, **66**, 1302–6.

Bernal, J. D. & Crowfoot, D. (1933). Crystalline phases of some substances studied as liquid crystals. *Trans. Faraday Soc.*, **29**, 1032–49.

Bernal, J. D. & Crowfoot, D. (1935). The structure of some hydrocarbons related to the sterols. *J. Chem. Soc.*, 93–100.

Clayton, A. F. D. (1982). *Structural Studies in a Series of Potentially Carcinogenic Cyclopenta[a]phenanthrenes*. Ph.D. Thesis, Council of National Academic Awards, London.

Clayton, A. F. D., Coombs, M. M., Henrick, K., McPartlin, M. & Trotter, J. (1983). X-ray structural studies and molecular orbital calculations (CNDO/2) in a series of cyclopenta[a]phenanthrenes: attempts at correlation with carcinogenicity. *Carcinogenesis*, **4**, 1569–76.

Coombs, M. M., Jaitly, S. B. & Crawley, F. E. H. (1970). Potentially carcinogenic cyclopenta[a]phenanthrenes. Part IV. Synthesis of 17-ketones by the Stobbe condensation. *J. Chem. Soc. (C)*, 1266–71.

Diels, O., Gadka, W. & Kording, P. (1927). Uber die Dehydrierung des Chlosterins. *Annalen*, **459**, 1–26.

DiGiovanni, J., Diamond, L., Harvey, R. G. & Slaga, T. J. (1983). Enhancement of skin-tumor initiating activity of polycyclic aromatic hydrocarbons by methyl substitution at non-benzo 'bay-region' positions. *Carcinogenesis*, **4**, 403–7.

Dixon, D. A., Klier, D. A. & Lipscomb, W. N. (1978). Localized molecular orbitals for polyatomic molecules. 6. Condensed aromatic ring systems. *J. Am. Chem. Soc.*, **100**, 5681–94.

Entwhistle, R. F., Ferrier, W. G. & Iball, J. (1954). Some similarities in the diffraction patterns of organic compounds. *Acta Crystallogr.*, **7**, 649.

Entwhistle, R. F. & Iball, J. (1961). The crystal and molecular structure of 1,2-cyclopenta[a]phenanthrene. *Z. Kristallogr.*, **116**, 251–62.

Fleming, I. (1976). *Frontier Orbitals and Organic Chemical Reactions*. Wiley: Chichester.

Glusker, J. P. (1981). X-ray crystallographic studies on carcinogenic polycyclic aromatic hydrocarbons and their derivatives. In *Polycyclic Hydrocarbons and Cancer*, ed. P. O. P. Ts'o & H. V. Gelboin, vol. 3, pp. 61–116. Academic Press: New York.

Glusker, J. P. & Trueblood, K. N. (1985). *Crystal Structure Analysis: a Primer*, 2nd edn. Oxford University Press: Oxford.

Hadfield, S. T., Abbott, P. J., Coombs, M. M. & Drake, A. F. (1984). The effect of methyl substituents on the *in vitro* metabolism of cyclopenta[a]phenanthren-17-ones: implications for biological activity. *Carcinogenesis*, **5**, 1395–9.

Harper, S. H., Kon, G. A. R. & Ruzicka, F. C. J. (1934). Syntheses of polycyclic compounds related to the steroids. Part II. Diels' hydrocarbon $C_{18}H_{16}$. *J. Chem. Soc.*, 124–8.

Hecht, S. S., Amin, S., Rivenson, A. & Hoffmann, D. (1979). Tumor initiating activity of 5,11-dimethylchrysene and the structural requirements favoring carcinogenicity of methylated polycyclic aromatic hydrocarbons. *Cancer Lett.*, **8**, 65–70.

Iball, J. (1935). The crystal structure of condensed ring compounds I: 1,2-cyclopentenophenanthrene. *Z. Kristallogr.*, **92**, 293–300.

Ibata, K., Shimanouchi, H., Sarada, Y. & Hata, T. (1975). Structural chemistry of the benzotropone system. II. The crystal and molecular structure of 4,5-benzotropone. *Acta Crystallogr.*, **B31**, 2313–21.

Iyer, R. P., Lyga, J. W., Secrist, J. A., Daub, G. H. & Slaga, T. J. (1980). Comparative tumor-initiating activity of methylated benzo[a]pyrene derivatives on mouse skin. *Cancer Res.*, **40**, 1073–6.

Kashino, S., Zacharias, D. E., Peck, R. M., Glusker, J. P., Bhatt, T. S. & Coombs, M. M. (1986). Bay region distortions in cyclopenta[a]-phenanthrenes. *Cancer Res.*, **46**, 1817–29.

Kay, M. I., Okaya, Y. & Cox, D. E. (1971). A refinement of the structure of the room temperature phase of phenanthrene, $C_{14}H_{14}$, from X-ray and neutron diffraction data. *Acta Crystallogr.*, **B27**, 26–33.

Libit, L. & Hoffmann, R. (1974). Towards a detailed orbital theory of substituent effects: charge transfer, polarization, and the methyl group. *J. Am. Chem. Soc.*, **96**, 1370–83.

Neidle, S. & Cutbush, S. D. (1983). X-ray crystallographic analysis of (±)-7β,8α-dihydroxy-9β,10β-epoxy-7,8,9,10-tetrahydrobenzo[a]pyrene: molecular structure of a 'syn'-diol-epoxide. *Carcinogenesis*, **4**, 415–18.

Neidle, S., Subbiah, A., Cooper, C. S. & Ribeiro, O. (1980). Molecular structure of (±)-7α,8β-dihydroxy-9β,10β-epoxy-7,8,9,10-tetrahydrobenzo[a]pyrene: an X-ray crystallographic study. *Carcinogenesis*, **1**, 249–54.

Newman, M. S. (1983). Synthesis of 7,11,12-trimethylbenz[a]anthracene. *J. Org. Chem.*, **48**, 3249–51.

Ribeiro, O., Hadfield, S. T., Clayton, A. F., Vose, C. W. & Coombs, M. M. (1983). Potentially carcinogenic cyclopenta[a]phenanthrenes. Part 11. Synthesis of 1-methyl, 1,11-methano, and 7,11-dimethyl derivatives of 15,16-dihydrocyclopenta[a]phenanthren-17-one. *J. Chem. Soc. Perkin Trans. I*, 87–91.

Pople, J. A., Santry, D. P. & Segal, G. A. (1965). Approximate self-consistent molecular orbital theory. Invariant procedures. *J. Chem. Phys.*, **43**, S129–S135.

Pople, J. A. & Segal, G. A. (1966). Approximate self-consistent molecular orbital theory. CNDO results for AB_2 and AB_3. *J. Chem. Phys.*, **44**, 3289–96.

Wiberg, K. B. (1968). Application of the Pople–Santry–Segal CNDO method to the cyclopropylcarbinyl and cyclobutyl cation and to bicyclobutane. *Tetrahedron*, **24**, 1083–96.

Zacharias, D. E., Kashino, S., Glusker, J. P., Harvey, R. G., Amin, S. & Hecht, S. S. (1984). The bay-region geometry of some 5-methylchrysenes: steric effects in 5,6- and 5,12-dimethylchrysenes. *Carcinogenesis*, **5**, 1421–30.

9

Conclusion

9.1   The occurrence of cyclopenta[a]phenanthrenes

From the beginning cyclopenta[a]phenanthrenes have been associated on the one hand with sterols and steroids, and on the other with polycyclic aromatic hydrocarbons. Related to this is the possibility of their occurrence in nature, particularly in animal tissues as a result of aberrant steroid metabolism. This idea was raised at an early stage (Cook, 1933) and has reappeared periodically on a number of occasions since (Steiner, 1943; Inhoffen, 1953; Haddow, 1958; Dannenberg, 1960; Bischoff, 1969; Coombs and Croft, 1969; Wilk and Taupp, 1969; Coombs *et al.*, 1973). However, to the best of the present authors' knowledge no definitive report of a cyclopenta[a]phenanthrene (i.e., a steroid derivative lacking both angular methyl groups) arising from such a source has yet appeared.

In contrast to this, recent studies indicate that cyclopenta[a]-phenanthrene hydrocarbons are widely distributed in several natural environments where they have probably arisen from sterols by microbiological dehydrogenation. This unexpected discovery has come to light as a result of the use of modern sophisticated analytical techniques such as gas chromatography–mass spectrometry with computer-assisted peak sorting. Nevertheless, Diels' hydrocarbon (**7**) was first identified in petroleum over 20 years ago (Mair and Martinez-Pico, 1962). In recent work (Ludwig *et al.*, 1981) aromatic components of shale oil were separated into classes containing 1,2,3 . . . aromatic rings, and these fractions were further separated by hplc. The nine cyclopenta[a]phenanthrenes shown in Fig. 86 were identified on the basis of their mass spectra, and the identity of five of them (**27**, **30**, **32**, **33**, **35**) was confirmed by comparison with authentic samples prepared from sterols by the method of Dannenberg, namely chloranil dehydrogenation to the

17*H*-cyclopenta[a]phenanthrene followed by catalytic hydrogenation to its 15,16-dihydro derivative. These hydrocarbons appear to be widespread constituents of petroleum-bearing sediments where they are formed by long-term degradation of sterols in the subsurface; they do not appear to occur in recent sediments. In an investigation of the hydrocarbons present in samples of Toarcian shales at different sites in the Paris basin, Mackenzie *et al.* (1981) identified the cyclopenta[a]phenanthrene (33) and also 15,16-dihydro-17-ethyl-17-methylcyclopenta[a]-phenanthrene (36), again by comparison with authentic specimens. The methyl ethyl hydrocarbon (36) has also been reported to occur in Chinese shales (Shi *et al.*, 1982). Mackenzie et al. found that the extent of steroid aromatization increased with burial depth, and therefore with maturity of the sample. The extent of carbon–carbon bond cracking in the side chain was found to be small in the shallow samples, and became significant only in the deepest specimens. It was suggested that these two reactions – aromatization and side-chain cracking – probably occur during petroleum formation and that steroid hydrocarbon distribution might serve as a useful indication of maturity in exploration studies. The parent hydrocarbon 16,17-dihydro-15*H*-cyclopenta[a]phenanthrene (1) has recently been identified in Australian brown coal where it was obtained as a minor component of the triaromatic hydrocarbon fraction separated by hplc. Its occurrence together with numerous other tetra- and pentacyclic hydrocarbons derived from phenanthrene establishes its probable origin from triterpene precursors (Chaffee and Johns, 1983).

A different cyclopenta[a]phenanthrene hydrocarbon, namely 16,17-dihydro-15-isopropyl-4-methyl-15*H*-cyclopenta[a]phenanthrene (37), has been identified by several groups in river and lake sediments. Wakeham *et al.* (1980) examined cores of recent sediment from Lake Lucerne, Lake Zurich and Grieifensee (Switzerland), and Lake Washington (north-west U.S.A.). Aromatic components were separated by hplc into groups according to the number of aromatic rings and these were subsequently analysed by gas chromatography–mass spectrometry; the cyclopenta[a]phenanthrene (37) was identified in the phenanthrene fraction. These authors considered that the variety of phenanthrenes and

Fig. 86. Cyclopenta[a]phenanthrenes which occur naturally in mineral oils.

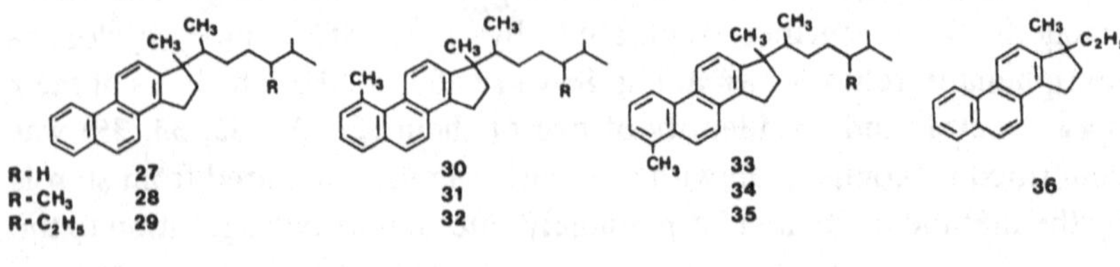

R = H   27
R = CH₃   28
R = C₂H₅   29

30
31
32

CH₃   33
       34
       35

36

chrysenes found pointed to short-term alteration of biogenic precursors and could in no way be linked to anthropogenic combustion or pyrolysis processes. It was proposed that the hydrocarbon probably arose as a result of dehydrogenation of sterols or triterpenes mediated by microorganisms The same cyclopenta[a]phenanthrene was also identified in sediment cores collected from two Adirondack lakes in New York state, remote from industrial activities (Tan and Heit, 1981), and from the Amazon river and Cariaco Trench (Laflamme and Hites, 1979). These authors suggested that it could be formed from a pentacyclic triterpene such as lupeol *via* cleavage of the oxygenated A-ring, followed by aromatization of the remaining six-membered rings, together with migration and loss of the angular methyl groups as shown in Fig. 87.

Whereas these cyclopenta[a]phenanthrenes can be considered as naturally occurring, others occur in edible oils which have been overheated. Heating above 200°C causes the formation of a small amount of fluorescent material, arising from aromatization of sterols which are always present naturally in both animal and vegetable fats. Schmid (1962) and Schmid and Waitz (1963) heated the potential sterol precursors, cholesterol, phytosterol, and ergosterol, at 400°C in a slow stream of nitrogen, and isolated from the products 16,17-dihydro-15*H*-cyclopenta[a]phenanthrene (1) and Diels' hydrocarbon (7) among other phenanthrene and chrysene derivatives. Pyrolysis of ergosterol (Hoffelner, Lisbet and Schmid, 1964) gave in addition 16,17-dihydro-3-hydroxy-15*H*-cyclopenta[a]phenanthrene (38). All these cyclopenta[a]phenanthrenes were obtained in the crystalline state and fully

Fig. 87. Suggested derivation of the cyclopenta[a]phenanthrene (37) found naturally in river and lake sediments from the triterpenoid lupeol. The phenol (38) was isolated from the products formed by heating sterols at 400°C in nitrogen, while the hydrocarbon (39) was obtained by exposing cholesterol adsorbed on silica gel to iodine vapour at ambient temperature.

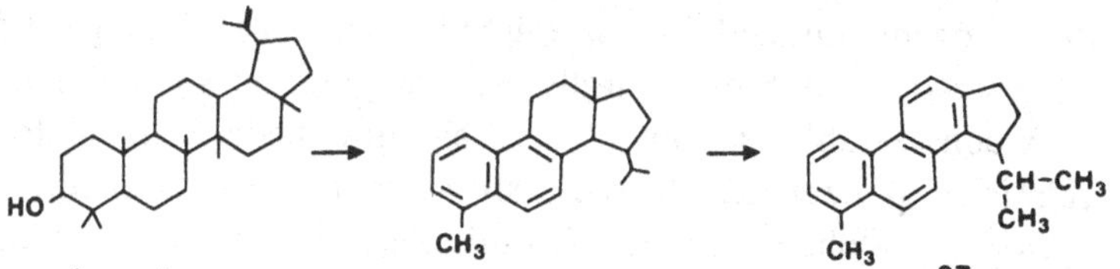

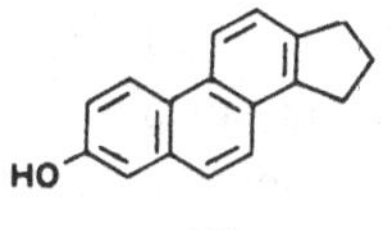

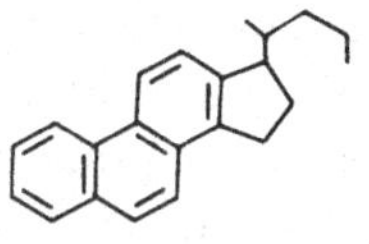

characterized. Earlier Falk *et al.* (1949) had studied the products obtained from heating cholesterol in air at 360°C, in connection with the report of Hieger (1947) that commercially obtained samples of this sterol were weakly carcinogenic. The products were separated chemically into acidic, basic, ketonic neutral, and non-ketonic neutral fractions, the last two fractions accounting for 23% and 75% of the whole, respectively. The non-ketonic neutral fraction was further separated by column chromatography, and the individual substances were identified by their ultraviolet absorption spectra. The phenanthrene derivative of cholesterol (33) and Diels' hydrocarbon (7) occurred in the fluorescent fractions from the column, but no trace of 3-methylcholanthrene was observed. The latter was carefully sought because theoretically it could have arisen through cyclization of the cholesteryl side chain; instead this side chain was apparently lost to yield Diels' hydrocarbon (7). Compounds (7) and (33) are not carcinogens, and Fieser considered that cholesterol itself, so widely distributed in nature, was most unlikely to be active. He therefore sought carcinogenic activity among the many known oxidation products of this sterol, eventually discovering definite activity in the 6β-hydroperoxy derivative of cholest-4-en-3-one (Fieser *et al.*, 1955).

The methods for producing cyclopenta[a]phenanthrenes from sterols all involve pyrolysis or quinone oxidation at elevated temperatures, conditions far removed from those encountered in living systems. It is therefore of considerable interest and possible significance that Wilk and Taupp (1969) found that 16,17-dihydro-17-isopentyl-15H-cyclopenta[a]phenanthrene (39), obtainable from cholesterol by selenium dehydrogenation at 350°C, was also formed when this sterol was adsorbed on silica gel and exposed to iodine vapour at room temperature for 20 h. The authors considered that the oxidation potential required in the adsorbed state was substantially lower than that normally required for dehydrogenation, and that this might be a model for biological dehydrogenation of steroids by naturally occurring quinones found in the cell.

A considerable amount of data has now been accumulated on the relationship between chemical structure and carcinogenicity among cyclopenta[a]phenanthrenes. On this basis it seems unlikely that any of the hydrocarbons so far identified from natural sources or as pyrolysis products would be active. However, the recently discovered widespread occurrence of cyclopenta[a]phenanthrenes indicates that this class of compound is rather prone to arise from sterols and steroids under a variety of conditions, and this again raises the unresolved question of whether they occur in animal tissues as a result of incorrect steroid biosynthesis or metabolism.

9.2 Do cyclopenta[a]phenanthrenes occur as a result of aberrant steroid metabolism in animals?

It is now well established that carcinogens are produced by a variety of microorganisms and plants, and there seems no *a priori* reason why animals should not also possess similar capabilities. The incidences of most common forms of cancer rise steeply with age, and in Great Britain about one in five people eventually die from one of the many forms of this disease. We now have extensive knowledge of the long latent periods encountered in animal experiments with weak carcinogens, or with very low doses of more potent carcinogens, and it seems entirely possible that at least some of this human disease might result from the prolonged action of minute amounts of an endogenous carcinogen formed in the body by aberrant steroid metabolism. The amount needed might only be small, and the potency not particularly high to produce this high cancer incidence observed in elderly people. This view, fashionable 40 years ago, led to experiments that failed to detect such a carcinogen, but in retrospect two reasons can now be advanced to account for this failure. The first has to do with the experimental methods available then. Quite astonishing advances have been made in analytical procedures in the intervening years, and as we have seen these are now beginning to disclose a whole range of unexpected cyclopenta[a]phenanthrenes in natural sources. The application of these new sensitive methods to animal tissues and extracts has not yet been undertaken. The second reason is undoubtedly connected with the history of this subject. As has already been pointed out, the straightforward synthesis in 1933 of the extremely potent carcinogen 3-methylcholanthrene from a simple derivative of cholic acid, coupled with the observations that Diels' hydrocarbon and other simple cyclopenta[a]phenanthrenes were inactive, for two decades strongly directed interest away from cyclopenta[a]phenanthrenes and towards the cholanthrenes. However, it now seems to be firmly established that sterol dehydrogenation does not lead to compounds of the latter class, but instead side-chain cleavage occurs to generate a variety of cyclopenta[a]phenanthrenes. The discovery of potent carcinogens among this class of sterol degradation products inevitably redirects attention to the possibility of the endogenous formation of carcinogenic cyclopenta[a]phenanthrenes by incorrect steroid metabolism in mammals.

244   *Conclusion*

In the older literature, reviewed by Steiner in 1943, there are a number of reports on the production of tumours in animals with various crude tissue extracts. Activity was generally found in association with lipids, and in most instances with the unsaponifiable fraction of these lipids. Crude extracts reported to be active were prepared from human cancer tissues, bile, urine, lung, and liver, but it was the latter source that was studied in greatest detail. Later, in an extensive comparison of extracts of human liver and other human and animal organs (Steiner *et al.*, 1947), considerable carcinogenic potential was detected with extracts of human liver from both normal and cancer patients. Extracts of the minced, frozen tissue were made by alkaline hydrolysis followed by extraction with ethylene dichloride; after removal of the solvent the unsaponifiable lipid was dissolved in warm tricaprylin and injected into C57Bl mice in groups of about 50. Sarcomas were induced at the site of injection in up to half the animals treated with some, but not all, of these liver extracts from both normal and cancer patients. Extracts prepared in the same way from human spleen, and even from livers of stillborn infants also gave some sarcomas, although fewer in number. It was felt these two sources reduced the possibility that all the carcinogenic activity was due to extrinsic, dietary carcinogens. Hieger (1946) also successfully induced sarcomas in mice with unsaponifiable lipid material from human liver, and from pooled lung, kidney, and muscle. He fractionated this lipid and determined that the most active fraction was the crystalline material obtained which consisted largely (85%) of cholesterol. The latent periods for these tumours were long (14–24 months) and he suggested that the carcinogen was probably of low potency. Bischoff (1963), in a thorough review of sterol carcinogenesis, pointed out that the cholesterol oxidation products $5\alpha,6\alpha$-epoxy-3β-cholesterol and 6β-hydroperoxycholest-4-en-3-one were known to produce local sarcomas on injection into mice. He felt that this should be taken into account when considering Hieger's results. With this in mind Higginson *et al.* (1964) attempted to reproduce the experiments of Des Ligneris (1940) who had found that non-saponifiable extracts obtained from the livers of Bantu subjects, both with and without primary liver cancer, were more carcinogenic in mice than similar extracts from white subjects. The extracts were prepared by the former authors by saponification of the livers in alcohol with potassium hydroxide, followed by extraction of the non-saponifiable lipid with peroxide-free ether, and care was taken to avoid aerial oxidation by carrying out the whole procedure under nitrogen. An extract was prepared from pooled mouse liver in the same way. None of these extracts yielded tumours when mice were repeatedly painted with them, but after injection all gave a low incidence of fibrosarcomas at the injection site, and this was not seen with the solvent (sesame oil or tricaprylin) alone. The authors concluded that while this experiment confirmed the existence of low-grade carcinogens in non-saponifiable extracts from human and mouse liver, it did not support the racial difference claimed by Des Ligneris. Deliberate exposure of these extracts to air and light for prolonged periods to produce peroxides, the presence of which was confirmed by analysis, did not increase this low sarcoma incidence, thus casting doubt on Bischoff's suggestion. It remains difficult to understand the reason for these results, but they cannot be ignored because they are the outcome of quite extensive experiments conducted by serious, capable workers. A whole battery of powerful methods is now available that could be employed to determine whether these crude extracts contain true endogenous carcinogens, or whether the activity is a result of artefacts, either exogenous carcinogens or carcinogens produced under the drastic conditions used in the extraction processes. For example, bacterial mutation assays could be used rapidly to pinpoint active fractions which could then be investigated by gas chromatography–mass spectrometry, a technique which has recently had spectacular success in identifying small molecules, including cyclopenta[a]phenanthrenes, in a variety of natural sources.

The net result of the various structure/carcinogenicity studies among cyclopenta[a]phenanthrenes outlined in this book can be readily summarized as follows:

(i) carcinogenicity is conferred on the parent hydrocarbon 16,17-dihydro-15*H*-cyclopenta[a]phenanthrene (**1**) by methyl substitution at C-7, and especially at C-11;

(ii) potency is increased by extending conjugation of the phenanthrene nucleus into the five-membered D-ring, either as an endocyclic carbon–carbon double bond or as an exocyclic carbon–oxygen double bond at C-17;

(iii) the 11-methyl group can be replaced by a methoxy group without marked loss of carcinogenicity, but longer side chains at this position reduce or abolish activity.

In contemplating possible structures for a hypothetical carcinogenic cyclopenta[a]phenanthrene which might be derived from a steroid *in vivo*, a difficulty is apparent. Whilst a 17-carbonyl group is a common feature of both androgens and oestrogens, rearrangements leading to an 11-methyl or 11-methoxy structure are without precedent; in all known examples rearrangement of the C-19 methyl group in steroids leads to 1-

or 4-methyl derivatives. It is therefore of considerable interest that introduction of an 11-hydroxy group was also found to lead to carcinogenicity in a cyclopenta[a]phenanthrene. Injection of the sparingly soluble phenol 15,16-dihydro-11-hydroxycyclopenta[a]phenanthren-17-one (**206**) suspended in olive oil into mice followed by repeated application of croton oil to their dorsal skin caused the appearance of skin tumours, both carcinomas and papillomas, at the site of promotion (Bhatt *et al.*, 1982), thus proving that this phenol is capable of systemic initiation. This compound was less potent than its 11-methyl analogue, but essentially the same result was obtained in two identical experiments separated in time by about a year. 11-Hydroxy steroids are, of course, well known and arise mainly if not entirely from the adrenal cortex. As we have already seen the 3-deoxy steroid androsta-3,5-dien-17-one has been isolated from the urine of both male and female patients with adrenal tumours (Burrows *et al.*, 1937; Wolfe *et al.*, 1941). This is important because the 3-hydroxy group present in the vast majority of steroids would probably inhibit activity in a cyclopenta[a]phenanthrene since the analogous synthetic phenol derived from 3-methylcholanthrene is not a carcinogen (Shear and Leiter, 1941). In this connection Marker and Rohrmann (1939) in their study which disclosed the presence of 3-deoxy equilenin in mares' pregnancy urine, also described a diketone $C_{18}H_{16}O_2$, mp 214°C. This compound was isolated from the non-crystalline carbinol fraction after mild oxidation with chromic acid and formed only a monosemicarbazone, from which the 11,17-diketone structure (see Fig. 88) was proposed for it. The close relationship between this 3-deoxy steroid and the carcinogenic cyclopenta[a]phenanthrene phenol (**206**) is apparent especially when one considers that the adrenal cortex is not only the centre of steroid 11-hydroxylation, but also of oxygenation at C-18, as in aldosterone biosynthesis. C-18 hydroxylation of this 11,17-diketone could lead to the loss of the angular methyl group and conversion to the 11-phenol (**206**). Whether this or any other cyclopenta[a]phenanthrene occurs in adrenal tissue or in tumours of this organ is, of course, at present unknown. Adrenal extracts were studied intensively during the isolation

Fig. 88.

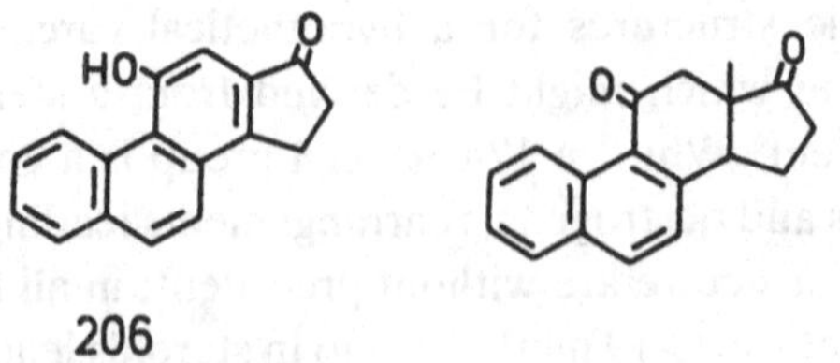

206

of the cortical hormones 40 years ago, but in almost all of this work only the more polar fractions were examined (Fieser and Fieser, 1959). In this work finely chopped frozen tissue was extracted with acetone, the latter was removed by evaporation, and the aqueous residue was extracted with petroleum ether to leave the adrenocortical hormone in the aqueous phase (Cartland and Kuizenga, 1936). Hieger (1946) tested adrenal extracts (prepared by the saponification and solvent extraction method used for liver) for carcinogenicity, but failed to induce sarcomas. It seems unlikely that either of these extraction methods would have isolated the phenol (**206**), although the petroleum extract might have contained cyclopenta[a]phenanthrene hydrocarbons, if they were present.

Modern cancer research is beginning to uncover the cause of some human tumours. By far the most important discovery is that cigarette smoking is causally related to the tragic increase in lung cancer observed during this century, a disease that now claims some 30 000 men each year in this country alone. Several other minor forms of cancer have been traced to industrial exposure to carcinogens. For example, bladder cancer is associated with exposure to aromatic amines previously used as dyestuff intermediates and as antioxidants in the manufacture of rubber. However, it still remains true that the cause of the majority of human tumours remains completely unknown. The case for the initiation of at least some of these by endogenous carcinogens formed in the body from steroids now seems as strong as it did 50 years ago. It is clear that a fresh approach to this whole question now needs to be made, fully utilizing both the splendid new analytical techniques and our deeper understanding of steroid biochemistry.

9.3   References

Bhatt, T. S., Hadfield, S. T. & Coombs, M. M. (1982). Carcinogenicity and mutagenicity of some alkoxy cyclopenta[a]phenanthren-17-ones: effect of obstructing the bay region. *Carcinogenesis*, **3**, 677–80.

Bischoff, F. (1963). Carcinogenesis through cholesterol and derivatives. *Prog. Exp. Tumor Res.*, **3**, 412–44.

Bischoff, F. (1969). Carcinogenic effects of steroids. *Adv. in Lipid Res.*, **7**, 165–244.

Burrows, H., Cook, J. W., Roe, E. M. F. & Warren, F. L. (1937). Isolation of $\Delta^{3,5}$-androstadiene-17-one from the urine of a man with a malignant tumour of the adrenal cortex. *Biochem. J.*, **31**, 950–61.

Cartland, G. F. & Kuizenga, M. H. (1936). The preparation of extracts containing the adrenal cortical hormone. *J. Biol. Chem.*, **116**, 57–64.

Chaffee, A. L. & Johns, R. B. (1983). Polycyclic aromatic hydrocarbons in Australian coals. 1. Angularly fused pentacyclic tri- and tetra- aromatic components of Victorian brown coal. *Geochim. Cosmochim. Acta*, **47**, 2142–55.

Cook, C. W. (1933). Discussion on experimental production of malignant tumours. *Proc. Roy. Soc. (B)*, **113**, 275–85.

Coombs, M. M. & Croft, C. J. (1969). Carcinogenic cyclopenta[a]-phenanthrenes. *Prog. Exp. Tumor Res.*, **11**, 69–85.

Coombs, M. M., Bhatt, T. S. & Croft, C. J. (1973). Correlation between carcinogenicity and chemical structure in cyclopenta[a]phenanthrenes. *Cancer Res.*, **33**, 832–7.

Dannenberg, H. (1960). Uber Beziechungen zwischen Steroiden und krebserzeugenden Kohlenwasserstoffen. *Z. Krebsforsch.*, **63**, 523–31.

Des Ligneris, M. J. A. (1940). The production of benign and malignant tumors in mice painted with Bantu liver extracts. *Am. J. Cancer*, **39**, 487–95.

Diels, O., Gadke, W. & Kording, P. (1927). Uber die Dehydrierung des Cholesterins. *Annalen*, **459**, 1–26.

Falk, H. L., Goldfein, S. & Steiner, P. E. (1949). The products of pyrolysis of cholesterol at 360°C and their relation to carcinogens. *Cancer Res.*, **9**, 438–47.

Fieser, L. F. & Fieser, M. (1959). *Steroids*, p. 726. Reinhold Publ. Corp.: New York.

Fieser, L. F., Green, T. W., Bischoff, F., Lopez, G. & Rupp, J. J. (1955). A carcinogenic oxidation product of cholesterol. *J. Am. Chem. Soc.*, **77**, 3928–9.

Haddow, A. (1958). The chemical and genetic mechanisms of carcinogenesis. In *Physiopathology of Cancer*, ed. F. Homberger, 2nd edn, pp. 570–2. Cassell: London.

Hieger, I. (1946). Carcinogenic substances in human tissues. *Cancer Res.*, **6**, 657–67.

Hieger, I. (1947). Carcinogenic activity of preparations rich in cholesterol. *Nature (London)*, **160**, 270–2.

Higginson, J., Dunn, J. A. & Sutton, D. A. (1964). The carcinogenicity of non-saponifiable extracts from livers of South African Bantu and white subjects. *Experimental & Molecular Pathology*, **3**, 297–303.

Hoffelner, K., Lisbet, H. & Schmidt, L. (1964). Aromatic cracking products from steroids. *Z. Ernaehungswiss.*, **5**, 16–21.

Inhoffen, H. H. (1953). The relationship of natural steroids to carcinogenic aromatic compounds. *Progress in Organic Chemistry*, vol. 2, pp. 131–55.

Laflamme, R. E. & Hites, R. A. (1979). Tetra- and pentacyclic, naturally occurring, aromatic hydrocarbons in recent sediments. *Geochim. Cosmochim. Acta*, **43**, 1687–91.

Ludwig, B., Hussler, G., Wehrung, P. & Albrecht, P. (1981). C_{26}–C_{29} triaromatic steroid derivatives in sediments and petroleum. *Tetrahedron Lett.*, **22**, 3313–16.

Mackenzie, A. S., Hoffmann, C. F. & Maxwell, J. R. (1981). Molecular parameters of maturation in the Toarcian shales, Paris Basin, France. III. Changes in aromatic steroid hydrocarbons. *Geochim. Cosmochim. Acta*, **45**, 1345–55.

Mair, B. J. & Martinez-Pico, J. L. (1962). Composition of the trinuclear aromatic portion of the heavy gas oil and light lubricating distillate. *Proc. Am. Petrol. Inst.*, **42**, 173–85.

Marker, R. E. & Rohrmann, E. (1939). The steroid content of mares' pregnancy urine. *J. Am. Chem. Soc.*, **61**, 2537–46.

Prelog, von V. & Fuhrer, J. (1945). Uber die Isolierung von 3-Deoxy-equilenin aus dem Harn trachtiger Stuten. *Helv. Chim. Acta*, **28**, 583–90.

Schmid, L. (1962). Cracking products of substances accompanying fats. *Mitt. Geb. Lebensmittelunter. Hyg.*, **53**, 507–10.

Schmid, L. & Waitz, W. (1963). Aromatic cracked products of steroids. *Z. Ernaehungwiss.*, *Suppl. 3*, 45–30.

Shear, M. J. & Leiter, J. (1941). Studies in carcinogenesis. XV. Compounds related to 20-methylcholanthrene. *J.N.C.I.*, **2**, 99–113.

Shi, J. Y., Mackenzie, A. S., Eglinton, R., Goward, G., Wolff, A. P. & Maxwell, J. R. (1982). A biological marker investigation of petroleums and shales from the Shengli Oilfield, The People's Republic of China. *Chem. Geol.*, **35**, 1–31.

Steiner, P. E. (1943). Cancer-producing agents from human sources. *Int. Abst. Surg.*, **76**, 105–12.

Steiner, P. E., Stanger, W. & Bolyard, M. N. (1947). Comparison of the carcinogenic activity in extracts of human liver and other human and animal organs. *Cancer Res.*, **7**, 273–80.

Tan, Y. L. & Heit, M. (1981). Biogenic and abiogenic polynuclear aromatic hydrocarbons in sediments from two remote Adirondack lakes. *Geochim. Cosmochim. Acta*, **45**, 2267–79.

Wakeham, S. G., Schaffner, C. & Giger, W. (1980). Polycyclic aromatic hydrocarbons in recent lake sediments. II. Compounds derived from biogenic precursors during early diogenesis. *Geochim. Cosmochim. Acta*, **44**, 415–19.

Wilk, M. & Taupp, W. (1969). Dehydrierung des Cholesterins in activiest adsorbierten Zustand unter Normalbedingungen, ein Beitrag zur Frage der endogenese carcinogener, polycyclischer Kohlenwasserstoffe. *Z. Naturforsch.*, **24B**, 16–23.

Wolfe, J. K., Fieser, L. F. & Friedgood, H. B. (1941). Nature of the androgens in female adrenal tumor urine. *J. Am. Chem. Soc.*, **63**, 582–93.

General index

Throughout this Index the word 'cyclopenta[a]phenanthren(e)' is abbreviated to 'cpp', but is indexed as the full word. The prefixes *cis*, *trans*, *syn*, *anti*, and *n* (= normal) are ignored for the purpose of indexing. Besides more general entries, the index also contains the chemical names of approximately 350 cpps, of which over 280 bear the serial numbers (in **bold type**) assigned to them in the text, tables, and figures. There is a brief guide to cpp nomenclature on pages 2–3 of this book, but in case of difficulty look up the serial number in the serial number-molecular formula index (pp. 122–5). Then using the molecular formula find the compound in the physical and spectral data compilation (pp. 85–122) which is arranged according to the Chemical Abstracts system and also contains the full chemical name used here. Author indexes are to be found at the end of each chapter.